Trauma: Evidence-Based Care and Treatment

Trauma: Evidence-Based Care and Treatment

Edited by Eliana Copeland

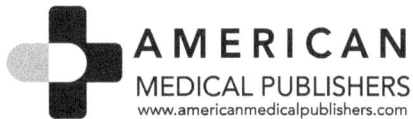

AMERICAN
MEDICAL PUBLISHERS
www.americanmedicalpublishers.com

American Medical Publishers,
41 Flatbush Avenue,
1st Floor, New York,
NY 11217, USA

Visit us on the World Wide Web at:
www.americanmedicalpublishers.com

ISBN: 978-1-63927-503-8

Cataloging-in-Publication Data

Trauma : evidence-based care and treatment / edited by Eliana Copeland.
    p. cm.
Includes bibliographical references and index.
ISBN 978-1-63927-503-8
1. Wounds and injuries. 2. Wounds and injuries--Surgery. 3. Wounds and injuries--Treatment.
4. Evidence-based medicine. 5. Medical care. I. Copeland, Eliana.
RD93 .T73 2022

617.1--dc23

Table of Contents

Preface

Trauma is an injury which can potentially cause prolonged disability or death. Trauma can be caused by falling, stabbing wounds, motor vehicle collisions and gunshot wounds. The quick management of the injury is necessary to prevent loss of life or limb. Injuries differ from one another based on their severity, and location of damage. Injury scales provide a measure of the physiological values, comorbidities, and damage to anatomical parts to measure the severity of the injury. The initial assessment of the condition is critical and therefore, involves physical evaluation and imaging. The management of trauma involves both pre-hospital and in-hospital management. Primary stabilization and spinal motion restriction are essential elements of pre-hospital trauma management. In-hospital trauma management requires the assistance of nurses, physicians, respiratory therapists, etc. The evaluation of the patient's airway, breathing, neurologic status and circulation is the first step. After the management of immediate life threats, surgical correction interventions are performed. This book is compiled in such a manner, that it will provide in-depth knowledge about the care and treatment of trauma. The aim of this book is to present researches that have transformed trauma care and aided its advancement. For someone with an interest and eye for detail, this book covers the most significant topics in trauma management.

This book is the end result of constructive efforts and intensive research done by experts in this field. The aim of this book is to enlighten the readers with recent information in this area of research. The information provided in this profound book would serve as a valuable reference to students and researchers in this field.

At the end, I would like to thank all the authors for devoting their precious time and providing their valuable contribution to this book. I would also like to express my gratitude to my fellow colleagues who encouraged me throughout the process.

Editor

Right-sided diaphragmatic rupture after blunt trauma

Ramon Vilallonga[1*], Vicente Pastor[2], Laura Alvarez[3], Ramon Charco[4], Manel Armengol[5], Salvador Navarro[6]

Abstract

Traumatic injuries of the diaphragm remain an entity of difficult diagnosis despite having been recognised early in the history of surgery, especially when it comes to blunt trauma and injuries of the right diaphragm. We report the case of a patient with blunt trauma with right diaphragmatic rupture that required urgent surgical treatment for hepatothorax and iatrogenic severe liver injury. Blunt trauma can cause substantial diaphragmatic rupture. It must have a high index of suspicion for diaphragmatic injury in patients, victims of vehicle collisions, mainly if they have suffered frontal impacts and/or side precipitates in patients with severe thoracoabdominal trauma. The diagnosis can be performed clinically and confirmation should be radiological. The general measures for the management of multiple trauma patients must be applied. Surgery at the time of diagnosis should restore continuity.

Introduction

Traumatic injuries of the diaphragm remain an entity of difficult diagnosis despite having been recognised early in the history of surgery. Sennertus, in 1541, performed an autopsy in one patient who had died from herniation and strangulation of the colon through a diaphragmatic gap secondary to a gunshot wound received seven months earlier [1]. However, these cases remain rare, and difficult to diagnose and care for. This has highlighted some of the aspects related to these lesions, especially when they are caused by blunt trauma and injuries of the right diaphragm [1,2].

Case report

We report the case of a man of 36 years of age, thrown from a height of 12 meters and was referred to our centre. The patient arrived conscious and oriented, and we began manoeuvring the management of the patient with multiple injuries according to the guidelines of the ATLS (Advanced Trauma Life Support) recommended by the American College of Surgeons. The patient had an unstable pelvic fracture (type B2) with hemodynamic instability and respiratory failure. Patient's Injury Severity Score (ISS) was 38. Pelvis and chest X-rays were

performed which confirmed the pelvic fracture and pathological elevation of the right hemidiaphragm was observed (Figure 1). We proceeded to stabilise the pelvic fracture and replace fluids, improving hemodynamic status. The patient continued with respiratory failure. For this reason, a chest tube was placed and Computerised Tomography (CT) was performed (Figure 2), showing a ruptured right hemidiaphragm, including chest drain in the right hepatic lobe and occupation of the lesser sac by blood. The patient underwent surgery, finding a right hemidiaphragm transverse rupture with a hepatothorax and an intrahepatic thoracic tube. We performed the suture of the diaphragm and liver packing, moved the patient to the intensive care unit, and after 48 hours, the liver packing was removed without problems. The patient evolved favourably.

Discussion

Currently, traumatic injuries of the diaphragm remain uncommon, and it is difficult to establish a global impact, but by autopsy studies, the incidence of these injuries range between 5.2% and 17% [3]. If we focus on patients with blunt trauma, we find that traumatic injuries of the diaphragm represent only 0.8% to 1.6% of the total lesions observed in these patients [4]. However, when we talk about open trauma, these injuries may represent up to 10% -15% of cases [3,5,6].

Road traffic collisions or lateral intrusions into the vehicle are the most frequent causes of diaphragm

* Correspondence: vilallongapuy@hotmail.com
[1]General Surgery Department. Endocrine, bariatric and metabolic Unit. Universitary Hospital Vall d'Hebron. Autonomous University of Barcelona. Spain

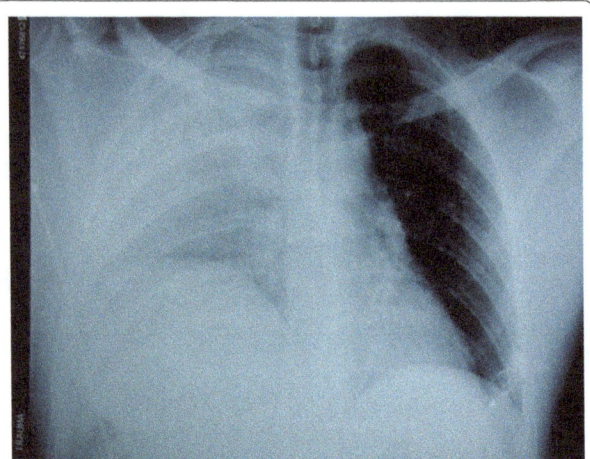

Figure 1 Chest radiograph of the patient showing an elevated right hemidiaphragm.

rupture [1,4,6,7]. Direct impacts depress the side of the rib cage, and can cause a tear in the diaphragm rib attachments, and even the transverse rupture of the diaphragm [8]. Also, serious slowdown pinching leads to a multiplication by ten times or more to the intra-abdominal pressure, especially if the patient holds his/her breath and contracts the abdominal wall at the time of impact, causing a muscle injury [2].

Classically, there has been a predominance of lesions of the left hemidiaphragm, with a ratio of 25:1. However, most modern series balance this data and show that right hemidiaphragm injuries can represent almost 35% of all diaphragm injuries [9]. This pattern may explain why the liver develops a protective cushioning pressure, although some authors believe that right hemidiaphragm injuries are associated with increased

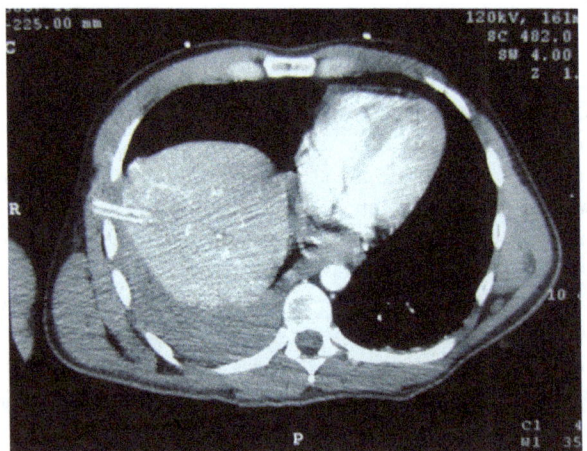

Figure 2 CT scan of the patient where hepatothorax is displayed with the drain inside.

mortality so would be undiagnosed, and for this reason would be found in equal proportion at autopsy [4,6,8].

Many authors have reviewed blunt diaphragmatic trauma over a period in their institutions. We do report the major reviewed series to our knowledge in which the do a specific mention to the blunt abdominal trauma associated with diaphragmatic rupture (Table 1).

The clinical presentation is defined by the overall assessment of the patient with multiple injuries. The injury must be suspected when any hemidiaphragm is not seen or not in the correct position in any chest radiograph [15]. The specific signs of diaphragmatic injury on plain radiographs are a marked elevation of the hemidiaphragm, an intrathoracic herniation of abdominal viscera, the "collar sign", demonstration of a nasogastric tube tip above the diaphragm [19]. Also, in the context of high-energy trauma, when combined with a head injury and pelvic fracture, diaphragmatic trauma should be suspected [7]. The diagnosis is based largely on clinical suspicion and a compatible chest radiograph or CT scan [10]. The biggest change in recent years in managing blunt diafragmatic trauma has been the use of high-resolution multislice CT angiography of the abdomen and chest. This is now a routine test performed in most blunt trauma patients. Ultrasound can also be diagnostic in patients with DR, especially if focused abdominal sonography for trauma (FAST) can be extended above the diaphragm looking for a hemothorax and assessing the diaphragmatic motions (using m-mode if possible). It adds little time to the examination but allows the operator to observe absent diaphragmatic movements, herniation of viscera, or flaps of ruptured diaphragm [19]. However, in the absence of a hernia, it may be difficult to identify traumatic diaphragmatic injury by conventional imaging. Blunt diaphragmatic rupture is often missed during initial patient evaluation. The initial chest radiograph can be negative and a repeat chest radiograph may be necessary. Other diagnostic modalities or even surgical exploration may be required to definitively exclude blunt diaphragmatic rupture. A midline laparotomy is the advocated approach for repair of acute diaphragmatic trauma because it offers the possibility of diagnosing and repairing frequently associated intra-abdominal injuries [11].

Closed diaphragmatic injuries should be treated as soon as possible. Special attention should be given to the placement of thoracic drainage tubes, especially if the radiograph is suspicious [3].

Midline laparotomy is the recommended approach because it allows for an exploration of the entire abdominal cavity [1,2,4,6,7]. Routine surgical repair of any diaphragmatic defect is accomplished by interrupted or continuous nonabsorbable sutures and placement of chest tube(s) in the affected thoracic cavity. In

Table 1 Major series reporting cases in the literature of blunt diaphragmatic rupture

Author	Number of cases	Trauma type	Location	Associated injuries	ISS*	Management	Mortality
Chughtai T et al. [9]	208 (1986-2003)	Blunt: 208	Right: 135 Left: 47 Bilateral: 4	Abdomen: liver (63,5%), spleen (52,9%), small bowel mesentery (46,2%)... Chest: Rib fracture (75,5%), pulmonary contusion (63,0%), hemothorax (40,4%), hemopneumothorax (22,1%)...	Mean ISS 38.0	93,3% laparotomy 1,4% thoracotomy	60 † within 28 days. Head injury: 25% Intra-abdominal bleeding: 23,2%
Ozpolat B et al. [7]	41 (1996-2007)	Blunt: 20 Penetrating: 21	Right: 12 Left: 28 Bilateral: 1	30 (73%): hemothorax, pneumothorax, liver and rib fractures	Not mentioned.	85% operated before 24 h	6 † (14,6%)
Lunca S et al. [12]	61 (1992-2003)	Blunt: 15 Penetrating: 46	Right: 15 Left: 45 Bilateral: 1	27 hemorrhagic shock	ISS = 24 (6-75)	100% operated before 12 h	9 † 15 complications
Cubukçu A et al. [13]	21 (1995-1998)	Blunt: 9 Penetrating: 12	Right: 12 Left: 9	20 patients with concomitants injuries (Liver in 10 patients) 7 patients with signs or symptoms related to diaphragmatic rupture	Not mentioned.	100% operated before 24 h	3 †
Dajee A et al. [14]	48 (1973-1978)	Blunt: 8 Penetrating: 40	Right: + Left: +++ Bilateral: 1	Intra-abdominal injuries involved the spleen, liver, stomach and colon. 8 patients herniations of intra-abdominal contents.	Not mentioned	100% laparotomy. No use of mesh.	3 † (6%)
Tan KK et al. [16]	14 (2002-2008)	Blunt: 14	Right: 5 Left: 9	8 Splenic laceration, 5 hemothorax and lung injuries, 4 long bone fracture, 4 pelvic fracture, 3 liver laceration, 3 colonic laceration, 3 injury major vessels, 2 kidney laceration, 2 small bowel laceration, 1 gastric perforation.	Median GCS: 14 (3-15) Median ISS: 41 (14-66).	85,7% laparotomy and repair 14,3% surgical intensive care unit.	5 † (33%) Extensive injuries
Matsevych OY. [19]	12 (4 years)	Blunt: 12	Right: 6 Left: 2 Bilateral: 1	100% associated injuries: 5 hemothorax, 4 head injuries, 3 extremity fracture, 3 pelvic fracture, 3 liver laceration, 3 retroperitoneal hematoma.	Not mentioned.	100% laparotomy. 1 patient thoracotomy.	3 † (25%) (Hypovolemic shock, 1 brain injury, 1 cardiac failure)
Bergeron E et al. [20]	160 (April 1, 1984, to March 31, 1999)	Blunt: 160	Right: 31 Left: 126 Bilateral: 3	Abdomen: liver (47%), spleen (50%), small bowel mesentery (38%)... Chest: Rib fracture (31%), pevi (41%), other orthopedic (50%).	ISS = 26.9 (+11.5)	100% operated between 60 minutes and 21.8 days after injury. 4 had repair of diaphragmatic rupture at a second laparotomy.	14,4%
Brasel KJ et al. [21]	32 (January 1987 through May 1994)	Blunt: 32	Right: 7 Left: 25 Bilateral: 0	Abdomen: liver (47%), spleen (50%), small bowel mesentery (38%)... Chest: Rib fracture (31%), pevi (41%), other orthopedic (50%).	ISS= 32	100% laparotomy. Sunning suture all patients and 1 patient polypropylene mesh repair.	22,0%
Shapiro MJ et al. [22]	20 (5 years period)	Blunt: 20	Right: 7 Left: 14 Bilateral: 0	Shock 16/20; hemo/pneumothorax 15/20; cerebral injury (12/20); pulmonary contusion 9/20; chest wall contusion 8/20; hepatic injury 8/20; splenic injury 8/20	36 (11-59)	Not mentioned	25,0%
Montresor E et al. [23]	17 (1970 to 1995)	Blunt: 17	Right: 7 Left: 14 Bilateral: 0	52.6% presented at operation with intrathoracic visceral herniation.	Not mentioned.	8 laparotomy. 7 laparotomy and thoracotomy. 4 thoracotomy	15,6%

Table 1 Major series reporting cases in the literature of blunt diaphragmatic rupture (*Continued*)

Esme H et al. [24]	14 (January 2000 and June 2005)	Blunt: 11 Penetrating: 3	Right: 4 Left: 10	Multiple associated injuries were observed in 12 patients (85%)	Not mentioned.	100% laparotomy.	Overall: 7%
Athanassiadi K et al. [25]	41 (1988 to 1997)	Blunt: 41	Right: 15 Left: 24 Bilateral: 2	In 34 patients (94%) involving: spleen (n = 18), rib fractures (n = 17), liver (n = 14), lung (n = 11), bowel (n = 7), kidney (n = 5) and other fractures (n = 21)	Not mentioned.	22 laparotomy 10 thoracotomy 4 laparo-thoracotomy	16.6% (6/36)
Gwely NN. [26]	44 (1998 and 2007)	Blunt: 44	Right: 12 Left: 30 Bilateral: 2		Not mentioned.	31 thoracotomy in 4 laparotomy 3 thoracolaparotomy	13.2% (5/38)
Yalçinkaya I et al. [27]	26 (1996-2005)	Blunt: 26	Right: 8 Left: 18	Multiple associated injuries were observed in patients (96%). Thorax herniation of organs (45%).	Not mentioned.	15 thoracotomy 7 laparotomy 4 thoraco-laparotomy	3 † (11.5%)

* Injury Severity Score.

hemodynamically stable patients with penetrating left thoracoabdominal trauma, the incidence of injury to the diaphragm is very high, and thoracoscopy or laparoscopy is recommended for the diagnosis and repair of a missed diaphragmatic injury. Laparoscopy or video-assisted thoracoscopic surgery (VATS) can be used in hemodynamically stable patients. VATS has greater accuracy (sensitivity and specificity close to 100%) and helps to avoid the risk of tension pneumothorax [19]. However, we feel that VATS is best reserved for stable patients when intraabdominal and contralateral diaphragmatic injuries are excluded.

Grimes, in 1974, described the three phases of the rupture of the diaphragm: an initial acute phase, at the time of the injury to the diaphragm; [17] a delayed phase associated with transient herniation of the viscera, thus accounting for absent or intermittent non-specific symptoms; and the obstruction phase involving the complication of a long-standing herniation, manifesting as obstruction, strangulation and posterior rupture [18]. The typical organs that herniate into the thoracic cavity include the stomach, spleen, colon, small bowel and liver, Repair with non-absorbable simple sutures is adequate in most cases, and the use of mesh should be reserved for chronic and large defects. Thus, all surgeons must be vigilant during any exploratory laparotomy to exclude any associated diaphragmatic injury.

Mortality strictly related to diaphragmatic rupture is minimal, and is usually caused by the associated injuries. The most common causes of death reported in the literature are shock, multiple organ failure and head injuries [9]. Outcomes of acute diaphragmatic hernia repair are largely dictated by the severity of concomitant injuries, with the Injury Severity Score being the most widely recognised predictor of mortality. Delayed diagnosis may increase mortality by up to 30% [8]. The rate of initially missed diaphragmatic ruptures or injuries in nonoperatively managed patients, therefore, ranges from 12 to 60% [3]. Blunt diafragmatic rupture can easily be missed in the absence of other indications for prompt surgery, where a thorough examination of both hemidiaphragms is mandatory. A high index of suspicion combined with repeated and selective radiologic evaluation is necessary for early diagnosis. Acute diaphragmatic hernia is a result of diaphragmatic injury that accompanies severe blunt or penetrating thoracoabdominal trauma. It is frequently diagnosed early on the trauma by chest radiograph or CT scan of the chest. Non-adverted diaphragmatic injury resulting from the chronic phase of a diaphragmatic hernia will probably require surgery to repair the defect.

Conclusions

Blunt diaphragmatic rupture can lead to important morbidity and mortality. It is a rare condition, usually masked by multiple associated injuries, which can aggravate the condition of patients. Therefore, there should be a high index of suspicion for diaphragmatic injury in those patients who are victims of vehicle collisions, especially if they have suffered frontal and/or lateral impacts, which have resulted in severe thoracoabdominal trauma. The diagnosis can be made clinically and radiologically. The general measures for the management of multiple trauma patients must be applied. Surgery at the time of diagnosis should restore continuity.

Acknowledgement of financial support
The authors acknowledge of the Dr. Ramon Vilallonga Foundation for its financial support in carrying out this work. http://www.fundacioramonvilallonga.org

Author details
[1]General Surgery Department. Endocrine, bariatric and metabolic Unit. Universitary Hospital Vall d'Hebron. Autonomous University of Barcelona. Spain. [2]General Surgery Department. Universitary Hospital Vall d'Hebron. Autonomous University of Barcelona. Spain. [3]HBP Surgery and Transplants Department. Universitary Hospital Vall d'Hebron. Autonomous University of Barcelona. Spain. [4]HBP Surgery and Transplants Department. Universitary Hospital Vall d'Hebron. Autonomous University of Barcelona. Spain. [5]General Surgery Department. Universitary Hospital Vall d'Hebron. Autonomous University of Barcelona. Spain. [6]General Surgery Department. Universitary Hospital Parc Tauli. Autonomous University of Barcelona. Spain.

Authors' contributions
VR has take care of the patient and has draft the manuscript. PV, AL, CR helped to the clinical assessment and draft of the manuscript. CR, AM and NS have been involved in drafting the manuscript or revising it critically for important intellectual content. All authors read and approved the final manuscript.

Competing interests
Dr. Ramon Vilallonga is president of the Dr. Vilallonga Foundation. The rest of authors, declare that they have no competing interests.

References
1. Asencio JA, Demetriades D, Rodriguez A: Injury to the diaphragm. In Trauma. 4 edition. Edited by: en Moore EE, Mattox KL, Feliciano DV. McGraw-Hill, New York; 2000:603-632.
2. Favre JP, Cheynel N, Benoit N, Favoulet P: Traitement chirurgical des ruptures traumatiques du diaphragme. Encycl. Méd. Chir. (Elsevier, Paris-France), Techniques chirurgicales- Appareil digestif, Paris 2005, 2:235-345.
3. Reber PU, Schmied B, Seiler CA, Baer HU, Patel AG, Büchler MW: Missed diaphragmatic injuries and their-long term sequelae. J Trauma 1998, 44:183-188.
4. Mansour KA: Trauma to the diaphragm. Chest Surg Clin N Am 1997, 7:373-383.
5. Scharff JR, Naunheim KS: Traumatic diaphragmatic injuries. Thorac Surg Clin 2007, 17:81-5.
6. Rosati C: Acute traumatic injury of the diaphragm. Chest Surg Clin N Am 1998, 8:371-379.

7. Ozpolat B, Kaya O, Yazkan R, Osmanoğlu G: **Diaphragmatic injuries: a surgical challenge. Report of forty-one cases.** *Thorac Cardiovasc Surg* 2009, **57**:358-62.

8. Boulanger BR, Mizman DP, Rosati C, Rodriguez A: **A comparision of right and left blunt traumatic diaphragmatic rupture.** *J Trauma* 1993, **35**:255-260.

9. Chughtai T, Ali S, Sharkey P, Lins M, Rizoli S: **Update on managing diaphragmatic rupture in Blunt trauma: a review of 208 consecutive cases.** *Can J Surg* 2009, **52**:177-81.

10. Ho ML, Gutierrez FR: **Chest radiography in thoracic polytrauma.** *AJR Am J Roentgenol* 2009, **192**:599-612.

11. Hanna WC, Ferri LE: **Acute traumatic diaphragmatic injury.** *Thorac Surg Clin* 2009, **19**:485-9.

12. Lunca S, Romedea NS, Moroşanu C: **Traumatic rupture of the diaphragm: diagnostic considerations, prognostic factors, outcomes.** *Rev Med Chir Soc Med Nat Iasi* 2007, **111**:416-22.

13. Cubukçu A, Paksoy M, Gönüllü NN, Sirin F, Dülger M: **Traumatic rupture of the diaphragm.** *Int J Clin Pract* 2000, **54**:19-21.

14. Dajee A, Schepps D, Hurley EJ: **Diaphragmatic injuries.** *Surg Gynecol Obstet* 1981, **153**:31-2.

15. ATLS: **Advanced Trauma Life Support for Doctors.** *American College of Surgeons* , 8 2008.

16. Tan KK, Yan ZY, Vijayan A, Chiu MT: **Management of diaphragmatic rupture from blunt trauma.** *Singapore Med J* 2009, **50**:1150-3.

17. Grimes OF: **Traumatic injuries of the diaphragm. Diaphragmatic hernia.** *Am J Surg* 1974, **128**:175-181.

18. Goh BK, Wong AS, Tay KH, Hoe MN: **Delayed presentation of a patient with a ruptured diaphragm complicated by gastric incarceration and perforation after apparently minor Blunt trauma.** *Canadian Journal of Emergency Medicine* 2004, **6**:277-280.

19. Matsevych OY: **Blunt diaphragmatic rupture: four year's experience.** *Hernia* 2008, **12**:73-8.

20. Bergeron E, Clas D, Ratte S, Beauchamp G, Denis R, Evans D, Frechette P, Martin M: **Impact of deferred treatment of Blent diaphragmatic rupture: a 15-year experience in six trauma centers in Quebec.** *J Trauma* 2002, **52**:633-40.

21. Brasel KJ, Borgstrom DC, Meyer P, Weigelt JA: **Predictors of outcome in Blent diaphragm rupture.** *J Trauma* 1996, **41**:484-7.

22. Shapiro MJ, Heiberg E, Durham RM, Luchtefeld W, Mazuski JE: **The unreliability of CT scans and initial chest radiographs in evaluating blunt trauma induced diaphragmatic rupture.** *Clin Radiol* 1996, **51**:27-30.

23. Montresor E, Mangiante G, Vassia S, Barbosa A, Attino M, Bortolasi L, Nifosi F, Modena S, Puchetti V: **[Rupture of the diaphragm caused by closed trauma. Case contributions and review of the literature.].** *Ann Ital Chir* 1997, **68**:297-303, discussion 303-5. Italian.

24. Esme H, Solak O, Sahin DA, Sezer M: **Blunt and penetrating traumatic ruptures of the diaphragm.** *Thorac Cardiovasc Surg* 2006, **54**:324-7.

25. Athanassiadi K, Kalavrouziotis G, Athanassiou M, Vernikos P, Skrekas G, Poultsidi A, Bellenis I: **Blunt diaphragmatic rupture.** *Eur J Cardiothorac Surg* 1999, **15**:469-74.

26. Gwely NN: **Outcome of blunt diaphragmatic rupture. Analysis of 44 cases.** *Asian Cardiovasc Thorac Ann* 2010, **18**:240-3.

27. Yalçinkaya I, Kisli E: **Traumatic diaphragmatic rupture: results of the chest surgery clinic.** *Ulus Travma Acil Cerrahi Derg* 2008, **14**:221-5.

2

Non operative management of abdominal trauma

Mohsin Raza[1,2*], Yasser Abbas[1], Vanitha Devi[1], Kumarapuram Venkatachalam Souriarajan Prasad[1], Kameel Narouz Rizk[1] and Permasavaran Padmanathan Nair[1]

Abstract

Introduction: Due to high rate of operative mortality and morbidity non-operative management of blunt liver and spleen trauma was widely accepted in stable pediatric patients, but the general surgeons were skeptical to adopt it for adults. The current study is analysis of so far largest sample (1071) of hemodynamically stable blunt liver, spleen, kidney and pancreatic trauma patients managed non operatively irrespective of severity of a single /multiple solid organ injury or other associated injuries with high rate of success.

Methods: Experience of 1071 blunt abdominal trauma patients treated by NOM at a tertiary care National Trauma Centre in Oman (from Jan 2001 to Dec 2011) was reviewed, analyzed to determine the indications, methods and results of NOM. Hemodynamic stability along with ultra sound, CT scan and repeated clinical examination were the sheet anchors of NOM. The patients were grouped as (1) managed by NOM successfully, (2) failure of NOM and (3) directly subjected to surgery.

Results: During the 10 year period, 5400 polytrauma patients were evaluated for abdominal trauma of which 1285 had abdominal injuries, the largest sample study till date. Based on initial findings 1071 patients were admitted for NOM. Out of 1071 patients initially selected 963 (89.91%) were managed non operatively, the remaining 108 (10.08%) were subjected to laparotomy due to failure of NOM. Laparotomy was performed on 214(19.98%) patients as they were unstable on admission or had evidence of hollow viscous injury.

Conclusion: NOM for blunt abdominal injuries was found to be highly successful in 89.98% of the patients in our study. Management depended on clinical and hemodynamic stability of the patient. A patient under NOM should be admitted to intensive care / high dependency for at least 48-72 hours for close monitoring of vital signs, repeated clinical examinations and follow up investigations as indicated.

Keywords: Non-operative management, Advanced Trauma life Support, Surgery

Introduction

Nearly six thousand men, women and children have lost their lives in road traffic crashes in Oman between 2000 and 2008. Seventy thousand injured and many disabled for life (Survey by German Institute of Technology in Oman).

Abdominal injuries occur in 31% patients of polytrauma with 13 and 16% spleen and liver injuries respectively, and pelvic injuries in 28% of cases, making differential diagnosis between pelvic or intractable abdominal injury difficult [1,2].The haemodynamically unstable patients with frank

signs of exsanguination have to undergo laparotomy, however, selecting these patients, especially in the polytrauma remains a challenge.

High rate of operative complications caused paradigm shift from operative to non-operative management (NOM) in hemodynamically stable blunt abdominal trauma patients [3,4]. NOM can be safely practiced in a Trauma Care Centre which has Trauma Surgeons, newer imaging modalities, High Dependency Unit (HDU), ICU and other supporting services [5]. Repeated clinical examination supplemented with modern imaging and laboratory investigations play a key role in reaching therapeutic decisions, thus preventing unnecessary laparotomies. Liver being a sturdy organ has a higher success NOM rate, exceeding

---
* Correspondence: drmohsinraza1@yahoo.com
[1]Surgery Department, Khoula Hospital, Muscat, Sultanate of Oman
[2]4/894, AikMinar Enclave, Near ShaukatManzil, Dodhpur, Aligarh, UP 202002, India

90% [6,7]. Haemodynamically stable liver and spleen injuries can be managed conservatively irrespective of the grade of injury [8-10]. NOM is also highly successful in case of renal trauma with success rates over 90% [11].

NOM of solid abdomen organ injuries is now established for hemodynamically stable patients. The present study is retrospective analysis and outcome of operative and NOM of blunt abdominal injuries in polytrauma at a Tertiary Care trauma Centre. Hemodynamically unstable patients with frank signs of exsanguination underwent urgent laparotomy, however, decision in polytrauma remains a challenge [12].

Material and methods

This is a ten year (January 2001 to December 2011) retrospective analysis of successful implementation of NOM for blunt abdominal trauma at a Tertiary Trauma Care Center in Oman. Oman has one of the highest incidences of Road traffic accidents in the world. Almost all the patients were victims of road traffic accidents. Being National trauma center, our hospital receives patients from all primary and secondary care hospitals in Oman, in addition to direct admission through accident and emergency.

On arrival all the patients were assessed and resuscitated if necessary, in accordance with ATLS protocol. History including the mechanism of injury formed an important part of the evaluation. All the patients underwent FAST/Abdominal sonography. Stable patients with positive FAST were further evaluated with chest, abdomen and pelvic CT scan. Patients with other associated injuries were examined by the respective specialists with close coordination. Patients with heart rate of <110/min, systolic BP of >90 mm Hg on arrival or following initial resuscitation were considered stable. Prior to the inclusion of the patients in the study an ethical clearance was sought from the competent authority of the Khoula Hospital, Oman. Written informed consent was obtained from the patient/close relatives for publication of this report and any accompanying images.

Among 5400 polytrauma patients, 1285 were diagnosed to have abdominal injuries. On secondary survey, based on hemodynamic stability, clinical findings and investigations, 1071(83%) patients were selected for NOM. The exclusion criteria for rejecting NOM in 214(17%) patients were signs of exsanguination, persistent hemodynamic instability and no response to initial resuscitation or obvious bowel injury. All stable patients were treated nonoperatively. The severity of head injury, associated orthopedic injuries, a high injury severity score or a higher radiological grading of the visceral injuries or multiple solid organ trauma were not considered as an exclusion criteria in haemodynamically stable patients.

NOM patients were admitted to HDU/ICU, closely monitored with repeated clinical assessment. The protocol included evaluation of vitals, Pulse, BP, temperature, urine output, 12 hourly hemoglobin, and hematocrit (HCT) estimation for the first 72 hrs. Follow up ultra sound abdomen or CT scan were done only if hemoglobin dropped despite 3 units of blood transfusion, progressive distension of abdomen, signs of infection, vomiting, hematuria or tachypnea. To detect occult bowel injuries, not able to diagnose otherwise, diagnostic peritoneal tap was notably successful.

NOM was successful in 963(89.91%) out of 1071 patients. Whereas, 108 patients showed signs of ongoing hemorrhage, delayed evidence of hollow viscous perforation, or intra-abdominal infection requiring laparotomy. They were grouped in NOM failed category.

Statistical analysis

The percent differences were calculated between the operated and nonoperated groups. Student's 't' test was used for statistical analysis, p values < 0.05 were considered to be statistically significant.

Results

A total of 5400 patients were evaluated for abdominal trauma during ten year period from January 2001 to December 2011. Various types of blunt abdominal injuries were found in 1285 patients. After initial evaluation, nonresponders to resuscitation, 214 hemodynamically unstable patients were operated, while, 1071 patients were initially selected for NOM, but NOM failed in 108 patients.

Males dominated in both groups with no significant difference in age, co-morbidities, and mechanism of injury (Table 1). Operated group presented with low systolic BP (<90 mm Hg), tachycardia, low haematocrit and higher blood transfusion requirement (Table 1). Intubation was done in 95% of patients in the Emergency Department.

Most of the patients had polytrauma, hence no significant difference in the Injury Severity Score (ISS) was appreciated between the two groups (Table 1). FAST was positive in 100% in the operated group. No significant difference was noted between the NOM and the operated group in relation to the liver, spleen and multiple abdominal injuries (Table 1). NOM failure group had multiple solid organ injuries in 92(85%) patients. We could easily manage the patients with severe isolated liver (Figure 1), spleen and kidney injuries (Figure 2). Both liver and spleen were injured in 15.6% patients (Figure 3), while 21 patients (1.9%) had three solid organs liver, spleen and kidney injured. One 6 year old girl had liver, spleen, pancreas, bilateral kidney injuries with bilateral hemothorax and bilateral pelvic acetabular fracture, was successfully managed non-operatively (Figure 4), 196 (18.3%) patients

Table 1 Comparison of various parameters in NOM-S, NOM-F and Operative groups and demographic, admission and injury characteristics

	NOM-S group	NOM-F group	Operative- group
	n = 963	n = 108	n = 214
Age	25.31#	35.21#	31.26*#
Male sex	558(58%)	73(68%)	132(62%)
RTA	895(93%)	99(92%)	201(93%)
ISS	37.09# ±1.58	41# ±2.25	40.93*# ±2.25
Haematocrit on admission	36.62# ±3.97	31.83# ±2.67	27.53*# ±2.89
SBP > 90mmhg	885(92%)	68(63%)	25(12%)
Heart rate < 110/min	799(83%)	92(85%)	203(95%)
Blood transfusion	2.77# ±0.85	5.10# ± 0.96	5.57*# ±0.87
Positive FAST	818(85%)	102(94.4%)	214(100%)
Co- morbidities	404(42%)	96(45%)	71(66%)
Liver Injury	320(33%)	0	29*(13.55%) ±1.64
Splenic injury	288(30%)	16(15%)	37*(17.3%) ±0.35
Others	355(37%)	92(85%)	148*(69.16%) ±1.92

RTA Road Traffic Accident, ISS Injury Severity Score, SBP Systolic Blood Pressure, FAST Focused Abdominal Sonography for Trauma.
Values are #Mean ± SEM. The *p < 0.05 were considered as significant as compared to NOM-S and Operative groups.

had multiple organ injury associated with retroperitoneal hematoma and fractures (Table 2).

The operated group had an ICU admission rate of 57%, with a longer period of hospitalization (23.31 days) and higher morbidity (16%) in comparison to the NOM with an ICU admission rate of 24%, length of stay (10.23 days) and morbidity of (<1%) (Table 1). In the operative group six patients died.

In the NOM failure group 16 patients had delayed splenic bleed presenting between 24 hours and 10 days. Delayed small bowel rupture was observed in 21 patients. Bowel injury was missed on the initial CT scan in 3 patients. Ongoing mesenteric vessel bleed with delayed bowel ischemia occurred in 37 patients. Intraperitoneal urinary bladder tear was missed in 5 cases, non-therapeutic laparatomies done in 28 cases of retroperitoneal hematoma. Sigmoid colon injury diagnosis was masked and delayed for 24 hours due to severe head injury associated with fracture femur in one patient, causing mortality.

Sub serous extravasations of dye in contrast CT (Figure 5), bowel wall thickening or mesenteric fat streaking may not be very reliable signs but suspicious of mesenteric injury. It causes ischemia but may take 2-3 days to cause perforation. We observed an unexplained tachycardia, while the ischemic process in the bowel goes on. Patients kept passing stools for 3-4 days after trauma until the ischemic bowel wall ruptured causing peritonitis (Figure 6).

Discussion

Sir McCormack in 1900 was the first to advocate "A man wounded in war in the abdomen dies if he is operated upon and remains alive if he is left in peace" [13]. This aphorism was a surgical doctrine to manage abdominal trauma in the warfield during early 20th century. This practice went into oblivion due to dogma of mandatory laparotomy in every case of hemoperitonium.

The advent of newer imaging techniques with high resolution CT scanners has enabled the clinicians to

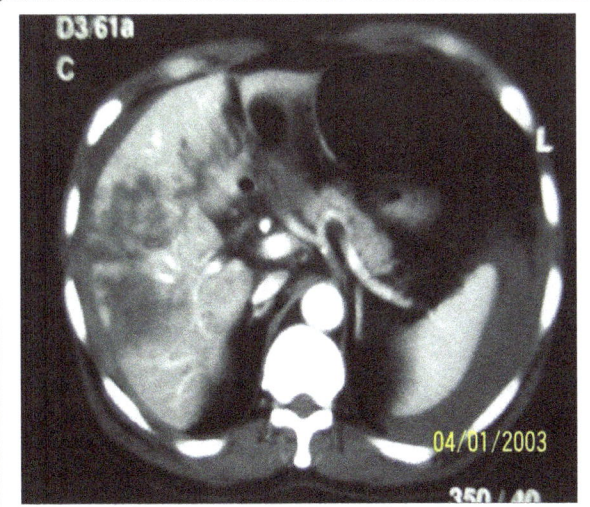

Figure 1 The picture shows severely injured liver.

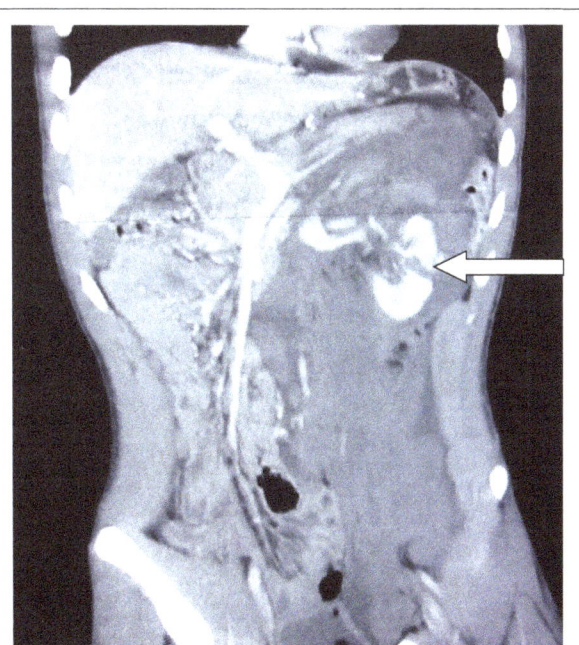

Figure 2 Severe renal injury with a midline shift, successfully managed non operatively, arrow showing injured kidney.

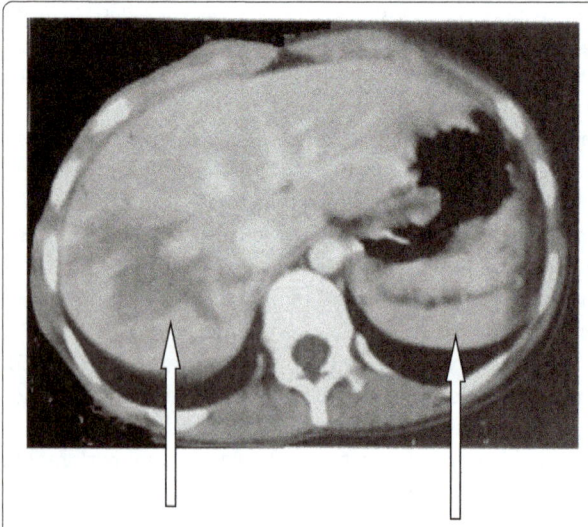

Figure 3 Shows both liver and splenic injuries indicated by arrows.

hemoperitoneum may not have any significant clinical findings. Hemodynamically stable patients with solid organ injury should be considered for NOM after ruling out bowel trauma. Published literatures and our study have shown that radiological grade of severity of injury is not a contraindication for NOM [15]. CT contrast blush from minor vessels in solid organs were managed by NOM with caution. However, a CT contrast blush of a major vessel in arterial / venous phase is indicative of ongoing hemorrhage, which portends NOM failure. Mesenteric injuries causing bowel ischemia remains a challenge [16]. Presence of fluid without solid organ injury is a significant marker of mesenteric or bowel injury [17]. Usefulness of CT in bowel injuries remains controversial [18].

Liver due to its firm texture is more confidently treated by NOM [19]. In our analysis NOM succeeded in all stable isolated liver injuries but failed in 15% isolated splenic trauma. Delayed splenic bleed occurred in 16 (1.5%) of total 1071 patients with other associated injuries. Most splenic injuries did not require close observation beyond 3 days [14,20].

In x-ray, absence of free air under diaphragm or oral contrast leak does not rule out bowel injury. In suspected stable patients we have done peritoneal tap to look for bowel contents. In absence of perforation and to ensure cessation of intraperitoneal bleed and subsequent resorption of blood breakdown products from the vast peritoneal surface, we left the catheter in situ to drain out collected blood from peritoneal cavity, until it stops draining.

We have very good success rate in the management of high grade renal injuries conservatively and the same is recorded in other centers [11,21]. All extraperitoneal

exactly diagnose the extent of intra-abdominal organ injury [2]. With the publication of many reports of success during the last 20 years, NOM has become an established and accepted management protocol for solid organ injuries in hemodynamically stable patients [9,14].

NOM poses challenge to Trauma Surgeons on account of varied clinical picture on arrival. The associated injuries, alcohol and drugs may mask abdominal signs and symptoms. Patients with short pre-hospital transport time have initial subtle clinical features affecting early diagnosis. Around 20 to 40% patients with radiologically significant

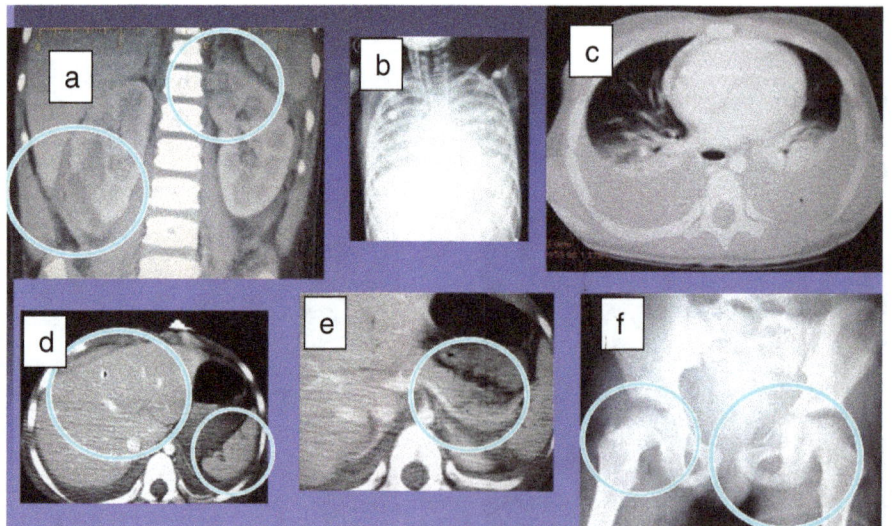

Figure 4 Shows all the solid organ injuries with bilateral haemothorax and fractures: A girl aged 6 years had injuries in all the solid organs (a) both kidneys,(b) and (c) bilateral haemothorax (d) liver and spleen, (e) body of pancreas, (f) bilateral acetabular fractures were treated non operatively except bilateral intercostal drains were inserted.

Table 2 Distribution of NOM patients according to their organ injury

Organs injured in nom patients	Number	Percentage
Liver Injury Isolated	320	29.8
Spleen Isolated Injury	304	28.3
Kidney Isolated Injury	052	05.2
Pancreatic injury	4	0.3
Ureteric Injury	3	0.2
Urinary Bladder (Intraperitoneal)	1	0.09
Liver/Spleen	168	15.6
Liver/Spleen/Kidney	21	1.9
Liver/Spleen/Kidney/Pancreas	1	0.09
Bilateral Kidney Injury	1	0.09
Others (Multiple organ injuries with associated retroperitoneal haematoma with pelvic fractures)	196	18.3

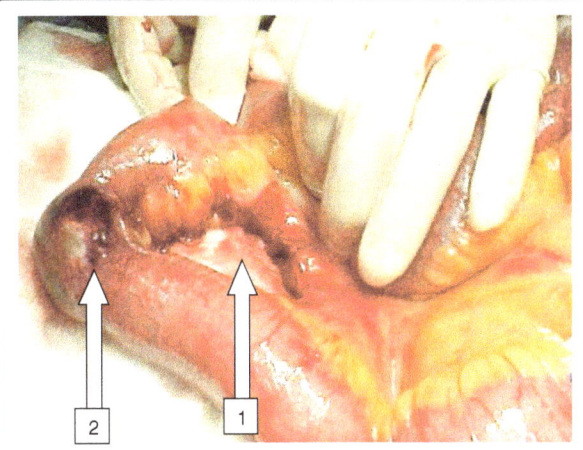

Figure 6 Mesentric vascular injury showing bowel wall necrosis and delayed perforation: Mesenteric injury (1) caused bowel ischemia but bowel wall necrosis and perforation occurred late on third day (2). Such patients have an unexplained high pulse rate.

urinary bladder injuries were treated with transurethral catheter, including 4 patients with small intraperitoneal leaks.

Blood transfusion requirement, morbidity, mortality and incidence of non-therapeutic laparotomy were significantly reduced with NOM. The successful management depends on repeated clinical assessment preferably by the same clinical team in HDU/ICU, hemodynamic stability, serial determination of hemoglobin, haematocrit, WBC and follow up ultrasound/CT scan, if indicated. However, routine repeate CT scan is not essential in clinically improving patients. Thumping of chest for physiotherapy is strictly forbidden in splenic and liver injuries. Conscious patients not having spine, lower limb or pelvic fractures were mobilized within 48 hours. Initially hospital authorities and even our surgical colleagues were critical about NOM, but following successful results, NOM has now been accepted as a standard method of managing hemodynamically stable blunt abdominal trauma patients in most of the Trauma Centres including ours with a success rate of above 80% [4]. Heyn etal [12] suggested that in patients with multiple injuries abdominal ultra sound and CT have complementary value. Anatomical CT grading is an ineffective exclusion criterion for NOM or embolisation for splenic or hepatic trauma [15].

Earlier NOM was not preferred in polytraumatised patients but recently several reports of successful results in polytrauma with strict monitoring irrespective of age or other concomitant injuries have been reported [7,22] and the same is reproduced in our study.

Higher amount of blood transfusions were given to maintain hemodynamic stability in patients with associated long bone, pelvic fractures, retroperitoneal hematomas and hemothorax etc. Isolated liver, spleen or kidney injuries did not receive more than 3-4 pints of blood.

In our analysis we did not find any significant differences between the operated and NOM group in relation to the age, co- morbidities and mechanism of injury. But the operated group presented with poor hemodynamic stability thus necessitating increased blood transfusion and higher rate of intubation in the Emergency Department as compared to the NOM group.

As we look ahead the NOM will play major role in management of patients with blunt abdominal trauma.

Conclusion

NOM for blunt abdominal trauma was found to be highly successful and safe in our analysis. Management by NOM depends on clinical and hemodynamic stability of the patient, after definitive indications for laparotomy are excluded. A patient under NOM should be admitted to

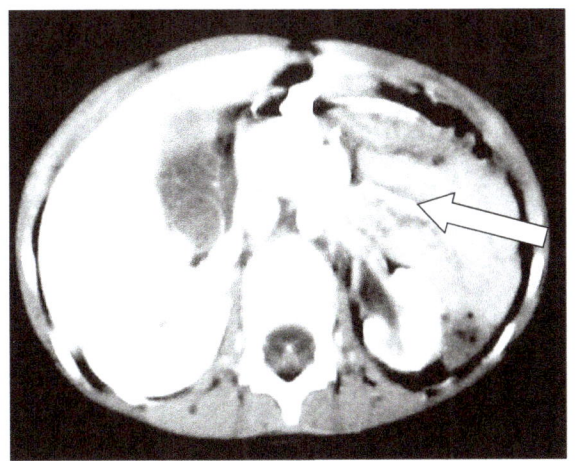

Figure 5 Subserous extravasation of dye causing a fuzzy mesentry is suspicious of mesenteric vascular disruption.

ICU / HDU for at least 48-72 hours for close monitoring of vital signs and repeated clinical examinations. Follow up radiological investigations to be done as indicated. Higher anatomical image grading [3-5] of solid organ injury is not a deterrent to NOM. Even patients with multiple abdominal injuries can be successfully managed by NOM provided they are closely monitored. NOM has a significant decrease in lengt of hospital stay and morbidity compared to patients who undergo surgery. Fully equipped trauma care centres with available trauma surgeons willing to operate at any time is very important. NOM to be terminated if patient develops haemodynamic instability and appearance of new peritoneal signs due to delayed hollow viscous or missed injuries.

No procedure /practice are free from risk. Admission to ICU and its related problems, delay in diagnosis and management of missed bowel and vascular injuries are few of the risks involved in NOM. With newer modalities of imaging the percentage of delay in diagnosis is negligible.

Abbreviations
HDU: High dependency unit; ICU: Intensive care unit; ATLS: Advanced life trauma support; FAST: Focused abdominal sonography in Trauma.

Competing interests
The authors declare that they have no competing interests.

Authors' contributions
MR Head of the unit conceived the idea of the study, and also performed and supervised the whole process and operated when required, written and corresponded the manuscript. YA assisted in managing the patients with strict vigilance and helped in the preparation of manuscript. VD, KVSP, PPN assisted in managing the patients, performed and recorded repeated clinical assessments, acted upon and notified alarming changes in clinical features of the patients. KNR closely collaborated and supported the study, helped in preparation of manuscript discussed and critically analyzed the non operative management of patients in grand rounds on day to day basis. All authors read and approved the final manuscript.

Acknowledgment
Thanks are due to Dr. Feras Al-lawaty, Former Director General, Khoula Hospital, Muscat, Oman for permission to conduct the study, support and assistance and also to our general surgery colleagues (Dr Helem Maskery ,Dr Atef Saqr and Dr Asrar Malik), Intensivists, Anaesthetists, Neurosurgery, Orthopedic, Obstetrics and Gynaecology colleagues of the hospital. Our thanks are also due to Prof. Dr. Naheed Banu for helping in preparation of the manuscript.

References
1. Luke PH, Leene K: Abdominal trauma: from operative to no-operative management. *Int J care Inj* 2009, **40S4**:S62–S68.
2. Deunk J, Brink M, Dekker H, *et al*: Predictors for the selection of patients for abdominal CT after blunt trauma: a proposal for a diagnostic algorithm. *Ann Surg* 2010, **251**(3):512–520.
3. Velmahos GC, Toutouzas KG, Radin R, Chan L, Demetriades D: Non-operative treatment of blunt injury to solid abdominal organs: a prospective study. *Arch Surg* 2003, **138**(8):844–851.
4. Giannopoulos GA, Katsoulis EI, Tzanakis NE, Panayotis AP, Digalakis M: Non-operative management of blunt abdominal trauma. Is it safe and feasible in a district general hospital? Scand. J. Trauma Resuscitation &. *Emerg Med* 2009, **17**:22–28.

5. van der Vlies CH, Olthof DC, Gaakeer M, Ponsen KJ, van Delden OM, Goslings JC: Changing patterns in diagnostic strategies and the treatment of blunt injury to solid abdominal organs. *Int J Emerg Med* 2011 Jul 27, **4**:47. doi:10.1186/1865-1380-4-47.
6. Velmahos GC, Toutouzas KG, Radin R, Chan L, Rhee P, Tillou A, Demetriades D: High success with non-operative management of blunt hepatic trauma:the liver is a sturdy organ. *Arch Surg* 2003, **138**(5):475–480.
7. Gwendolyn M, Van der Wilden, George CV, Timothy E, Samielle B, *et al*: Successful nonoperative management of the most severe blunt liver injuries: a multicenter study of the research consortium of New England centers for trauma. *Arch Surg* 2012, **147**(5):423–428. doi:10.1001/archsurg.2012.147.
8. Marmorale C, Guercioni G, Siquini W: Non-operative management of blunt abdominal injuries. *Chir Ital* 2007, **59**(1):1–15.
9. Peitzman A, Ferrada P, Puyana J: Nonoperative management of blunt abdominal trauma: have we gone too far? *Surg Infect (Larchmt)* 2009 Oct, **10**(5):427–433.
10. Swift C, Garner J: Non-operative management of liver trauma. *J R Army Med Corps* 2012 Jun, **158**(2):85–95.
11. Santucci RA, Wessells H, Bartsch G, Descotes J, Heyns CF, McAninch JW, Nash P, Schmidlin F: Evaluation and management of renal injuries: consensus statement of the renal trauma subcommittee. *BJU Int* 2004, **93**:937–954.
12. Heyn J, Ladurner R, Ozimek A, *et al*: Diagnosis and preoperative management of multiple injured patients with explorative laparotomy because of blunt abdomina trauma. *Eur J Med Res* 2008, **13**:517–524.
13. McCormack: *J. Royal Soc. Medicine.* 84th edition. Derbyshire Royal Infirmary Derby DEI 2 QY: 555 JDC Bennett FRCS DCH Department of ENT; 1991.
14. Stassen N, Bhullar I, Cheng J, *et al*: Selective nonoperative management of blunt splenic injury: an Eastern Association for the Surgery of Trauma practice management guideline. *J Trauma Acute Care Surg* 2012 Nov, **73**(5 Suppl 4):S294–S300.
15. Cohn SM, Arango JI, Myers JG, *et al*: Computed tomography grading systems poorly predict the need for intervention after spleen and liver injuries. *Am Surg* 2009, **75**:133–139.
16. Sherck JP, Oakes DD: Intestinal injuries missed by computed tomography. *J Trauma* 1990, **30**:1–5.
17. Chen ZB, Zhang Y, Liang ZY, Zhang SY, Yu WQ, Gao Y, Zheng SS: Incidence of unexplained intra-abdominal free fluid in patients with blunt abdominal trauma. *Hepatobiliary Pancreat Dis Int* 2009 Dec, **8**(6):597–601.
18. Magu S, Agarwal S, Ravinder G: Multi Detector Computed Tomography in the Diagnosis of Bowel Injury. *Indian J Surg* 2012, **74**(6):p445.
19. Bouras A, Truant S, Pruvot F, *et al*: Management of blunt hepatic trauma. *J Visc Surg* 2010, **147**(6):e351–e358.
20. Beuran M, Gheju I, Venter M, *et al*: Non-operative management of splenic trauma. *J Med Life* 2012, **5**(1):47–58.
21. Baverstock R, Simons R, McLoughlin M: Severe blunt renal trauma: a 7-year retrospective review from a provincial trauma centre. *Can J Urol* 2001, **8**:1372–1376.
22. Sartorelli, Kennith H, Frumiento, Carmine R, Frederick B, Osler, Turner M: Nonoperative management of hepatic, splenic, and renal injuries in adults with multiple injuries. *Journal of Trauma-Injury Infection & Critical Care* 2000, **49**(1):56–62. 56.

3

Blunt trauma induced splenic blushes are not created equal

Clay Cothren Burlew[1,2]*, Lucy Z Kornblith[1], Ernest E Moore[1], Jeffrey L Johnson[1] and Walter L Biffl[1]

Abstract

Background: Currently, evidence of contrast extravasation on computed tomography (CT) scan is regarded as an indication for intervention in splenic injuries. In our experience, patients transferred from other institutions for angioembolization have often resolved the blush upon repeat imaging at our hospital. We *hypothesized* that not all splenic blushes require intervention.

Methods: During a 10-year period, we reviewed all patients transferred with blunt splenic injuries and contrast extravasation on initial postinjury CT scan.

Results: During the study period, 241 patients were referred for splenic injuries, of whom 16 had a contrast blush on initial CT imaging (88% men, mean age 35 ± 5, mean ISS 26 ± 3). Eight (50%) patients were managed without angioembolization or operation. Comparing patients with and without intervention, there was a significant difference in admission heart rate (106 ± 9 *vs* 83 ± 6) and decline in hematocrit following transfer (5.3 ± 2.0 *vs* 1.0 ± 0.3), but not in injury grade (3.9 ± 0.2 *vs* 3.5 ± 0.3), systolic blood pressure (125 ± 10 *vs* 115 ± 6), or age (38.5 ± 8.2 *vs* 30.9 ± 4.7). Of the 8 observed patients, 3 underwent repeat imaging immediately upon arrival with resolution of the blush. In the intervention group, 4 patients had ongoing extravasation on·repeat imaging, 2 patients underwent empiric embolization, and 2 patients underwent splenectomy for physiologic indications.

Conclusions: For blunt splenic trauma, evidence of contrast extravasation on initial CT imaging is not an absolute indication for intervention. A period of observation with repeat imaging could avoid costly, invasive interventions and their associated sequelae.

Keywords: Trauma, Injury, Spleen, Blush, Contrast extravasation, Angioembolization

Introduction

A contrast blush on computed tomography (CT) scan has been identified as a risk factor for failure of nonoperative management (NOM) of splenic injuries [1-3], prompting many centers to perform routine splenic artery angioembolization in the presence of a blush [4,5]. Using evidence of contrast extravasation on CT scan as an indication for angioembolization, however, has never been subjected to rigorous analysis. In our experience, patients with splenic injuries transferred from other institutions specifically for angioembolization have often resolved the blush upon repeat imaging at our hospital. This made us question whether all

postinjury splenic blushes were equivalent. Is evidence of contrast blush a mandate for intervention, or are there some injuries that cease active bleeding due to "internal tamponade" within the substance of the spleen? And how does one differentiate such patients? We *hypothesized* that not all splenic blushes require intervention and that patients may be selectively observed based upon physiologic status.

Materials and methods

During a 10 year period, all patients transferred from an outside hospital with blunt splenic injuries and evidence of active contrast extravasation on initial postinjury CT scan were evaluated. Patients undergoing intervention (angioembolization or splenectomy) were compared to those managed without intervention. Demographic data, laboratory values, vitals, intervention, and outcome were

* Correspondence: clay.cothren@dhha.org
[1]From The Department of Surgery, Denver Health Medical Center, Denver CO, USA

analyzed. Patients with identified pseudoaneurysms were excluded. Statistical analysis was performed using SAS for Windows (SAS Institute, Cory, NC); *p-value* < 0.05 was considered statistically significant. The Colorado Multi-Institutional Review Board approved this study.

Results

During the study period, 241 patients with splenic injuries were transferred from an outside hospital, of which 16 had a contrast blush on CT imaging. All contrast blushes were intraparenchymal. The majority (88%) of patients were men with a mean age of 35 ± 5 and mean ISS of 26 ± 3. Mean time of transfer to Denver Health following injury and evaluation at an outside hospital was 6.4 ± 1.5 h. One patient received 1 unit of packed red blood cells during transfer. No patient reported use of anticoagulant or antiplatelet medications. Eight (50%) of these sixteen patients were managed without angioembolization or operation. In the group not undergoing intervention, Focused Abdominal Sonography for Trauma (FAST) examination was positive in six and negative in two patients. In patients undergoing intervention, FAST was positive in two patients and was not performed in the remainder. The two groups of patients had similar splenic AAST injury grades, age, injury severity scores, and emergency department systolic blood pressure (Table 1). The amount of intraperitoneal blood did not appear to be different between the two groups. The group managed without intervention had 1 patient with left upper quadrant (LUQ) blood, 5 patients with bilateral upper quadrant (BUQ) free fluid, and 2 patients with blood extending into the pelvis. In the group undergoing intervention, 3 patients had BUQ free fluid, and 3 patients had blood extending into the pelvis; the remaining 2 patients had no comment of intraperitoneal free fluid noted. In patients undergoing intervention there was a significant difference in admission heart rate and decline in hematocrit following transfer compared to patients who did not require operation or angioembolization (Table 1).

In the 8 (50%) patients managed with observation, 3 underwent repeat imaging immediately after transfer; CT scan revealed the blush had resolved (Figure 1). None

required blood product transfusion. Of these 8 patients there was 1 complication; a 49 year-old man with a grade III splenic laceration which had been stable without extravasation on repeat CT scan imaging had a delayed bleed on hospital day #4 treated with angioembolization. Eight (50%) patients underwent intervention following transfer (5 angioembolizations and 3 splenectomies). Two patients underwent immediate angiography without repeat CT scanning; although there was no evidence of contrast extravasation they underwent empiric main splenic artery embolization. Four patients had evidence of ongoing extravasation on repeat CT scan imaging and underwent intervention (3 angioembolization and 1 splenectomy). Two patients underwent immediate splenectomy upon arrival to DHMC based upon clinical indices. The eight patients received a mean of 3 ± 1.6 units of packed red cells during hospitalization. None of the eight patients had a splenic related complication. There were no significant differences in ventilator days, ICU length of stay, or hospital length of stay between the intervention and observation groups.

Discussion

Angioembolization has been reported to increase the success rates of NOM of splenic injuries [5-10]. One scenario which is considered by some to be an absolute indication for angioembolization is the hemodynamically stable patient demonstrating a contrast blush on admission CT scan. It is a logical presumption that evidence of arterial bleeding, a contrast blush, seen on CT imaging would decrease the likelihood of spontaneous hemostasis. In fact, patients with a splenic injury and an associated contrast blush are reportedly 24 times more likely to fail NOM [1]. Further study by Federle et al. noted a 19% incidence of contrast blush in their patient population of which only 7% were successful in NOM [2]. Therefore, angiography for patients manifesting a blush associated with their splenic injury has been recommended [11]. However, these data do not answer the question of whether all patients with evidence of contrast extravasation from splenic injury mandate intervention. Angioembolization is invasive, costly, and complications occur in over 20% of patients [8,12-14].

Table 1 Patient demographics and injury characteristics stratified by management technique

	Injury Grade	Age	ISS	SBP in the ED	HR in the ED	Decline in hematocrit following transfer
Nonoperative Management (N = 8)	3.5 ± 0.3	30.9 ± 4.7	26.8 ± 4.2	115 ± 6	83 ± 6	1.0 ± 0.3
Intervention (N = 8)	3.9 ± 0.2	38.5 ± 8.2	25.5 ± 4.6	125 ± 10	106 ± 9*	5.3 ± 2.0*

ISS Injury Severity Score, *SBP* systolic blood pressure, *HR* heart rate **p-value* < 0.05
ED Emergency Department

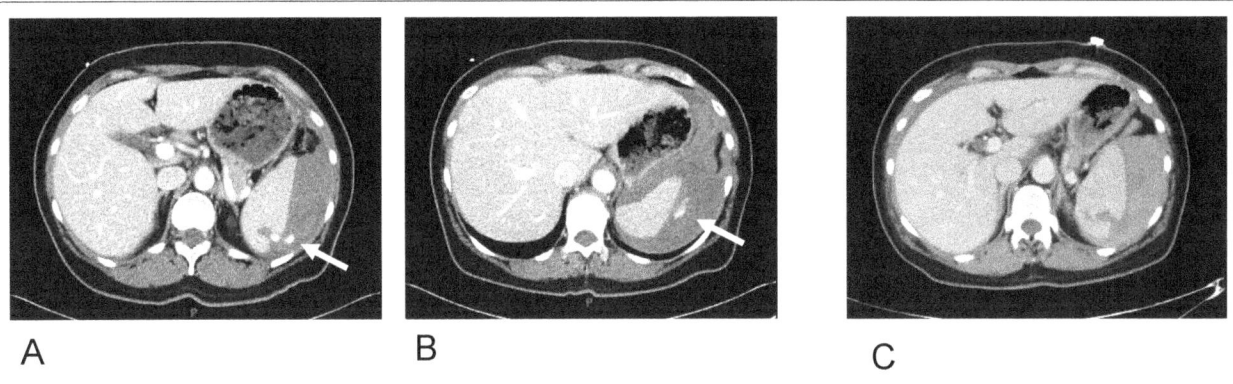

Figure 1 CT scans from the outside hospital demonstrate contrast extravasation from the spleen (A,B). Repeat imaging at Denver Health reveals the blush has resolved (c).

In our experience, half of patients with a contrast blush on initial postinjury CT scan did not require intervention, either operative or catheter based, following transfer to our hospital for intended angioembolization. This number may, in fact, have been higher if the two patients who did not show evidence of extravasation at angiography but underwent empiric embolization were considered in this group rather than the treatment group. Those patients that underwent intervention had significantly higher ED heart rates and decline in their post-transfer hematocrit. Similar to our findings, Omert et al. reported that a patient's hemodynamics are more predictive of the need for intervention than contrast blush alone [15]. They describe the successful NOM of nine patients with splenic injuries and contrast blush, concluding that the mere presence of a contrast blush was not an absolute indication for intervention. Similar conclusions in children have also been reported [16]. Unlike other studies that have shown a correlation between increasing AAST splenic injury grade, increased incidence of contrast blush, and need for intervention [1], our group showed similar injury grades between those undergoing NOM and those requiring intervention.

There are inherent limitations in any retrospective evaluation. Additionally, the numbers in this series may be considered small, hence precluding broad generalization. However, this study serves to underscore that the surgical dictum, all blushes require embolization, may not be supported by scientific evidence once evaluated. This study is small due to the catchment population - only those patients with outside facility imaging demonstrating a blush associated with a splenic injury were included. We purposefully excluded those patients whose first evaluation was in our own emergency department with subsequent admission as management along the "surgical dictum" was more probable. By analyzing those patients who underwent transport times and hence permitted a repeated and delayed evaluation, gave us a time-frame

without intervention. Finally, specifics of CT imaging technique at the outside hospital were not obtained, such as contrast volume, rate of infusion, slice thickness, and presence of delayed images; if the outside facility's physicians felt the imaging supported a diagnosis of a splenic blush mandating transport to a level I trauma center we felt specifics were of secondary importance.

Conclusions

With increases in technology and high resolution CT imaging, it is likely that more contrast blushes will be detected. Assuming that a hemodynamically stable patient requires angiography for investigation of a contrast blush is not based on scientific evidence. Based upon our experience, albeit limited in numbers and retrospective in nature, we do not feel evidence of contrast extravasation on initial CT imaging alone is a definitive indication for intervention. A period of close observation, serial examination, repeat laboratory evaluation, repeat FAST for those with an initial negative FAST, and selective repeat CT imaging, should be considered. A clinically based approach, similar to that used in all patients to determine operative versus NOM of blunt splenic injuries, rather than immediate angiography could avoid costly, invasive interventions and their associated sequelae. Future prospective trials would help delineate patients with splenic blushes who can be managed non-operatively, and could help develop treatment algorithms.

Author details
[1]From The Department of Surgery, Denver Health Medical Center, Denver CO, USA. [2]Surgical Intensive Care Unit, Trauma & Acute Care Surgery Fellowship, Department of Surgery, Denver Health Medical Center, 777 Bannock Street, MC 0206, Denver, CO 80204, USA.

Authors' contributions
Study Design: B Data Collection/Analysis/Interpretation: B, K, M. Manuscript Drafting: B, K, M. Critical Review: B, J. All authors read and approved the final manuscript.

Competing interests
The authors declare that they have no competing interests.

References
1. Schurr MJ, Fabian TC, Gavant M, et al: Management of blunt splenic trauma: computed tomographic contrast blush predicts failure of nonoperative management. J Trauma 1988, 28:828-831.
2. Federle MP, Courcoulas AP, Peitzman AB, et al: Blunt splenic injury in adults: clinical and CT criteria for management, with emphasis on active extravasation. Radiology 1998, 206:137-142.
3. Bee TK, Croce MA, Miller PR, Pritchard FE, Fabian TC: Failures of splenic nonoperative management: is the glass half empty or half full? J Trauma 2001, 50(2):230-236.
4. Haan JM, Bochicchio GV, Kramer N, Scalea TM: Nonoperative management of blunt splenic injury: a 5-year experience. J Trauma 2005, 58:492-498.
5. Wei B, Hemmila MR, Arbabi S, Taheri PA, Wahl WL: Angioembolization reduces operative intervention for blunt splenic injury. J Trauma 2008, 64:1472-1477.
6. Sclafani SJ, Shaftan GW, Scalea TM, et al: Nonoperative salvage of computed tomography-diagnosed splenic injuries: utilization of angiography for triage and embolization for hemostasis. J Trauma 1995, 39:818-827.
7. Davis KA, Fabian TC, Croce MA, et al: Improved success in nonoperative management of blunt splenic injuries: embolization of splenic artery pseudoaneurysms. J Trauma 1998, 44:1008-1015.
8. Haan JM, Biffl W, Knudson MM, et al: Splenic embolization revisited: a multicenter review. J Trauma 2004, 56:542-547.
9. Dent D, Alsabrook G, Erickson BA, et al: Blunt splenic injuries: high nonoperative management rate can be achieved with selective embolization. J Trauma 2004, 56:1063-1067.
10. Rajani RR, Claridge JA, Yowler CJ, et al: Improved outcome of adult blunt splenic injury: a cohort analysis. Surgery 2006, 140(4):625-631.
11. Moore FA, Davis JW, Moore EE Jr, Cocanour CS, West MA, McIntyre RC Jr: Western Trauma Association (WTA) critical decisions in trauma: management of adult blunt splenic trauma. J Trauma 2008, 65(5):1007-1011.
12. Wu SC, Chen RJ, Yang AD, Teng CC, Lee KH: Complications associated with embolization in the treatment of blunt splenic injury. World J Surg 2008, 32:476-482.
13. Smith HE, Biffl WL, Majercik SD, Jednacz J, Lambiase R, Cioffi WG: Splenic artery embolization: Have we gone too far? J Trauma 2006, 61(3):541-544.
14. Ekeh AP, McCarthy MC, Woods RJ, et al: Complications arising from splenic embolization after blunt splenic trauma. Am J Surg 2005, 189:335-339.
15. Omert LA, Salyer D, Dunham CM, Silva A, Protetch J: Implications of the 'contrast blush' finding on computed tomographic scan of the spleen in trauma. J Trauma 2001, 51(2):272-277.
16. Cloutier DR, Baird TB, Gormley P, McCarten KM, Bussey JG, Luks FI: Pediatric splenic injuries with a contrast blush: successful nonoperative management without angiography and embolization. J Pediatr Surg 2004, 39:969-971.

4

Therapeutic anticoagulation can be safely accomplished in selected patients with traumatic intracranial hemorrhage

Matthew C Byrnes[1,2,3*], Eric Irwin[1], Robert Roach[1], Molly James[2], Patrick K Horst[2] and Patty Reicks[1]

Abstract

Introduction: Therapeutic anticoagulation is an important treatment of thromboembolic complications, such as DVT, PE, and blunt cerebrovascular injury. Traumatic intracranial hemorrhage has traditionally been considered to be a contraindication to anticoagulation.

Hypothesis: Therapeutic anticoagulation can be safely accomplished in select patients with traumatic intracranial hemorrhage.

Methods: Patients who developed thromboembolic complications of DVT, PE, or blunt cerebrovascular injury were stratified according to mode of treatment. Patients who underwent therapeutic anticoagulation with a heparin infusion or enoxaparin (1 mg/kg BID) were evaluated for neurologic deterioration or hemorrhage extension by CT scan.

Results: There were 42 patients with a traumatic intracranial hemorrhage that subsequently developed a thrombotic complication. Thirty-five patients developed a DVT or PE. Blunt cerebrovascular injury was diagnosed in four patients. 26 patients received therapeutic anticoagulation, which was initiated an average of 13 days after injury. 96% of patients had no extension of the hemorrhage after anticoagulation was started. The degree of hemorrhagic extension in the remaining patient was minimal and was not felt to affect the clinical course.

Conclusion: Therapeutic anticoagulation can be accomplished in select patients with intracranial hemorrhage, although close monitoring with serial CT scans is necessary to demonstrate stability of the hemorrhagic focus.

Introduction

Injury represents one of the most common causes of morbidity and mortality in children and young adults. Although many complications can be seen after injury, venous thromboembolic disease can be among the most vexing. Virchow's triad involves venous stasis, endothelial injury, and hypercoaguability, which are often seen in this patient population [1-3]. Injured patients often require immobility as a result of critical illness or skeletal fractures. Endothelial injuries are caused by fractures or venous stretching, and hematologic alterations associated with trauma result in hypercoagulability. The risk of venous thromboembolism (VTE) is dependent upon the specific injuries present in individual patients. While a single site arm fracture is unlikely to lead to VTE, a multisystem injury that includes a spinal cord injury, head injury, and multiple long bone fractures is very likely to lead to VTE [1]. The actual risks of VTE have been estimated to vary between 7%–58% [4].

A significant amount of study has been directed at preventing VTE in injured patients. Prophylactic doses of heparin or low molecular weight heparin have been demonstrated to significantly reduce the risk of VTE [4,5]. This intervention has been demonstrated to be safe within days of the initial injury, with only a small risk of bleeding complications. Once a thrombosis or embolus has occurred, however, prophylactic doses of anticoagulation are no longer adequate.

Injured patients are also at risk of arterial thromboembolism (ATE). Patients with mitral valve replacements

* Correspondence: mbyrnes150@yahoo.com
[1]Department of Trauma, North Memorial Medical Center, Robbinsdale, MN, USA
[2]Division of Critical Care and Acute Care Surgery, University of Minnesota, Minneapolis, MN, USA

are at risk of cerebrovascular accidents without anticoagulation. Patients with traumatic blunt cerebrovascular injury are also at risk without anticoagulation.

The traditional treatment of VTE has been therapeutic levels of anticoagulation [3]. The primary complication of therapeutic anticoagulation is hemorrhage, which is a significant consideration in injured patients. Patients with intracranial hemorrhagic diatheses (traumatic and nontraumatic) have been felt to be at an especially high risk of developing complications of anticoagulation [2,6]. Extension of an intracranial bleed can be especially troublesome and can potential lead to death or severe disability. In the presence of a contraindication to anticoagulation, inferior vena cava filters have been recommended to prevent embolus of thrombi from the lower extremity venous system to the pulmonary vasculature [3]. While this approach is reasonable for many injured patients, there are certain patient populations who would benefit from anticoagulation. As such, it is important to know the risks of therapeutic anticoagulation in patients with intracranial hemorrhage. Unfortunately, there is very literature to guide clinical decisions. Expert recommendations have suggested that therapeutic anticoagulation should be avoided, but no studies to date have reported the safety profile of this intervention.

Herein, we developed a study with the following objectives: (1) to evaluate the likelihood of extension of intracranial bleeding after the introduction of therapeutic anticoagulation; and (2) to evaluate the time course associated with introduction of therapeutic anticoagulation after the initial injury.

Methods

Medical records of patients admitted to a university affiliated Level I trauma center were reviewed. Patients who had both a thrombotic complication and an intracranial hemorrhage were selected for inclusion. The thrombotic events that were incorporated in the study included: deep venous thrombosis (DVT), pulmonary embolus (PE), and blunt cerebrovascular injury. Patient demographics and CT scan results were noted. Patients were stratified according to the decision to use therapeutic anticoagulation vs. another treatment modality. Mortality and expansion of hemorrhage on CT scan were compared between the groups.

All patients were admitted to the trauma service. All patients received a head CT on admission and neurosurgery was subsequently consulted. There were four trauma surgeons during the study period that served as the core of the program and there were two neurosurgeons that were consulted on all patients with neurologic injuries. Patients who had leg swelling or unexplained hypoxia were evaluated for DVT or PE. This was done with bedside sonography and CT angiography.

During the study period, we did not perform screening sonography, so all the DVT in the study were initially suspected based upon symptoms. We currently screen patients who do not receive prophylactic anticoagulation every four days, but this protocol was developed after this study was completed. We developed a formal screening criterion to evaluate for blunt cerebrovascular injury during the study time period. These criteria included a fracture of C1 through C4, LeFort 3 fracture, unexplained neurologic deficit, and fracture through the vascular foramen.

All patients in this study were regularly discussed with the neurosurgical service. When a diagnosis of DVT, PE, or blunt cerebrovascular injury was made, a discussion was held regarding the appropriateness of anticoagulation. After reviewing the radiologic images and the clinical course, the neurosurgeon determined whether or not anticoagulation could be safely administered. These decisions were made on a case by case basis. There was not a specific protocol for obtained follow up head CT scans after anticoagulation was started, but this was typically done 1–4 days later.

Data were analyzed with Analyse-It (Leeds, England). Categorical data were analyzed with chi-square tests and continuous data were analyzed with t-tests. Permission to conduct the study was obtained from the institutional review board at North Memorial Medical Center, which includes an ethical review of the research protocol.

Results

During the study period, there were 42 patients who had both an ICH and an indication for anticoagulation. The average patient age was 50 years. 31% were female. The average injury severity score was 30.7.

Patients who received therapeutic anticoagulation were compared with patients who were treated without anticoagulation (Table 1). Twenty-six patients received anticoagulation, and 16 patients were treated without anticoagulation. The average age was similar in both groups. The gender distribution was identical in each group. The average length of stay was higher in the patients receiving anticoagulation (30 days vs. 20.9 days, p = 0.01). The thrombotic events were primarily composed of DVT and PE, with two cases of blunt cerebrovascular injury in each group.

As noted by the high injury severity scores, most of the patients had significant injuries beyond the traumatic head injury. Concomitant injuries included 16 patients with skull fractures, 17 with spinal cord injuries, 8 with long bone fractures, 20 with at least one known rib fracture, 2 blunt liver injuries and 5 splenic injuries.

Overall, 62% of patients received therapeutic anticoagulation for treatment of their thrombotic complication (Table 2). All patients receiving anticoagulation received

Table 1 Patient characteristics

	Anticoagulation	No Anticoagulation	p
N	26	16	
Mean Age	51	48	0.43
Gender**			
–M	18 (69%)	11 (69%)	1.0
–F	8 (31%)	5 (31%)	
Mean ISS	31.1	30.1	0.95
Mortality	2 (7.7%)	2 (12.5%)	0.63
Mean LOS	30.0	20.9	0.01
Thrombosis*			
–PE	16	8	0.53
–DVT	15	9	1.0
–BCVI	2	2	0.63

*some pts had more than one type of thrombosis (DVT and PE). Blunt cerebrovascular injury (BCVI).

either enoxaparin at a dose of 1 mg/kg BID or a heparin drip with a goal PTT between 60 and 80 s (our high intensity protocol). The average time to instituting anticoagulation was 11.9 days after admission. Nearly one-quarter of the patients received full anticoagulation within the first 7 days of admission. Among these patients, two were anticoagulated within 24 h of injury, two were anticoagulated on day 4, and two were anticoagulated on day 6. Approximately 30% of patients were not anticoagulated until two weeks after their injury.

The decision to anticoagulate was not protocolized. Rather, the decision was left to the discretion of the attending neurosurgeon, in discussion with the trauma surgeon. The distribution of intracranial hemorrhage is listed in Table 3. The frequency of epidural, subdural, and intraparenchymal hemorrhage was similar between the groups. The average size of extra-axial hemorrhage was 9.48 mm in the group receiving anticoagulation and 9.89 mm in the group that did not receive anticoagulation. There was not a difference in rate of craniotomy for the treatment of the intracranial hemorrhage between the groups (30.8% vs. 56.6%, p = 0.19).

There was extension of intracranial hemorrhage after institution of anticoagulation in only one patients. 96% of patients had no change in the volume of intracranial bleeding after initiation of anticoagulation. The extension of bleeding was very minor in one patient

Table 2 Anticoagulation characteristics

Percent receiving anticoagulation	62%
Mean time until anticoagulation	11.9 days (range: 0–24)
Percent <7 days	23.1%
Percent 7–14 days	46.2%
Percent >14 days	30.7%

Table 3 Decision to anticoagulate

	Anticoagulation	No Anticoagulation	p
Epidural	1	2	0.54
Subdural	13	9	0.75
SAH	20	13	1.0
Contusion	14	12	0.21
Marshall Score			

(1-2 mm growth in intraparenchymal hemorrhage), and the clinical course was felt to be unaffected. This was noted on follow up imaging 6 days after initiation of anticoagulation.

There were two deaths in each group of patients. The causes of death related to brain injury and multisystem organ failure. There were no deaths strictly from the thrombotic complications.

Discussion

Injured patients are at significant risk of both hemorrhagic and thrombotic complications. These divergent risks create a therapeutic conundrum for trauma surgeons. Use of anticoagulation can lead to potential exsanguination and death, while avoidance of anticoagulation can lead to thrombotic complications and death [7]. Our data represents a novel report that suggests that therapeutic anticoagulation can be safely accomplished in select patients with intracranial hemorrhage.

There is very little to guide trauma surgeons in the safety profile of therapeutic anticoagulation. A recent review by Golob, et. al. evaluated the safety of initiating therapeutic anticoagulation in multi-injured trauma patients [7]. They noted that 21% of patients had complications from the therapy. The most common complication was an acute drop in hemoglobin requiring a blood transfusion; three patients died as a result of hemorrhage. Clinical factors associated with a higher risk of complications were COPD, low platelet count before therapy, and the use of unfractionated hemorrhage. This study, however, did not include any patients with head injuries, so extrapolation to this population is difficult.

Injured patients are at significant risk of thrombotic complications. Patients with multisystem trauma may develop DVT at a rate of 58%, while a quarter of patients with isolated intracranial hemorrhage may develop DVT [1]. This has led to significant study evaluating medical DVT prophylaxis in head injured patients. These studies have evaluated both low dose heparin and low molecular weight heparin. Norwood, et.al. noted that enoxaparin could be safely administered to select patients within 24 h of craniotomy for trauma [8]. In a separate report, this group noted a 3.4% progression rate of intracranial hemorrhage after institution of prophylactic doses of anticoagulants [2].

These reports were highly important in that they dispelled the traditional viewpoint that prophylactic anticoagulation is unsafe after brain trauma. They do not, however, speak to the safety profile of therapeutic anticoagulation. Traditional recommendations suggest that therapeutic anticoagulation is unsafe after traumatic intracranial hemorrhage. Textbooks have noted that anticoagulation should be delayed for 3 days to 6 weeks after injury "depending on local customs" (although no references were cited to support this recommendation) [9]. Our data suggests that anticoagulation in the earlier portion of this window may be safe.

Much of the hesitation to use therapeutic anticoagulation after brain trauma likely stems from studies on pre-injury use of anticoagulants. Cohen, et.al. reported mortality rates of 84%–91% among patients who were anticoagulated prior to an intracranial bleed [10]. Mina, et.al. compared anticoagulated patients to matched controls and found an absolute increase in mortality of 30% among the anticoagulated patients [11]. Another study evaluated the effect of rapid reversal of coagulopathy. Patients who underwent a rapid, protocolized reversal of coagulopathy had a 38% absolute reduction in mortality compared to historical controls [12]. Although these studies clearly indicated higher risks of death and disability among patients exposed to anticoagulants before the time of injury, they do not speak to the risks of administration of anticoagulants in a delayed fashion.

While many thrombotic complications can be treated without anticoagulation, there are specific scenarios in which anticoagulation has the potential to markedly improve a treatment regimen. Inferior vena cava (IVC) filters are the mainstay of treatment of both DVT and PE in patients with a contraindication to anticoagulation [3]. There are certain situations, however, in which IVC filters are not adequate. The filters do not prevent propagation of a thrombus that has already embolized to the pulmonary vasculature. A saddle PE requires very little propagation to result in lethal shock, so anticoagulation in this population is critical. Similarly, the long term morbidity of phlegmasia cerulean dolens is reduced with anticoagulation. Further, there is a small, but defined, risk of thrombosis of the IVC after placement of a filter [6]. This situation also requires anticoagulation. A final venous thrombosis that that is not amenable to treatment with an intravascular filter is an upper extremity DVT. Superior vena cava filters are uncommon and would lead to fatal intracranial swelling in the event of filter thrombosis.

There is only one report that has attempted to define the optimal treatment regimen of DVT or PE after intracranial hemorrhage [6]. This report focused on non-traumatic hemorrhage, so the generalizability may be limited. The authors conducted a review of the literature and were unable to develop firm recommendations.

Blunt cerebrovascular injury is another event that may require anticoagulation despite the presence of an intracranial hemorrhage [13]. Dissection of the carotid or vertebral arteries can lead to disabling or fatal stroke events, which may be prevented by adequate anticoagulation. Although much of the focus of treatment has shifted to antiplatelet regimens, there is a role for heparin in select cases. Our data suggests that therapeutic anticoagulation can be safely given to select patients with blunt cerebrovascular injury and intracranial hemorrhage.

Patients with mechanical cardiac valves represent a significant challenge to trauma surgeons [14-17]. The risk of artificial valves appears to be the highest in patients with a cage/ball valve in the mitral position. Atrial fibrillation and reduced left ventricular function add to the risk of stroke without anticoagulation. The natural history of these patients is unclear, as they are generally on anticoagulants, but we can glean some estimate of risk from studies that have evaluated temporarily discontinuing anticoagulation after intracranial hemorrhage. It appears safe to discontinue anticoagulation for brief periods of time [14,15]. Most of this work has been conducted in patients with spontaneous intracranial hemorrhage. It is possible that traumatic hemorrhage is a different entity, as injured patients are more hypercoaguable than then general population. Our data represents an important adjunct to these studies, in that we have demonstrated that early reintroduction of anticoagulation can be safely accomplished.

There are limitations of this study worth noting. We did not have a protocolized approach to management of anticoagulation. Rather, we consulted with the neurosurgeons on a daily basis and we started anticoagulation when their clinical judgment indicated it was safe to do so. As such, we are likely dealing with a highly select patient population. Additionally, our sample size is limited. It is possible that we would have yielded different results with a larger sample size. Finally, some of our patients received anticoagulation for uncomplicated PE rather than the extreme examples listed in this discussion. This does not detract from our results demonstrating safety of anticoagulation, however.

In conclusion, selected patients with brain injury may safely be anticoagulated to prevent the propagation of thrombotic complications. Our data does not provide definitive evidence of the safety profile. Rather, this manuscript provides initial evidence that suggests that traditional beliefs about anticoagulation in patients with brain injuries may be incorrect. Our data should be used a springboard to develop further study on this issue, so that the specific groups that would most benefit from anticoagulation could be defined.

Competing interests

None of the authors have any conflicts of interest or special declarations to make regarding the contents of this manuscript.

Therapeutic anticoagulation can be safely accomplished in selected patients with traumatic...

21

Authors' contribution

MB directed the design of the study, data interpretation, and was involved in the drafting and revision of the manuscript. EI was involved in the study design and the manuscript revision. PR was involved in the data acquisition, study planning, and manuscript revision. RR was involved in the data interpretation and manuscript revision. PH was involved with the data acquisition and the data interpretation. All authors read and approved the final manuscript.

Author details

[1]Department of Trauma, North Memorial Medical Center, Robbinsdale, MN, USA. [2]Division of Critical Care and Acute Care Surgery, University of Minnesota, Minneapolis, MN, USA. [3]North Memorial Medical Center, Division of Trauma, 3300 Oakdale Avenue, Robbinsdale, MN 55422, USA.

References

1. Geerts WH, Code KI, Jay RM, Chen E, Szalai JP: A prospective study of venous thromboembolism after major trauma. *N Engl J Med* 1994, **331**(24):1601–1606.
2. Norwood SH, Berne JD, Rowe SA, Villarreal DH, Ledlie JT: Early venous thromboembolism prophylaxis with enoxaparin in patients with blunt traumatic brain injury. *J Trauma* 2008, **65**(5):1021–1026. discussion 6–7.
3. Bates SM, Ginsberg JS: Clinical practice. Treatment of deep-vein thrombosis. *N Engl J Med* 2004, **351**(3):268–277.
4. Geerts WH, Heit JA, Clagett GP, Pineo GF, Colwell CW, Anderson FA Jr, *et al*: Prevention of venous thromboembolism. *Chest* 2001, **119**(1 Suppl):132S–175S.
5. Knudson MM, Morabito D, Paiement GD, Shackleford S: Use of low molecular weight heparin in preventing thromboembolism in trauma patients. *J Trauma* 1996, **41**(3):446–459.
6. Kelly J, Hunt BJ, Lewis RR, Rudd A: Anticoagulation or inferior vena cava filter placement for patients with primary intracerebral hemorrhage developing venous thromboembolism? *Stroke* 2003, **34**(12):2999–3005.
7. Golob JF Jr, Sando MJ, Kan JC, Yowler CJ, Malangoni MA, Claridge JA: Therapeutic anticoagulation in the trauma patient: is it safe? *Surgery* 2008, **144**(4):591–596. discussion 6–7.
8. Norwood SH, McAuley CE, Berne JD, Vallina VL, Kerns DB, Grahm TW, *et al*: Prospective evaluation of the safety of enoxaparin prophylaxis for venous thromboembolism in patients with intracranial hemorrhagic injuries. *Arch Surg* 2002, **137**(6):696–701. discussion -2.
9. Feliciano DV, Mattox KL, Moore EE: *Trauma*. 6th edition. New York: McGraw-Hill Medical; 2008.
10. Cohen DB, Rinker C, Wilberger JE: Traumatic brain injury in anticoagulated patients. *J Trauma* 2006, **60**(3):553–557.
11. Mina AA, Knipfer JF, Park DY, Bair HA, Howells GA, Bendick PJ: Intracranial complications of preinjury anticoagulation in trauma patients with head injury. *J Trauma* 2002, **53**(4):668–672.
12. Ivascu FA, Howells GA, Junn FS, Bair HA, Bendick PJ, Janczyk RJ: Rapid warfarin reversal in anticoagulated patients with traumatic intracranial hemorrhage reduces hemorrhage progression and mortality. *J Trauma* 2005, **59**(5):1131–1137. discussion 7–9.
13. Wahl WL, Brandt MM, Thompson BG, Taheri PA, Greenfield LJ: Antiplatelet therapy: an alternative to heparin for blunt carotid injury. *J Trauma* 2002, **52**(5):896–901.
14. Ananthasubramaniam K, Beattie JN, Rosman HS, Jayam V, Borzak S: How safely and for how long can warfarin therapy be withheld in prosthetic heart valve patients hospitalized with a major hemorrhage? *Chest* 2001, **119**(2):478–484.
15. Garcia DA, Regan S, Henault LE, Upadhyay A, Baker J, Othman M, *et al*: Risk of thromboembolism with short-term interruption of warfarin therapy. *Arch Intern Med* 2008, **168**(1):63–69.
16. Wijdicks EF, Schievink WI, Brown RD, Mullany CJ: The dilemma of discontinuation of anticoagulation therapy for patients with intracranial hemorrhage and mechanical heart valves. *Neurosurgery* 1998, **42**(4):769–773.
17. Phan TG, Koh M, Wijdicks EF: Safety of discontinuation of anticoagulation in patients with intracranial hemorrhage at high thromboembolic risk. *Arch Neurol* 2000, **57**(12):1710–1713.

5

Enhancing trauma education worldwide through telemedicine

Antonio C Marttos[1], Fernanda M Kuchkarian[1*], Phillipe Abreu-Reis[2], Bruno MT Pereira[3], Francisco S Collet-Silva[4], Gustavo P Fraga[3]

Abstract

Advances in information and communication technologies are changing the delivery of trauma care and education. Telemedicine is a tool that can be used to deliver expert trauma care and education anywhere in the world. Trauma is a rapidly-evolving field requiring access to readily available sources of information. Through videoconferencing, physicians can participate in continuing education activities such as Grand Rounds, seminars, conferences and journal clubs. Exemplary programs have shown promising outcomes of teleconferences such as enhanced learning, professional collaborations, and networking. This review introduces the concept of telemedicine for trauma education, and highlights efforts of programs that are utilizing telemedicine to unite institutions across the world.

Introduction

Advances in telemedicine now allow trauma specialists to remotely care for patients anywhere in the world. Telemedicine is the use of telecommunications technology to provide healthcare services at a distance [1] Telehealth, a closely related term, encompasses a broader definition to include activities beyond clinical services such as education and administrative services [2]. Telemedicine provides unique opportunities to meet some of the challenges of contemporary trauma education. At the core of such technologies is videoconferencing, which is frequently used to deliver trauma care and education in real-time. In addition to meeting trauma educational needs, telemedicine is promoting international collaborations that promise to revolutionize the way trauma care is delivered on a population-based level. This paper will review the use of telemedicine in trauma, with emphasis on education. Experience implementing trauma tele-educational activities from our respective institutions will be highlighted.

Telemedicine for trauma

In recent years, there has been tremendous growth in the field of telemedicine. Due to a combination of technology-driven market forces, as well as increasing demands for improvements in the global health sector; these advances are providing the tools necessary to enhance medical care and education. Telemedicine in trauma can be used for the routine monitoring of patients [3], to austere environments and large-scale disasters [4]. Examples of telehealth services include specialist consultations, remote patient monitoring, continuing education, and referral services. Wide adoption of telemedicine and telehealth promises increased access to quality trauma care, while simultaneously reducing costs. At its fundamental core, telemedicine is based on the ethical principle that quality care should be made available to all people, anywhere and at anytime.

The trauma, emergency and critical care fields are facing multiple challenges worldwide. Issues with overcrowding, increased demands for trauma care, lack of funding, and a lack of disaster preparedness have been identified as chief concerns [5]. Of particular concern is the continued workforce shortage, including shortage of specialists and nurses. Researchers estimate that there will be significant shortages of physicians across several

* Correspondence: fkuchkarian@med.miami.edu
[1]University of Miami Miller School of Medicine, Surgery Department (D40), PO Box 016960 Miami, FL 33101, USA

surgical specialties [6]. As population increases, it is estimated that there will be a deficit of 6,000 general surgeons by 2050 [7]. Several factors have been identified as contributors to the shortage; including barriers to recruitment of medical students into general surgery residencies, and general dissatisfactions with lifestyle concerns. In trauma care there are inherent discrepancies, particularly between rural and urban areas. Inadequate access to trauma is a reality for many populations. Despite research that patients have better outcomes when treated at designated trauma centers, many hospitals around the world that provide injury care are not such facilities [8]. Providers often lack the resources and experience to treat trauma patients, due to either low volume of severely injured patients and/or limited training opportunities. In addition, rural hospitals do not have sufficient access to subspecialty care for instance orthopedics and neurosurgery. These factors can cause unintended delays in the diagnosis and treatment of trauma patients, resulting in poorer outcomes such as increased morbidity and length of stay. At these moments, the ability to have a more experienced trauma specialist available through telemedicine for a consultation is invaluable.

The advent of telemedicine use for trauma and emergency care developed out of the need to address such disparities. Telemedicine facilitates access to care for traditionally underserved populations in remote areas with fewer health services. Trauma surgeons can now remotely assist in the evaluation and care of patients. There are many studies demonstrating the clinical effectiveness of teletrauma applications in rural settings [9-11]. Perhaps the most significant effect is the decrease in time to treat trauma patients. Patients can be either treated locally with the assistance of a remote expert or quickly transferred to an appropriate center. This has significant cost-reducing potential for healthcare systems as well as patients and their families; as costly transfers can be minimized when appropriate avoiding further financial and social burdens.

Rationale

Technology is revolutionizing how health professionals obtain information. The constantly evolving state of medicine makes efficiently obtaining information a necessity. In trauma care, teams of physicians and other clinicians frequently rely on a flow of information using a multitude of communication modes. New surgical techniques and procedures, heavy emphasis on trauma care protocols and evidence-based medicine naturally lead to the use of telemedicine to disperse new knowledge in a timely fashion. This is especially beneficial when resident education and rural providers are considered. Due to the geographical misdistribution of health professionals, rural providers often face professional isolation that can result in

knowledge and skill attrition [12]. Physical distance from other specialists, regional hospitals, and continuing education programs prevent remote practitioners from staying up-to-date. Work-hour limitations and changes in training duration for residency programs have challenged educators to find innovative solutions to overcome limited faculty resources and time while also improving the quality of medical education [13].

Telemedicine in surgical education

There are considerable applications of telemedicine for surgical education and training. At the center of such applications is the use of videoconferencing (VC). VC first was first used to broadcast a surgical procedure overseas in 1962 [14]. Since then, VC has been embraced as an effective tool among surgeons to discuss surgical procedures as well as to conduct telementoring and teleconsultations [15]. The educational process in surgery is essentially composed of training and manual abilities development supervised by a more experienced surgeon who acts as a teacher [16]. However, many surgical procedures (i.e. open abdominal/thoracic trauma surgery) are difficult for learners to visualize the maneuvers of the surgeon due to field view limitations. The introduction of laparoscopy was a milestone in the teaching of surgery mainly by allowing images shared between observers, tutors and residents in real time [17]. The use of robot-observers is a paradigm shift for open surgery teaching, in which cameras can be used for images transmission as a new tool in surgeons' training [18]. Through telemedicine, students and residents can observe the procedure from a remote classroom [15]. Studies show that students feel more comfortable to ask questions, learn more, and have fewer questions not answered by faculty [19]. Furthermore, reducing the number of people in the OR results in is less noise and distraction for the surgical team [20]. VC has also been examined for surgical follow-up care, burns, and wound management.

Interactive remote support can help health staff improve the management of patients as well as enhance the educational value of daily patient care activities, such as with patient rounds. At the University of Miami/Ryder Trauma Center in Miami, FL, use of telemedicine for daily morning rounds is currently standard operating procedure in the Trauma Intensive Care Unit (TICU) [21]. In replacement of traditional bedside rounds, the TICU team uses a mobile videoconferencing telemedicine system (Figure 1). The technology used for daily rounds is the InTouch Health's RP-7 System, a wireless mobile robotic platform that includes a remote Control Station. The Control Station software consists of a joystick that can be used to maneuver the robot remotely. Clinicians are able to remotely view the patient, look at vital signs, ventilator settings, and examine laboratory

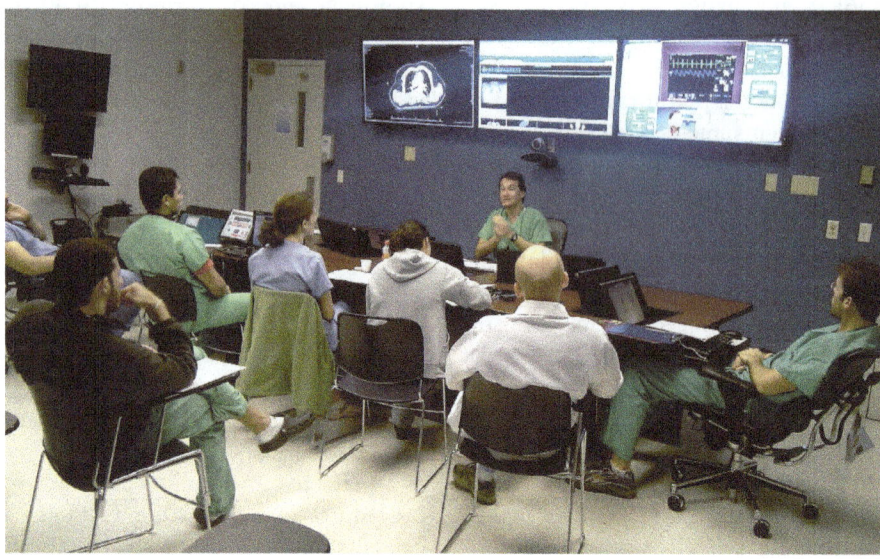

Figure 1 Use of telemedicine during daily rounds at University of Miami/Ryder Trauma Center in Miami.

and imaging data—all from one single location. The remote location is fitted with multiple large screens and computers to display patient information to an audience of clinicians. An important outcome of tele-rounds is that it helps reduce the spread of infections associated with heavy bedside traffic, while maintaining the educational integrity of traditional rounds [22].

Examples of current initiatives in trauma tele-education

The experiences gained through the use of VC in surgical education have paved the way to incorporate its use in other areas of trauma education. There are several initiatives to expand trauma education through telemedicine occurring at multiple international sites. Earlier initiatives consisted of using integrated services digital networks (ISDN) for data transmission modes. Through the use of ISDN videophones, a "virtual residency" was established in Canada between a rural and urban hospital [23]. Their collaborations include teleconsultations and biweekly trauma rounds to provide continuing medical education to rural providers. In Europe, six University hospitals in four countries (Switzerland, Belgium, Germany and France) held weekly surgical teleconferences and reported their experiences over a two-year period [24]. The authors measured the accuracy of telediagnosis by randomly selecting surgical cases to be reviewed by a panel of surgeons. The authors found that the real-time transmission of documents, combined with interactive discussion increased diagnostic accuracy.

In recent years, VC via ISND use has been reduced considerably due to declining equipment costs and increases in Internet protocol (IP)-based and 3G mobile

phones solutions. Since then, several small to large-scale networks that link trauma centers, academic center, tertiary care hospitals and clinics have been developed. It is estimated that in the United States alone, there are currently 200 existing telemedicine networks, each with varying degrees of activity and capacity [25] Some networks are local, while others are statewide. Notable examples are seen in Florida [26], Utah [27], Arizona [28] and California [29]. Through telemedicine networks, health professionals at multiple sites can interact with one another, collaborate on projects, and attend professional meetings. Continuing education activities can occur such as Grand Rounds, case presentations and seminars. In Brazil, the telemedicine network named RUTE (University Network of Telemedicine, available from http://rute.rnp.br) has been connecting university hospitals around the country, with the objective to create a more uniform surgical medical education of these health professionals [30]. This national network supports existing telemedicine projects as well as provides incentives for inter-institutional collaborations.

Together with several institutions around the world, the University of Miami/Ryder Trauma Center has established the International Trauma Tele-Grand Rounds. Through videoconferencing, complex trauma case presentations and advanced trauma and critical care topics are discussed on a weekly basis. Case presentations provide students, residents, fellows and attending physicians with an outstanding tool for education and sharing of medical expertise across borders. Continuing medical education (CME) credits are available to eligible physicians. To date, there have been 42 participating institutions from the United States, Brazil, Colombia, Bahamas,

Haiti, Canada, Venezuela, Argentina, Panama, Puerto Rico, Dominican Republic, British Virgin Islands, Spain, Thailand, Turkey and Iraq; ranging from academic medical centers to urban trauma centers, military, community and rural hospitals. The Panamerican Trauma Society has adopted the Tele-Grand Rounds as one of their educational activities (Figure 2). The Clinical Hospital of University of Campinas (Unicamp), in Campinas, Brazil, reported their experiences participating in 100 videoconferencing meetings over a one-year period in all specialities [31]. Trauma surgery meetings accounted for the majority of the teleconferences. Through the results of the program's success, telemedicine is now an integral part of their trauma surgical residency curriculum.

An additional innovative use of telemedicine for education is with the rise of remote "journal clubs". With the huge number of articles published daily worldwide, it is a challenge to surgeons with a busy practice to keep themselves up-to-date. Through telemedicine, the Brazilian Society of Integrated Trauma Care (SBAIT) and the Brazilian College of Surgeons (CBC) have joined forces with the University of Toronto, Canada to promote Evidence-Based Telemedicine – Trauma and Acute Care Surgery (EBT-TACS) [32]. These are regular meetings for literature review of topics most relevant to surgeons. Participants select ahead of time a scientific article for review, and conduct in-depth analysis of the study design, outcomes, strengths and limitations. Subsequently recommendations are disseminated in the Journal of the CBC. These meetings make it possible for non-academic physicians who practice in smaller centers to stay up-to-date, as well as promote critical analysis of evidence-based surgical topics.

Discussion

Telemedicine, as an expanding technology, is creating previously unimagined possibilities for the reality of health care providers. There is now a way to extend the reach of a trauma surgeon anywhere in the world. This extension reduces limitations imposed on distant providers as well as patients. With high-speed data linked to video units, specialists can now take care of patients in distant hospitals who normally would not have access to such services. This ability has tremendous cost-saving potential, as well as for improved patient outcomes. Patients who do not require transfer can be treated locally when a remote expert can assist the local team. In addition, if the patient does need to be transferred, the remote expert can also ensure that the patient is stable.

Telemedicine also offers a solution to address the disparities in access to trauma education. Experiences from using VC for surgical education have broadened its use to a wider scope and audience. Today VC can be used for consultations, patient rounding, mentoring and continuing medical education. Providers in rural or remote areas can have access to educational opportunities available to those in large, urban academic settings. Studies have shown that the use of telemedicine for trauma education

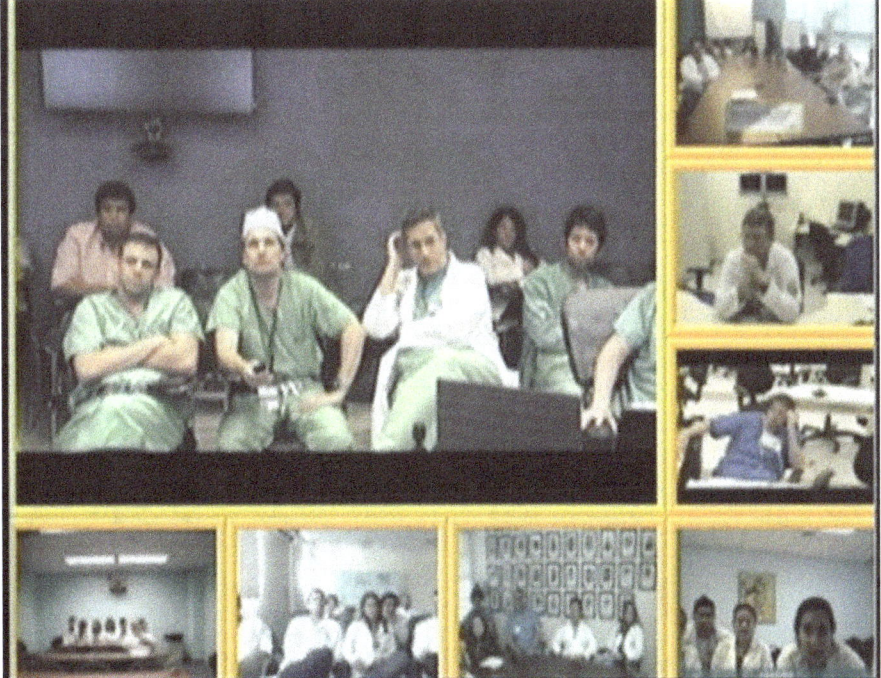

Figure 2 Tele-Grand Rounds organized every Friday discussing trauma cases from different institutions.

facilitates resident training, enhances communication and enriches the educational experience. The diversity of institutional settings allows participants to learn from others on how to best treat trauma patients, despite differences in resources and expertise. In addition to serving as an educational tool, the series provides a mechanism for physicians to network and collaborate on future endeavors. All of this leads will lead to a more robust, educated workforce.

Many telehealth programs have been developing across the world. Some of them however, find difficulties in sustaining their activities once program funding ends. Adding an educational component to a telehealth program may ensure its sustainability in the long-run. The synergy created by different institutions participating in teleconferences for example, can lead to other collaborations in the future. In addition, as physicians become more accustomed to being on video, they can then be better prepared to communicate with patients in the same way.

Conclusion

The development and advancement of telemedicine over the past years have opened doors to an immense number of possibilities. Not only has telemedicine been used for consultation, diagnosis and treatment purposes; it is also being used in distance and continuing medical education. Institutions are developing a variety of web-based distance learning programs as well as formal grand rounds and lectures using telemedicine technology. In particular, telemedicine can be used to overcome disparities in training and education and to deliver higher-quality health care to patients in remote locations. Telemedicine will not only extend the reach of the trauma education but it will also help bridge the gap between limited resources, lack of available staff and reduced budget across many specialties in medicine.

Acknowledgements
This article has been published as part of World Journal of Emergency Surgery Volume 7 Supplement 1, 2012: Proceedings of the World Trauma Congress 2012. The full contents of the supplement are available online at http://www.wjes.org/supplements/7/S1.

Author details
[1]University of Miami Miller School of Medicine, Surgery Department (D40), PO Box 016960 Miami, FL 33101, USA. [2]Federal University of Parana, Rua XV de Novembro, 1299, CEP 80.060-000, Curitiba, Parana, Brazil. [3]University of Campinas (Unicamp), Faculty of Medical Sciences, Division of Trauma Surgery, (FCM/Unicamp), R. Alexander Fleming, 181, Cidade Universitaria "Prof. Zeferino Vaz", CEP: 13.083-970, Campinas, São Paulo, Brazil. [4]Hospital das Clínicas da Faculdade de Medicina Universidade de Sao Paulo, Av. Dr. Arnaldo, 455, Cerqueira Cesar, CEP: 01.246-903, São Paulo, Brazil.

Authors' contributions
AM, GF, FC, and BP provided subject matter expertise and assistance with the literature. FK was responsible for preparing and editing the manuscript. All authors read the manuscript.

Competing interests
The authors declare that they have no competing interests.

References
1. Telemedicine: A Guide to Assessing Telecommunications for Health Care. In Institute of Medicine. Committee on Evaluating Clinical Applications of Telemedicine. Washington, D.C.:National Academy Press;Field MJ 1996:.
2. American Telemedicine Association: Telemedicine Defined. [http://www.americantelemed.org/i4a/pages/index.cfm?pageid=3333], Accessed April 2012.
3. Thomas EJ, Lucke JF, Wuest L, Weavind L, Patel B: Association of telemedicine for remote monitoring of intensive care patients with mortality, complications, and length of stay. JAMA 2009, 302(24):2671-8.
4. Simmons S, Alverson D, Poropatich R, D'Iorio J, DeVany M, Doarn C: Applying telehealth in natural and anthropogenic disasters. Telemed J E Health 2008, 14(9):968-71.
5. Napolitano LM, Fulda GJ, Davis KA, et al: Challenging issues in surgical critical care, trauma, and acute care surgery: A report from the critical care committee of the American association for the surgery of trauma. J Trauma 2010, 69(6):1619-33.
6. Williams TE Jr., Ellison EC: Population analysis predicts a future critical shortage of general surgeons. Surgery 2008, 144(4):548-56.
7. Williams TE, Satiani B: The Coming Shortage of Surgeons: Why They Are Disappearing and What That Means for Our Health. Santa Barbara, CA: Praeger; 1999.
8. Demetriades D, Martin M, Salim A, Rhee P, Brown C, Chan L: The effect of trauma center designation and trauma volume on outcome in specific severe injuries. Ann Surg 2005, 242(4):512-9.
9. Duchesne JC, Kyle A, Simmons J, Islam S, Schmieg RE, Olivier J, McSwain NE: The impact of telemedicine upon rural trauma care. J Trauma 2008, 64:92-8.
10. Ricci MA, Caputo M, Amour J, Rogers F, Sartorelli K, Callas PW, Malone PT: Telemedicine reduces discrepancies in rural trauma care. Telemed J E Health 2003, 9(1):3-11.
11. Latifi R, Hadeed GJ, O'Keefe T, Friese RS, Wynne JL, Ziemba ML, Judkins D: Initial experiences and outcomes of telepresence in the management of trauma and emergency surgical patients. Am J Surg 2009, 198(6):905-10.
12. Jukkala AM, Henly SJ, Lindeke LL: Rural perceptions of continuing professional education. J Contin Educ Nurs 2008, 39(12):555-63.
13. Zollo SA, Kienzle MG, Henshaw Z, Crist LG, Wakefield DS: Tele-Education in a telemedicine environment: implications for rural health care and academic medical centers. J Med Syst 1999, 23(2):107-22.
14. Merell RC, Doarn CR, Michael E, DeBakey MD: . Telemed J E Health 2008, 14(6):503-4.
15. Ereso AQ, Garchia P, Tseng E, Gauger G, Kim H, Dua MM, Victorino GP, Guy TS: Live transference of surgical subspecialty skills using telerobotic proctoring to remote general surgeons. J Am Coll Surg 2010, 211(3):400-11.
16. Doarn CR: The power of video conferencing in surgical practice and education. World J Surg 2009, 33(7):1366-7.
17. Masic I, Pandza H, Kulasin I, Masic Z, Valjevac S: Tele-education as method of medical education. Med Arh 2009, 63(6):350-3.
18. Patel K: Robotics the future of surgery. Int J Surg 2008, 6(6):441-2.
19. McIntyre TP, Monahan TS, Villegas L, Doyle J, Jones DB: Teleconferencing surgery enhances effective communication and enriches medical education. Surg Laparosc Endosc Percutan Tech 2008, 18(1):45-8.
20. Pereira BM, Pereira AM, Correia Cdos S, Marttos AC Jr, Fiorelli RK, Fraga GP: Interruptions and distractions in the trauma operating room: understanding the threat of human error. Rev Col Bras Cir 2011, 38(5):292-8.
21. Marttos A, Wilson K, Krauthamer S, Augenstein J, Schulman C, Baquero S, Vara A: Telerounds in a Trauma ICU (TICU) department. Poster presented at the 38th Critical Care Congress of the Society for Critical Care Medicine 2009.
22. Lilly CM, Cody S, Zhao H, Landry K, Baker SP, McIlwaine J, Chandler MW, Irwin RS: Hospitality mortality, length of stay, and preventable complications among critically ill patients before and after tele-ICU reengineering of critical care processes. JAMA 2011, 305(21):2175-83.
23. Ho K, Brown R, Bradley C, Gareau A, Harrison D, Kirkpatrick A, McLouglin M, Pursell R, Simons R: Virtual residency" in continuing health education:

turning trauma telemedicine consultations into continuing health education opportunities. *Proc AMIA Symp* 2001, 820.

24. Dermartines N, Mutter D, Vix M, Leroy J, Glatz D, Rosel F, Harder F, Marescaux J: **Assessment of telemedicine in surgical education and patient care.** *Ann Surg* 2000, **231**(2):282-91.

25. American Telemedicine Association: **Delivery Mechanisms.** [http://www.americantelemed.org/i4a/pages/index.cfm?pageid=3333], Accessed April 2012.

26. Marttos A: **Ryder Trauma Center/Florida DOH Disaster Management Telemedicine Projects.** [http://www.americantelemed.org/files/public/membergroups/PICATA/Marttos.pdf].

27. **Utah Telehealth Network.** [http://www.utahtelehealth.net/], Accessed April 2012.

28. **Arizona Telemedicine Program.** [http://www.telemedicine.arizona.edu/], Accessed April 2012.

29. **California Telehealth Network.** [http://www.caltelehealth.org/], Accessed April 2012.

30. **Rute Rede Universitaria de Telemedicine.** [http://rute.rnp.br/], Accessed April 2012.

31. Pereira BM, Calderan TR, Silva MT, Silva AC, Marttos AC Jr, Fraga GP: **Initial experience at a university teaching hospital from using telemedicine to promote education through video conferencing.** *Sao Paulo Med J* 2012, **130**(1):32-6.

32. Fraga GP, Nascimento B Jr, Rizoli S: **Evidence-based telemedicine: trauma & acute care surgery (EBT-TACS).** *Rev Col Bras Cir* 2012, **39**(1):3.

6

Analytical review of 664 cases of penetrating buttock trauma

Raimundas Lunevicius[*] and Klaus-Martin Schulte

Abstract

A comprehensive review of data has not yet been provided as penetrating injury to the buttock is not a common condition accounting for 2-3% of all penetrating injuries. The aim of the study is to provide the as yet lacking analytical review of the literature on penetrating trauma to the buttock, with appraisal of characteristics, features, outcomes, and patterns of major injuries. Based on these results we will provide an algorithm. Using a set of terms we searched the databases Pub Med, EMBASE, Cochran, and CINAHL for articles published in English between 1970 and 2010. We analysed cumulative data from prospective and retrospective studies, and case reports. The literature search revealed 36 relevant articles containing data on 664 patients. There was no grade A evidence found. The injury population mostly consists of young males (95.4%) with a high proportion missile injury (75.9%). Bleeding was found to be the key problem which mostly occurs from internal injury and results in shock in 10%. Overall mortality is 2.9% with significant adverse impact of visceral or vascular injury and shock ($P < 0.001$). The major injury pattern significantly varies between shot and stab injury with small bowel, colon, or rectum injuries leading in shot wounds, whilst vascular injury leads in stab wounds ($P < 0.01$). Laparotomy was required in 26.9% of patients. Wound infection, sepsis or multiorgan failure, small bowel fistula, ileus, rebleeding, focal neurologic deficit, and urinary tract infection were the most common complications. Sharp differences in injury pattern endorse an algorithm for differential therapy of penetrating buttock trauma. In conclusion, penetrating buttock trauma should be regarded as a life-threatening injury with impact beyond the pelvis until proven otherwise.

Keywords: buttock injury, penetrating trauma, shot wound, stab wound

Background

The buttock comprises the lateral half of the lower most sagittal zone of the torso [1] where there is a particularly high density of vital structures above and below the peritoneum in the pelvis [2,3]. Sparse evidence points to the frequency of life-threatening visceral and vascular injuries in patients with penetrating trauma to the buttock [2,4,5]. Pelvic anatomy results in the possibility of major complications or death following penetrating buttock injury in any path of trajectory and in absence of hard vascular, abdominal, or pelvic signs [4].

A comprehensive review of data has not yet been provided as penetrating injury to the buttock is not a common condition accounting for 2-3% of all penetrating injuries [3,6-10]. Four previous reviews of the literature

do however require additional research in terms of consistent patterns, peculiarities, and management [6-9].

The purpose of this study is to provide an analytical review of the literature on penetrating trauma to the buttock and to appraise the characteristics, features, outcomes, and patterns of major injuries. Recognition of specific patterns should enhance management of this trauma.

Methods

The Entrez PubMed interface of MEDLINE database, EMBASE, Cochran, and CINAHL databases were searched using the following Medical Subject Heading (MeSH) keywords: "Injuries", "Wounds and Injuries", "Wound Penetrating"; each of these keywords was combined with the keyword "Buttocks". The term 'Penetrating Gluteal Injuries' was also used. This resulted in 1021 titles and abstracts of studies related to these terms

* Correspondence: rlunevichus@yahoo.com
Major Trauma Centre, King's College Hospital NHS Foundation Trust, King's Health Partners Academic Health Sciences Centre, Denmark Hill, London, SE5 9RS, UK

which were then read on the basis of English language and relevance.

Commentaries and literature reviews were also taken into account. We excluded articles relating to blunt injury, acupuncture injury, intragluteal injection injury, needle stick accidents, iatrogenic injury of the gluteal arteries, wound closure, reconstructive surgery of gluteal defects, wound botulism, bone fracture complications, injury from ultraviolet light, burn injury, true aneurisms, malignancies, and animal studies.

Relevant studies on penetrating buttock injury in acute trauma setting were grouped and categorised chronologically. Clustered and individual data regarding the demographic characteristics, mechanism of injury, clinical mode of presentation, imaging, buttock zone wounded, injuries, management strategy, complications, and final outcome were accumulated from all the studies, either prospective or retrospective, and case reports. When calculations in main series were impossible due to the lack of particular data, they were performed through the use of informative subset with indication of the exact number of entered cases.

In order to assess outcomes of visceral, vascular, skeletal, nerve injuries as well as outcomes of major surgery after stabbing or shootings, the 95% confidence intervals of odds ratios were calculated. In order to detect differences in injury related with stabbing or shooting patterns and outcomes between two independent proportions a Z-test was chosen and employed as both sample sizes were greater than 30. The two-tailed test was used to assess the null hypothesis. Chi-square test with Yates' correction was employed to compare categorical "alive - dead" outcome. Two-tailed p values were calculated where by $P < 0.05$ was considered to indicate statistical significance. Microsoft Office XP Excel 2007 Worksheets were used for accumulation and analysis of data.

Results

Literature search

We identified four literature reviews [6-9], two prospective studies [11,12], twelve retrospective reviews [2-5,10,13-19], seventeen papers with case reports [6,8,20-33], and three commentaries [34-36]. 31 publication contributed patient data on a total of 664 patients. Although individual studies chosen for review had some variations in specific measures, they were conceptually similar. No articles reported population-based data on overall and type-specified buttock injury in relation to incidence and mortality. There were no systematic reviews or prospective randomised controlled trials identified. A summary of two prospective and twelve retrospective studies are shown in Table 1.

Patient data

The analysis includes 664 patients for whom the minimal dataset was identified. Overall, 95.4% of cases (621/654) were males, and the median age was 29 (range 12-70). Missile injury accounted for 75.9% (504/664) and was mainly due to shooting (68.8%, 457/664), and rarely blasting (7.1%, 47 cases). Injury rate for stabbings was 23.8% (158/664). Impalement was rare with only 0.3% of cases (2/664). For 97 patients the zonal distribution was known, where by 66.0% (n = 64) were related to the upper zone of the buttock.

Clinical presentation on admission was known in 654 patients. 74 patients (11.3%) were regarded haemodynamically unstable and 56 (8.6%) were diagnosed to be in haemorrhagic shock. Peritoneal irritation was present in 48 (7.3%), gross rectal blood in 41 (6.3%), and gross haematuria in 27 (4.1%) patients. Massive external bleeding was documented in 15 patients, false aneurysm formation in 12, absence of distal pulse or cold painful leg in two, groin hematoma in two, and severe bone pain in three patients.

Initial diagnostic procedures were described by the authors as follows: diagnostic proctosigmoidoscopy in 295 (45.1%), angiography in 47 (7.2%), urology imaging (cystography, intravenous pyelography, urethrography) in 27 (4.1%) patients, and CT-scan for 10 (1.5%) patients. Retrograde irigoscopy and diagnostic peritoneal lavage were mentioned in a few reports.

Treatment modalities

The treatment approaches were described in 654 patients. 176 (26.9%) patients underwent emergency laparotomy. 40 (6.1%) patients required extended gluteal surgery. The interventional radiology procedures were used as sole modality to control bleeding or target bullets in 12 patients (1.8%). 356 (54.4%) patients were observed without major procedure. Other surgical procedures such as debridement under general anaesthesia were performed in 16.5% (n = 108) of patients.

Laparotomy and extended gluteal surgery was performed for 207 patients in the subset of 615 patients with gunshot or stab trauma (33.7%). Laparotomy was performed on 12.0% of stabbed patients (19/158) and 32.4% (148/457) of patients that were shot (OR, 0.29; CI, 0.17-0.48; Z value 4.857; $P < 0.001$). Extended gluteal surgery was more often performed in the group of patients with stab injuries to the buttock: 33/158 (21.0%) operations in contrast to 7/457 (1.5%) operations in gunshot victims (OR, 16.97; CI, 7.33-39.29; Z value 8.32; $P < 0.001$).

Outcomes

Mortality

Overall mortality rate was 2.9% (19/664). In terms of stabbing injury the mortality rate was 3.8% (6/158) and

Table 1 Major endpoints of two prospective [11,12] and twelve retrospective reviews on penetrating buttock injury in acute trauma setting

Study/reference	Period years	Patients	Male	Mean age	Viscus/major vessel injury	Bony ring injury	Mean ISS	Major surgery*	Overall mortality	Morbidity in survivals	Concomitant injuries	Hospital stay†	Cited articles	Contribution/concern
Velmahos et al. [11] (1997)	1	59	58	23	17 (29%)	5 (8%)	-	19(32.2%)	0	3 (15.8%)	High	7.2	11	Clinical examination is very accurate
Velmahos et al. [12] (1998)	1	10	-	-	-	-	-	-	0	-	-	-	14	Clinical examination is a reliable predictor
Maull et al. [13] (1979)	5	15	11	29	6 (54.5%)	-	-	12	0	5 (33%)	0	12	0	Liberal laparotomy advocated
Ivatury et al. [4] (1982)	4	60	57	-	16 (26.7%)	3 (5%)	-	16 (26.7%)	2 (3%)	14 (23%)	-	2 vs 18	3	Aggressive management
Vo et al. [5] (1983)	5	20	18	32	5 (25%)	2 (10%)	-	12 (60%)	0	5 (25%)	10 (50%)	-	2	Bullet's trajectory is important
Fallon et al. [14] (1988)	-	51	43	28.9	16 (31%)	0	-	25 (49%)	0	4 (8%)	High	-	4	Thorough evaluation and all investigations
Gilroy et al. [15] (1992)	6	8	7	33	8	-	-	8	2 (25%)	0	0	-	9	Danger of gluteal incision: vessels
Mercer et al. [3] (1992)	6	81	75	26	18 (22%)	4 (5%)	-	26% (21)	1 (1.2%)	-	-	-	6	Two zones of buttock: upper vs lower
Ferraro et al. [16] (1993)	2	70	68	25	34 (49%)	7 (17%)	11(1-45)	34 (49%)	3 (4%)	-	-	-	8	Sigmoidoscopy advocated
DiGiacomo et al. [2] (1994)	3	73	71	-	24 (33%)	10 (14%)	-	27 (37%)	1 (1.4%)	9 (12%)	-	-	10	Transpelvic bullet trajectory: surgery
Makin et al. [17] (2001)	5	17	17	27	4 (23.5%)	0	-	2 (11.8%)	0	1 (6%)	0	4 (1-16)	5	Upper zone wounds carry higher risk
Susmallian et al. [18](2005)	5	39	38	-	4 (10.5%)	-	-	2 (5.1%)	0	0	0	-	6	Meticulous observation
Ceyran et al.[19] (2009)	17	27	27	-	-	0	-	25 (93%)	3 (11.1%)	1 (4.2%)	0	8 (7-11)	7	Surgical approach and technique, if needed
Lesperance et. [10] (2009)	1.33	115	113	28	36 (31%)	40 (35%)	13 (1-75)	87 (76%)	7 (6%)	16 (14%)	66 (57%)	-	24	Military surgery experience
Summary	1 - 17	8 - 115	Most	Young	10.5 - 54.5%	0 - 35%	11 - 13	5.1 - 93%	0 - 25%	0 - 33%	High	Long	0 - 24	Dangerous injury/ Contingencies possible

*Major surgery: laparotomy, suprapubic cystostomy, massive/operating room gluteal surgery (massive debridement included). †Hospital stay - mean/average. Values in parenthesis are percentages.

2.6% (13/504) following missile injuries. Mortality rate due to gunshot injuries was 2.2% (10/457). 6.4% (3/47) of patients admitted for blast injuries had died. Both patients treated for impalement survived. Details related to each fatality due to penetrating injuries to the buttock are demonstrated in Table 2. Hypovolaemic shock, major surgical intervention, and visceral and/or vascular injury are all factors which have a significant impact on a lethal outcome (Table 3).

Morbidity

The authors described 18 specific postoperative complications. As they did not adhere to a set of auditable complications, the following figures have mere descriptive value: wound infection (n = 16), sepsis or multiorgan failure (n = 10), small bowel fistula (n = 7 via laparotomy; n = 1 via gluteal wound), prolonged ileus or transient obstruction (n = 6), rebleeding (n = 5), local neurologic dysfunction or weakness of leg (n = 5), urinary tract infection (n = 4), myocardial infarction (n = 3), sacral decubitus (n = 3), stroke (n = 2), pleuropulmonary dysfunction (n = 2), thrombophlebitis/thrombosis (n = 2), and compartment syndrome of the lower extremity, perirectal hematoma, acute renal failure,

paraplegia, malignant hypothermia, impotence (n = 1 for each complication). The seven most common complications constituted 75% of all complications (54 cases). 17 (2.6%) patients needed early postoperative reintervention.

Patterns of major injuries

Pattern of major injuries related with penetrating trauma to the buttock

There were 615 cases of penetrating buttock injuries caused by stabbing or shooting after exclusion of blasting (n = 47) and impaled injuries (n = 2). There were 292 injuries to viscera, named vessels, bony pelvis, and nerves. Injuries of viscera (n = 173; 28.1%) prevail over injuries to major vessels (n = 81; 13.2%), bony pelvis (29 cases; 4.7%), or regional nerves (n = 9; 1.5%). Lumbosacral (n = 4) and sciatic nerve injuries (n = 5) were rare.

The details of major injuries due to penetrating trauma to the buttock is shown in Figure 1. 30 anatomical terms were used to describe a particular injury type. The small bowel (8.3%), colon (6.3%), superior gluteal artery (5.4%), rectum (4.9%), bony pelvis (4.4%), bladder (3.7%), and iliac artery (2.0%) were on the top of the

Table 2 Deaths due to penetrating injuries to the buttock in series of 664 cases

Author	Case no	Age	Gender	Injury Mechanism	Buttock or zone	Major finding on admission	Shock presentation	Bleeding	Surgical approach	Injuries	Surgical procedure	Cause of death
Ivatury [4]	1	15	Male	Stabbing	Left	Hypovolemic shock	ED	Internal	Laparotomy	IA	na	Shock
	2	26	Male	Stabbing	Left	Wound	Ward	Internal	Laparotomy	IA	Repair	Shock†
Gilroy [15]	3	45	Male	Shooting	Left	Hypovolemic shock	ED	External	Laparotomy	GA, bowels, bladder	Ligation, repair	Shock
	4	36	Male	Stabbing	Left	False aneurysm	Theatre	External	*Laparotomy	SGA	Ligation	Sepsis
Mercer [3]	5	17	Male	Shooting	Upper	Hypovolemic shock	ED	External & internal	Laparotomy	EIV	Repair	Shock
Ferraro [16]	6	na	na	Shooting	na	Hypovolemic shock	ED	na	Laparotomy	Pelvic veins	Pelvic packing	Shock
	7	na	na	Shooting	na	na	na	na	na	na	na	na
	8	na	na	Shooting	na	na	na	na	na	na	na	na
DiGiacomo [2]	9	na	na	Shooting	na	Hypovolemic shock	ED	Internal	Laparotomy	CIA, CIV Sigmoid colon	na	Shock
Ceyran [19]	10	na	Male	Stabbing	Left	Hypovolemic shock	ED	Internal	No surgery	IA	No	Shock
	11	na	Male	Stabbing	Right	Hypovolemic shock	ED	External	Gluteal	SGA	No	Shock†
	12	na	Male	Stabbing	Right	Hypovolemic shock	ED	External	Gluteal	SGA	No	Shock†
Lesperance [10]	13-16	na	na	Shooting	na	na	na	na	na	na	na	na
	17-19	na	na	Blast	na	na	na	na	na	na	na	na

IA - iliac artery, GA - gluteal artery, SGA - superior gluteal artery, EIV - external iliac vein, IIA - internal iliac artery, CIA - common iliac artery, CIV - common iliac vein, * Embolization was performed before laparotomy, † intraoperative deaths

Table 3 The impact of gender, injury mechanism, injury severity, and intervention on survival of patients with penetrating trauma to the buttock (n = 240)

Factor	Groups	Alive/Death	p*
Gender	male *vs* female	228/9 *vs* 12/0	0.4917
Injury mechanism	stabbing *vs* shooting	64/5 *vs* 176/4	0.1281
Hypovolemic shock	present *vs* not present	17/8 *vs* 224/1	< 0.0001
Visceral/vascular injury	present *vs* not present	61/9 *vs* 179/0	< 0.0001
Intervention extent	major *vs* minor/no surgery	89/9 *vs* 151/0	0.0006

* Chi²-test with Yates' correction

drawing scale of damaged anatomical structures. Summing up data on large bowel and major junctional vessel injury demonstrated that prevalence of injury to large bowel was 11.2% (n = 69); it was 2.9% for iliac artery or vein injury (n = 18), and 1.3% (n = 8) for femoral artery or vein injury. 10 major vessels injured due to penetrating buttock trauma were not named. Gluteal arteries were damaged in 37 patients (6.0%).

Pattern of major injuries related to stabbing

99 (63%) major injuries were identified in the subset of 158 patients with stab wounds (Figure 2). The prevalence of major vessel, visceral, sciatic nerve, and

ligament/joint injury was 34.8% (n = 55), 24.1% (n = 38), 2.5% (n = 4), and 1.3% (n = 2), respectively. Rectum, superior gluteal artery, and iliac artery were the most frequently damaged major structures accounting for 19.0%, 17.7%, and 7.0%. In total, there were 32 injuries to gluteal arteries (20.3%), 13 injuries to iliac artery or vein (8.2%), and 6 injuries to femoral artery or vein (3.8%).

Pattern of major injuries related to shot wounds

225 major injuries were identified in the subset of 457 patients with gunshot injury (Figure 3). There were 166 visceral injuries (36.3%), 27 injuries to the bony pelvis

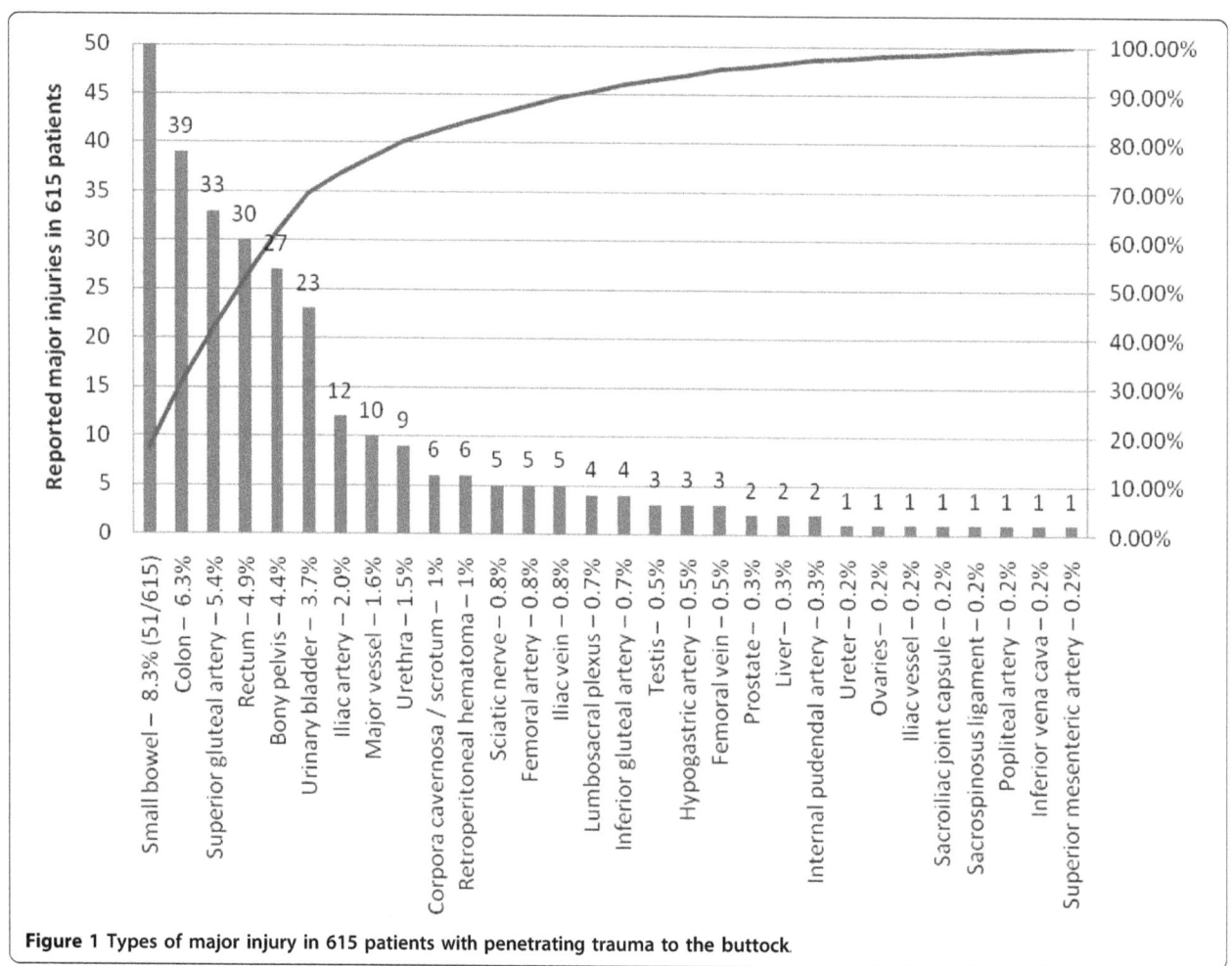

Figure 1 Types of major injury in 615 patients with penetrating trauma to the buttock.

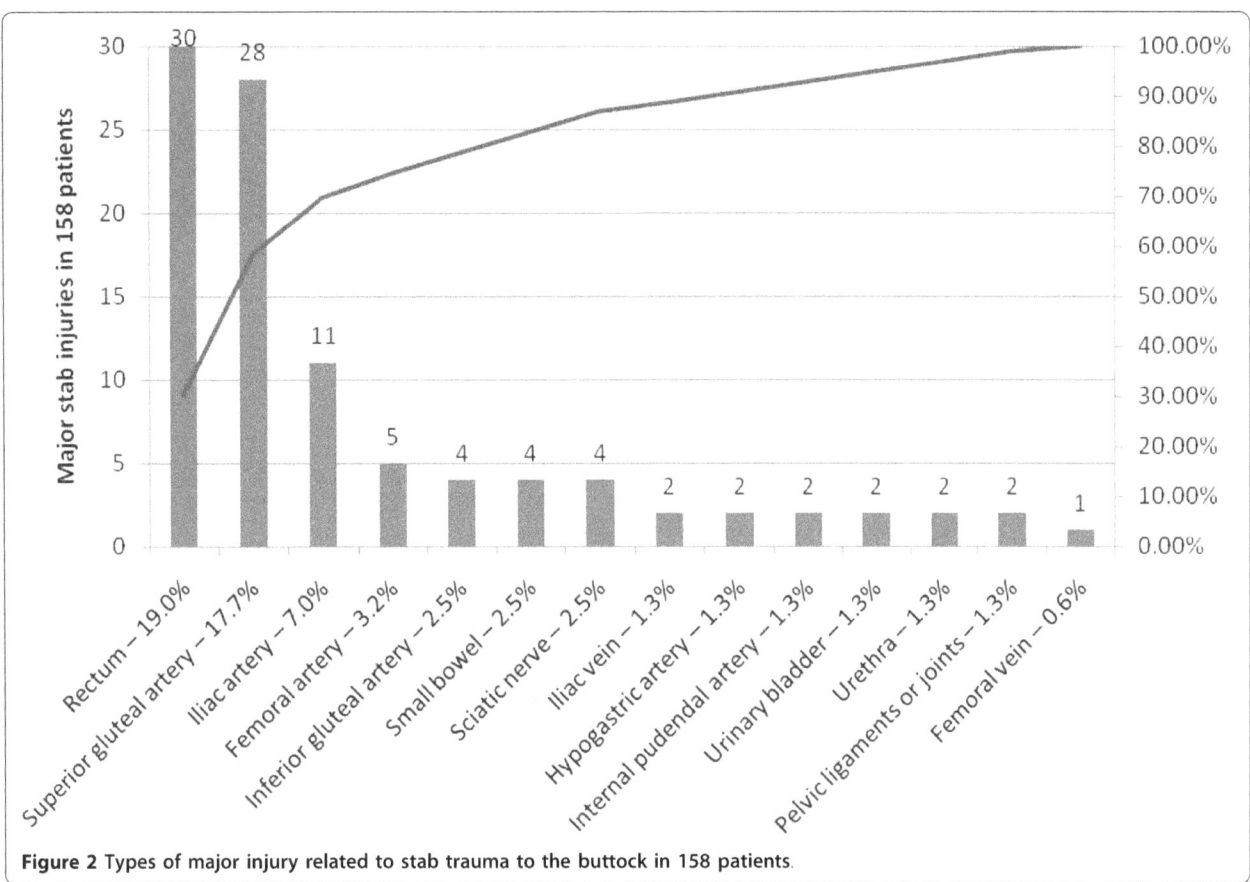

Figure 2 Types of major injury related to stab trauma to the buttock in 158 patients.

(5.9%), 26 injuries to major vessel (5.7%), 6 cases of retroperitoneal hematoma (1.3%), and 5 neurologic injuries (1.1%). The spectrum of major injuries associated with gunshot trauma to the buttock comprised 21 different types of injury. Injury of small bowel, colon, rectum, bony pelvis, and bladder were most frequent with 10.3%, 8.5%, 8.1%, 5.9%, and 4.6%, respectively. When colon and rectal injuries were collated, the prevalence of large bowel injury increased to 16.6% (n = 76).

The pattern of major injury relating to injury mechanism

Table 4 demonstrates a higher frequency for all visceral and skeletal pelvic injuries in the patients with shot wounds. Injuries to the organs located more distally from the wound site (colon, small bowel, and bladder) were far more frequently damaged in patients with shot wounds to the buttock. Rectum and major vessels of the region (iliac vessels, femoral vessels, and gluteal arteries) were damaged more frequently in patients with stab wounds to the buttock.

Penetrating injuries to the upper *vs* lower zone of the buttock

A subset including 97 cases from two retrospective studies [3,17] and six case reports [21,22,25,27,29] provided

data to assigns the main wound site to the upper or lower buttock region. Statistical results regarding penetrating injuries above and below the intertrochanteric line are shown in Table 5. There were 64 wounds to the upper zone (66.0%): 26 of them were related to stabbing and 38 to shooting. The lower zone of the buttock was targeted 33 times (34.0%): 15 subjects had stab wounds and 18 subjects had shot wounds. A prevalence of major injuries, either visceral/vascular, bony pelvis or sciatic nerve, was higher in patients with the entrance wound position above the intertrochanteric line. Visceral/vascular injuries were more frequent in patients with penetrating wounds in the upper zone of the buttock (25/64, 39.1% *vs* 6/33, 18.2%; OR, 2.88; CI, 1.04-7.98; *P* < 0.05). The sensitivity of this test was 0.81, the positive predictive value was 0.39. Injury of soft tissue alone was more frequent in patients with penetrating injury to the lower zone of the buttock (32/64, 50.0% *vs* 26/33, 78.8%; *P* < 0.05). The sensitivity of this test was 0.55, positive predictive value was 0.5.

Discussion

It may be helpful to remind ourselves of the former surgical perspective on buttock trauma. Feigenberg (1992) reviewed four papers on stab wounds to the buttock

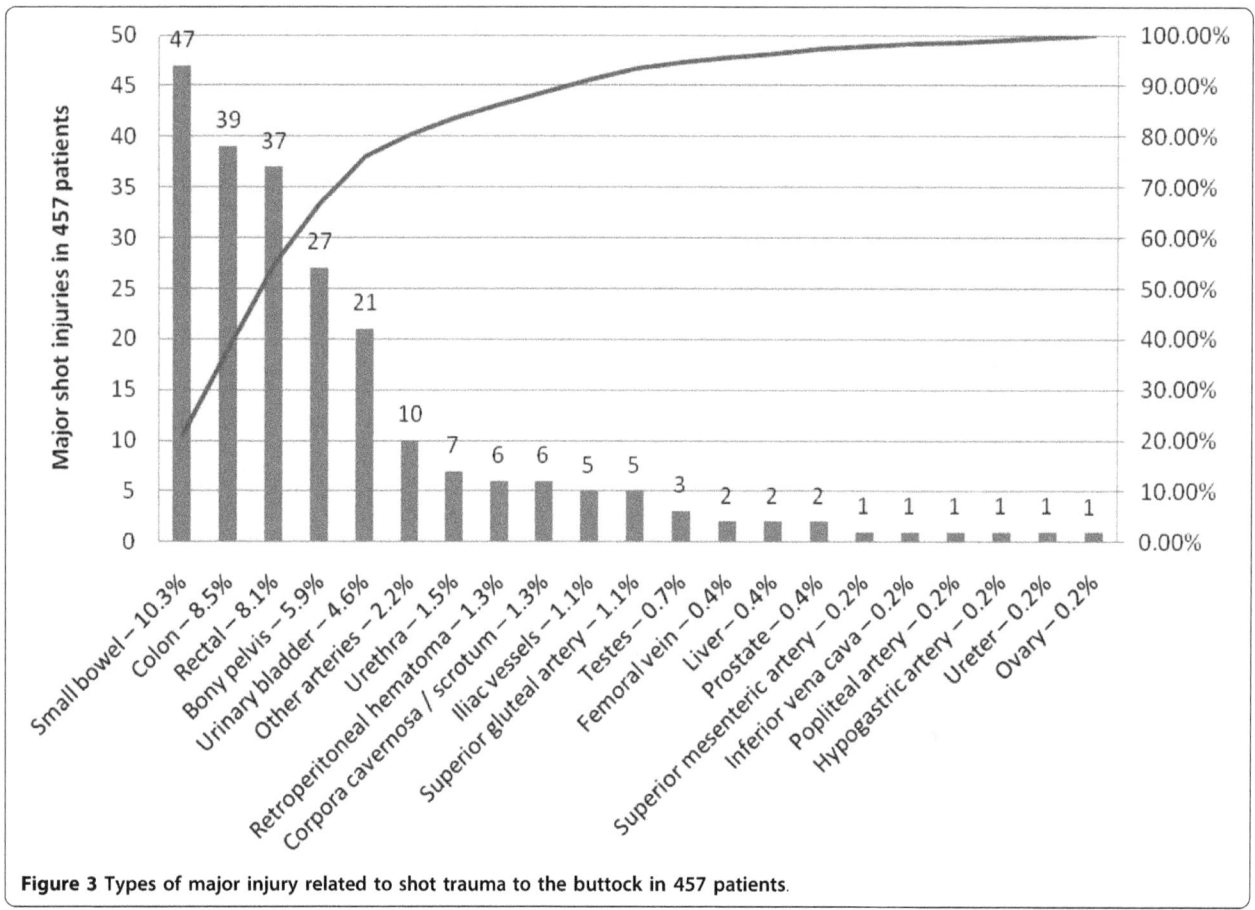

Figure 3 Types of major injury related to shot trauma to the buttock in 457 patients.

and concluded that any stab wound to this body region should be regarded as potentially dangerous and every effort should be made to locate possible injuries [6]. Salim and Velmahos' review (2002) on abdominal gunshot wounds contains only one chapter regarding injury to the buttocks [7] and refers to one reference [11] pointing out that haemodynamically stable patients should be triaged (operation *vs* adjunct investigations) according to findings of physical examination. Aydin (2007) highlighted the importance of placing an acute

Table 4 Stabbing *vs* shooting related major injuries of the buttock

Injuries	Stab wound n = 158	Shot wound n = 457	Odds Ratio	95% Confidence Internal	P*
Visceral:	38 (24%)	166 (36%)	0.56	0.37-0.84	0.006
Colon	0	39 (9%)	0.24	0.11-0.50	0.0003
Small bowel	4 (3%)	47 (10%)	0.23	0.08-0.64	0.004
Rectal	30 (19%)	37 (8%)	2.66	1.58-4.48	0.0003
Bladder	2 (1%)	21 (5%)	0.33	0.08-1.42	0.0097
Major vessel:	55 (35%)	26 (6%)	8.85	5.30-14.80	0.0001
Gluteal arteries:	32 (20%)	5 (1%)	22.96	8.76-60.14	0.0001
Superior gluteal artery	28 (18%)	5 (1%)	19.47	7.37-51.43	0.0001
Inferior gluteal artery	4 (3%)	0	49.97	5.28-473.4	0.005
Iliac vessels:	13 (8%)	5 (1%)	8.10	2.84-23.12	0.0001
Iliac artery	7 (4%)	1 (0.2%)	8.10	2.84-23.12	0.0003
Internal iliac artery	4 (3%)	0	49.97	5.28-473.4	0.0046
Femoral vessels:	6 (4%)	2 (0.4%)	8.98	1.79-44.96	0.005
Femoral artery	5 (3%)	0	50.30	6.72-376.39	0.001
Sciatic nerve	4 (3%)	1 (0.2%)	11.84	1.31-106.78	0.023
Bony pelvis	0	27 (6%)	0.25	0.10-0.59	0.004

Values in parenthesis are percentages. *Z test.

Table 5 Penetrating injuries to the upper zone *vs* lower zone of the buttock

Injuries	Upper zone* n = 64	Lower zone† n = 33	Odds Ratio	95% Confidence Internal	P‡
Buttock soft tissue	32 (50%)	26 (79%)	0.27	0.10-0.71	0.012
SW	13 (50%)	10 (67%)	0.5	0.13-1.87	0.478
GSW	19 (50%)	16 (89%)	0.13	0.03-0.62	0.012
Visceral/Vascular/Bony	29 (45%)	6 (18%)	3.73	1.35-10.26	0.016
SW	11 (42%)	4 (27%)	2.02	5.51-8.05	0.506
GSW	18 (47%)	2 (11%)	7.2	1.45-35.73	0.019
Visceral/Vascular	25 (39%)	6 (18%)	2.88	1.04-7.98	0.063
SW	11 (42%)	4 (27%)	2.02	5.51-8.05	0.506
GSW	14 (37%)	2 (11%)	4.67	0.93-23.37	0.094
Bony pelvis	4 (6%)	0	4.78	0.58-39.10	0.353
SW	0	0	-	-	-
GSW	4 (11%)	0	4.90	0.58-41.69	0.383
Sciatic nerve	3 (5%)	1 (3%)	1.57	0.16-15.75	0.882
SW	2 (8%)	1 (7%)	1.17	0.10-14.06	0.616
GSW	1 (3%)	0	4.37	0.07-290.2	0.700

* 26 stab wounds, and 38 gunshot wounds, † 15 stab and 18 gunshot wounds. Values in parenthesis are percentages. ‡Z test . SW - stab wound, GSW - gunshot wound

false aneurysm in the differential diagnosis of an indurate, fluctuant, warm, erythematous posttraumatic gluteal mass [8]. The key statements of the review provided by Butt (2009) [9] are based on the summary of three papers [11,12,37] on gunshot wounds to the buttocks, back, and pelvis: firstly, the management of gunshot wounds of the buttocks should follow the same principles with anterior abdomen gunshot wounds; secondly, clinical examination is a reliable predictor for the need of an operation; thirdly, a rigid sigmoidoscopy is introduced per routine for all patients.

Case reports on penetrating buttock injury [6,8,19-33] highlight the importance of a thorough and aggressive evaluation of the patient [6], observation [23,27], prompt differential diagnosis [8,21,30,31], immediate assessment of the lower urinary tract [21,22], and lately the value of dynamic 2D and 3D CT-scanning and angiography [28]. They also highlight rare complications following high-velocity or low-velocity gunshot injury to the buttock where the bullet or pellet migrates to major veins such as inferior cava vein and hepatic veins [29] or if it reaches the right ventricle of the heart [23], needing a broad range of approaches ranging from open surgery to angioembolization [6,21,22], transjugular extraction of bullet from middle hepatic vein [29], image navigation surgery [33], gluteal surgery [28,32], laparoscopy [24], and laparotomy [6,20,21,25].

Our analytical review demonstrates that penetrating trauma to the buttock is a serious diagnostic and clinical concern with a mortality rate of 2.9%. Mortality of penetrating stab injuries to the buttock is comparable to that of extra-buttock regions of the body, such as penetrating injury to the posterior abdomen is 0-2% [37-39], the anterior abdomen 0-4.4% [40-43], the thoracoabdominal area 2.1% [44], and the chest 2.5-5.6% [44-46]. Mortality may be less in cohorts with isolated stab injury to the chest (1.46%) [45], or after exclusion of cardiac injuries (0.8%) [44]. Regarding pelvic or transpelvic gunshot trauma, mortality rates vary from 0-12.2% [11,47,48]. Cohorts with gunshot wounds to the limbs may show no mortality [49,50]. We conclude that penetrating injuries to the buttock poses a similar threat to the patient as penetrating trauma of any other body region.

Despite the fact that stab wound primarily cause locoregional damage, whilst gunshot trauma is associated with frequent extraterritorial injury, stab wounds (3.8% mortality rate) are even more dangerous than missile wounds *per se* or gunshot wounds specifically (2.6% and 2.2% mortality rate, respectively). Injury of buttock due to impalement remains uncommon [26,51]. It is therefore recommended to classify impalement related injuries as a separate category of penetrating injuries [52].

Analysis of the associated major injuries due to penetrating trauma to the buttock reveals several unexpected particularities. The most commonly damaged particular organs and vessels were, in descending order, small bowel, colon, superior gluteal artery, and rectum. Injury of iliac artery and/or vein was a rare, but relevant finding with 2.9%. This counterintuitive finding is better understood on analysis of subgroups created according to injury mechanism.

As expected, stabbings were most frequently associated with injuries to gluteal arteries (20.3%), rectum (19.0%), and iliac vessels (8.2%). The prevalence of injuries to femoral artery or vein was 3.8%. Gunshot injuries frequently result in wider organ damage involving small bowel (10.3%), colon (8.5%), rectum (8.1%), bony pelvis (5.9%), and bladder injuries (4.6%). Table 4 provides ample evidence that gunshot and stab trauma of the buttock are actually two separate clinical entities. They require different diagnostic and surgical approaches which are summarised in Figure 4. In our view, such an approach based on empiric evidence might usefully supersede former algorithms by trying to address particular aspects of buttock trauma [2,5,14,17].

This review confirms the conclusion of two other authors [3,17] suggesting that injuries of upper zone of the buttock are associated with higher probability of viscus or major vessel injury comparing with injuries to the lower zone of the buttock. Table 5 reveals significant differentiation of injury patterns according to zone of primary injury site. However, the low positive predictive value does not recommend to rely on this criterion, for management strategies based on division of the buttock. On any account, the frequency of extraregional injury should prompt an aggressive and speedy computed tomography imaging approach to the entire abdomen and pelvis, complemented by a chest x-ray in all gunshot wounds to the buttock.

The current review contains a significant amount of historical data, bringing the use of endovascular approaches to only 1.8% in the current cohort. The advent of interventional radiological techniques should enable embolisation of pelvic vessels beside the level of the common or external iliac vessels [36,53].

Selective non-operative management of penetrating trauma to the buttock in stable patients without evidence of major organ injury is a successful approach [11]. Serial clinical examination should include per rectal examination, rigid sigmoidoscopy, and urinanalysis because of quite high probability of colorectal (11.2%) as well as bladder, urethra, and ureter injury (5.4%).

A classification of CT findings into three main groups of subset in relation to stable patients (abdominal/pelvis injury, gluteal vessel injury, and femoral vessel injury) is another feature of the algorithm (Figure 4). The rationale of this is the following: the buttocks should be regarded as a distinct anatomical/junctional zone in trauma surgery because patterns of penetrating injury and clinical characteristics as well as implications of buttock trauma disclosed in this paper correspond with general hallmarks of junctional trauma [54].

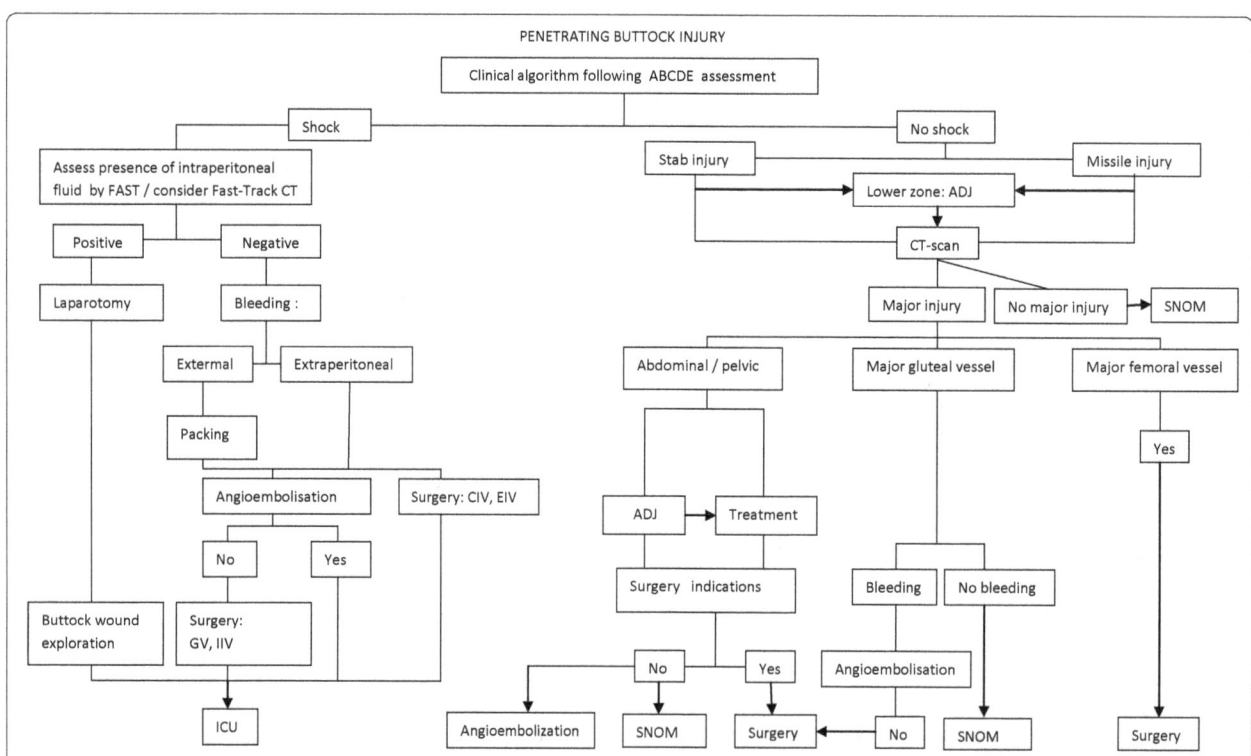

Figure 4 Algorithm for management of penetrating trauma to the buttock. FAST - Focused assessment with sonography for trauma. SNOM - Selective non-operative management. SE - Serial examination. ADJ - Adjuncts. Surgery indications: haemoperitoneum, injury of major or junctional vessel (CIV, EIV), perforation of bowel, peritonitis, not-stable bony pelvis, sciatic nerve transsection, necrotic/dirty soft tissue, urethra/ ureter transsection, intraperitoneal bladder rupture (consider on individual basis). CIV - common iliac vessel. EIV - external iliac vessel. IIV - internal iliac vessel. ICU - Intensive care unit

In terms of injury severity score, only Ferraro [16] and Lesperance [10] used the ISS scale. It is important to emphasise coding technique for penetrating buttock injury according to newest AIS 2005©Update 2008 [55]. It indicates that superficial (minor) penetrating injury to the buttock should be regarded as grade 1 (code 816011.1). When there is tissue loss >25 cm^2, it should be regarded as grade 2 injury (code 816012.2), and when it is associated with blood loss >20% by volume, it has to be regarded as grade 3 injury (816013.3). Such injuries should be assigned to the external body region when calculating the ISS. However, if underlying anatomical structures are involved, documented diagnoses should be coded only, and they should be assigned to either the lower extremity body region or abdomen. Penetrating injuries involving a bone is coded as open fracture to the specific bone.

There are several limitations of this review. Publication bias, retrospective approach, clustered data, complexity of some injuries, and constrained nature of this study are the factors which undoubtedly cause our bias views. Prospective networked studies would be a better approach to the problem. The current review may help to design such studies.

In conclusion, penetrating buttock trauma should be regarded as a life-threatening injury with impact beyond the pelvis until proven otherwise.

Authors' contributions

RL and KMS equally participated in the design of the study and interpretation of data. RL performed the literature review, statistical analysis of data, and drafting. KMS carried out the critical revision of the manuscript. Both authors read and approved the final manuscript.

Competing interests

The authors declare that they have no competing interests.

References

1. Trunkey D: Torso trauma. Curr Probl Surg 1987, 24:4.
2. DiGiacomo JC, Schwab CW, Rotondo MF, Angood PA, McGonigal MD, Kauder DR, Phillips GR: Gluteal gunshot wounds: who warrants exploration? J Trauma 1994, 37:622-628.
3. Mercer DW, Buckman RF Jr, Sood R, Kerr TM, Gelman J: Anatomic considerations in penetrating gluteal wounds. Arch Surg 1992, 127:407-410.
4. Ivatury RR, Rao PM, Nallathambi M, Gaudino J, Stahl WM: Penetrating gluteal injuries. J Trauma 1982, 22:706-709.
5. Vo NM, Russell JC, Becker DR: Gunshot wounds to the buttocks. Am Surg 1983, 49:579-581.
6. Feigenberg Z, Ben-Baruch D, Barak R, Zer M: Penetrating stab wound of the gluteus-a potentially life-threatening injury: case reports. J Trauma 1992, 33:776-778.
7. Salim A, Velmahos GC: When to operate on abdominal gunshot wounds. Scand J Surg 2002, 91:62-66.
8. Aydin A, Lee CC, Schultz E, Ackerman J: Traumatic inferior gluteal artery pseudoaneurysm: case report and review of literature. Am J Emerg Med 2007, 25:488.e1-3.
9. Butt MU, Zacharias N, Velmahos GC: Penetrating abdominal injuries: management controversies. Scand J Trauma Resusc Emerg Med 2009, 17:19.
10. Lesperance K, Martin MJ, Beekley AC, Steele SR: The significance of penetrating gluteal injuries: an analysis of the Operation Iraqi Freedom experience. J Surg Educ 2008, 65:61-66.
11. Velmahos GC, Demetriades D, Cornwell EE, Asensio J, Belzberg H, Berne TV: Gunshot wounds to the buttocks: predicting the need for operation. Dis Colon Rectum 1997, 40:307-311.
12. Velmahos GC, Demetriades D, Cornwell EE III: Transpelvic gunshot wounds: routine laparotomy or selective management? World J Surg 1998, 22:1034-1038.
13. Maull KI, Snoddy JW, Haynes BW Jr: Penetrating wounds of the buttock. Surg Gynecol Obstet 1979, 149:855-857.
14. Fallon WF Jr, Reyna TM, Brunner RG, Crooms C, Alexander RH: Penetrating trauma to the buttock. South Med J 1988, 81:1236-1238.
15. Gilroy D, Saadia R, Hide G, Demetriades D: Penetrating injury to the gluteal region. J Trauma 1992, 32:294-297.
16. Ferraro FJ, Livingston DH, Odom J, Swan KG, McCormack M, Rush BF Jr: The role of sigmoidoscopy in the management of gunshot wounds to the buttocks. Am Surg 1993, 59:350-352.
17. Makrin V, Sorene ED, Soffer D, Weinbroum A, Oron D, Kluger Y: Stab wounds to the gluteal region: a management strategy. J Trauma 2001, 50:707-710.
18. Susmallian S, Ezri T, Elis M, Dayan K, Charuzi I, Muggia-Sullam M: Gluteal stab wound is a frequent and potentially dangerous injury. Injury 2005, 36:148-150.
19. Ceyran H, Akçali Y, Özcan N, Tasdemir K: Isolated penetrating gluteal injuries. Perspect Vasc Surg Endovasc Ther 2009, 21:253-256.
20. Knight RJ: Resuscitation of battle casualties in South Vietnam: experiences at the First Australian Field Hospital. Resuscitation 1973, 2:17-31.
21. Mamode N, Reid AW: Haemorrhage following penetrating gluteal trauma. Br J Surg 1994, 81:203-204.
22. Rub R, Madeb R, Kluger Y, Chen T, Avidor Y: Posterior urethral disruption secondary to a penetrating gluteal injury. Urology 2000, 56:509.
23. Obermeyer RJ, Fecher A, Erzurum VZ, DeVito PM: Embolization of bullet to the right ventricle. Am J Surg 2000, 179:189.
24. Kalimi R, Angus LD, Gerold T, DiGiacomo JC, Weltman D: Bullet embolization from the left internal iliac vein to the right ventricle. J Trauma 2002, 52:772-774.
25. Carrick MM, Morel AN, Pham HQ: Shotgun wounds to the buttocks, sacrum, and rectum. J Trauma 2007, 62:552.
26. Napier F, Fountain-Polley S, Kallapa C: Images in paediatrics: Ironing board impalement. Arch Dis Child 2007, 92:758.
27. van Oldenrijk J, Unlü C, van Wagensveld BA: Perforation of the ileum after a stab wound of the gluteal region: a case report. Emerg Med J 2007, 24:737-738.
28. Ramasamy A, Hinsley DE, Brooks AJ: The use of improvised bullet markers with 3D CT reconstruction in the evaluation of penetrating trauma. J R Army Med Corps 2008, 154:239-241.
29. Raikar SS, Jureidini SB, Balfour IC, Tinker K: The fantastic journey of a bullet: out with a snare. Pediatr Cardiol 2010, 31:108-110.
30. Demetriades D, Rabinowitz B, Sofianos C: Gluteal artery aneurysms. Br J Surg 1988, 75:494.
31. Holland AJ, Ibach EG: False aneurysm of the inferior gluteal artery following penetrating buttock trauma: case report and review of the literature. Cardiovasc Surg 1996, 4:841-843.
32. Culliford AT, Cukingham RA, Worth MH Jr: Aneurysms of the gluteal vessels: their etiology and management. J Trauma 1974, 14:77-81.
33. Chappell ET, Pare L, Salepour M: Fluoroscopic image guidance for minimally invasive extraction of a bullet from the gluteus maximus. J Trauma 2006, 60:664-667.
34. Scalea TM: Invited commentary on Velmahos, G.C., et al: Transpelvic gunshot wounds: routine laparotomy or selective management? World J Surg 1998, 22:1038.
35. DiGiacomo JC, Schwab CW, Kauder DR, Rotondo MF: Re: Velmahos, G.C., et al: Transpelvic gunshot wounds: routine laparotomy or selective management? World J Surg 1999, 23:619-620.

36. Rasmussen TE: **Commentary on "Isolated penetrating gluteal injuries: a potentially life-threatening trauma".** *Perspect Vasc Surg Endovasc Ther* 2009, **21**:257-258, discussion 258.

37. Velmahos GC, Demetriades D, Foianini E, Tatevossian R, Cornwell EE, Asensio J, Belzberg H, Berne TV: **A selective approach to the management of gunshot wounds to the back.** *Am J Surg* 1997, **174**:342-346.

38. Peck JJ, Berne TV: **Posterior abdominal stab wounds.** *J Trauma* 1981, **21**:298-306.

39. Demetriades D, Rabinowitz B, Sofianos C, Charalambides D, Melisas J, Hatzitheofilou C, Da Silva J: **The management of penetrating injuries of the back. A prospective study of 230 patients.** *Ann Surg* 1988, **207**:72-74.

40. Shaftan GW: **Indications for operation in abdominal trauma.** *Am J Surg* 1960, **99**:657-664.

41. Goins WA, Anderson BB: **Abdominal trauma revisited.** *J Natl Med Assoc* 1991, **83**:883-888.

42. Leppäniemi A, Haapiainen R: **Diagnostic laparoscopy in abdominal stab wounds: a prospective, randomized study.** *J Trauma* 2003, **55**:636-645.

43. Ohene-Yeboah M, Dakubo JCB, Boakye F, Naeeder SB: **Penetrating abdominal injuries in adults seen at two teaching hospitals in Ghana.** *Ghana Med J* 2010, **44**:103-108.

44. Mandal AK, Oparah SS: **Unusually low mortality of penetrating wounds of the chest. Twelve years' experience.** *J Thorac Cardiovasc* 1989, **97**:119-125.

45. Inci I, Ozçelik C, Taçyildiz I, Nizam O, Eren N, Ozgen G: **Penetrating chest injuries: unusually high incidence of high-velocity gunshot wounds in civilian practice.** *World J Surg* 1998, **22**:438-442.

46. Fullum TM, Siram SM, Righini M: **Stab wounds to the chest: a retrospective review of 100 consecutive cases.** *J Nat Med Assoc* 1999, **82**:109-112.

47. Duncan AO, Philips TF, Scalea TM, Maltz SB, Atweh NA, Sclafani SJ: **Management of transpelvic gunshot wounds.** *J Trauma* 1989, **29**:1335-1340.

48. Navsaria PH, Edu S, Nicol AJ: **Nonoperative management of pelvic gunshot wounds.** *Am J Surg* 2011, **201**:784-788, Epub 2010 Sep 29.

49. Stewart MP, Kinninmonth A: **Shotgun wounds of the limbs.** *Injury* 1993, **24**:667-670.

50. Burg A, Nachum G, Salai M, Haviv B, Heller S, Velkes S, Dudkiewicz I: **Treating civilian gunshot wounds to the extremities in a level 1 trauma center: our experience and recommendations.** *IMAJ* 2009, **11**:546-551.

51. O'Leary ST, Waterworth P, Fountain SW: **Multiple impalement injury-a remarkable survival.** *Injury* 1996, **27**:589-590.

52. Eachempati SR, Barie PS, Reed RL: **Survival after transabdominal impalement from a construction injury: a review of the management of impalement injuries.** *J Trauma* 1999, **47**:864-866.

53. Guven K, Rozanes I, Ucara A, Poyanli A, Yanarb H, Acunas B: **Pushable springcoil embolization of pseudoaneurysms caused by gluteal stab injuries.** *Eur J Radiol* 2010, **73**:391-395.

54. Tai NRM, Dickson EJ: **Military junctional trauma.** *JR Army Med Corps* 2009, **155**:285-292.

55. Association for the Advancement of Automotive Medicine:Edited by: Gennarelli TA, Wodzin E. Barrington, IL, USA; 2008:, Abbreviated Injury Scale ©2005. Update 2008..

7

A population based study of hospitalised seriously injured in a region of Northern Italy

Osvaldo Chiara[1*], Cristina Mazzali[3], Sofia Lelli[2], Anna Mariani[1] and Stefania Cimbanassi[1]

Abstract

Background: Injury is a public health problem in terms of mortality, morbidity and disability. The implementation of a regionalised trauma system has been proved to significantly reduce the social impact of severe trauma on population. A population-based registry may be useful to obtain reliable epidemiologic data.

Aim: To perform an exhaustive analysis of severe trauma patients hospitalised in Lombardia, a region of northern Italy.

Materials and methods: The regional Hospital Discharge Registry (HDR) was used to retrieve data of all patients who suffered from serious injuries from 2008 to 2010. ICD9-CM codes of discharge diagnoses were analysed and patients coded from 800.0 to 939.9 or from 950.0 to 959.9 have been retrieved. Femur fractures in elderly and patients with length of hospital stay less than 2 days were excluded. Patients have been considered seriously injured if discharged dead or any of followings: admission or transit in ICU, need of mechanical ventilation, tracheotomy, invasive hemodynamic monitoring. Average reimbursement based on DRG has been evaluated.

Statistics: Student's t test, ANOVA for continuous data, chi-square test for categorical data were used, and a p value less than 0.05 was considered significant.

Results: The severely injured patients hospitalised in Lombardia in three years were 11704, 391 per million per year. Overall mortality was 24.17% and increased with age. Males aging from 18 to 64 years had more occupational injuries, trauma on the road and violence by others. Females were more susceptible to domestic injuries and self inflicted violence, mostly in older ages. Acute mortality was higher after traffic accidents, while late mortality was increased in domestic trauma. Pediatric cases were unusual. A significant increase (+10.18%) in domestic trauma, with a concomitant decrease (−17.76%) in road-related accidents was observed in the three years study period. Reimbursement paid to hospitals for seriously injured was insufficient with regard to estimated costs of care.

Conclusion: Serious injury requiring hospitalisation in Lombardia is still an healthcare problem, with a trend toward a decrease of traffic accidents, increase in domestic trauma and involvement of older people. These results may help to plan a new regionalised Trauma System.

Keywords: Epidemiology, Major trauma, Population-based study, Trauma registry, Trauma system

Introduction

Injury is a major public health problem in terms of mortality, morbidity and disability and it has been largely demonstrated that the organisation of a regionalised Trauma System significantly decreases the deleterious impact of severe trauma on population [1,2]. In Europe the inclusive trauma system model has gained dominance. In this model a network of hospitals with different resources takes care of trauma patients suffering from any among the full spectrum of injuries [3]. Epidemiologic information based on the entire population in a given region and understanding the number of severely injured that need to be admitted to a level one hospital, is of pivotal importance in the design of an inclusive Trauma System. With this objective, methodological approaches in measuring incident rates should use large representative samples of the whole population, to offer the potential to observe data on all the people living in a region or a

* Correspondence: osvaldo.chiara@ospedaleniguarda.it
[1]Trauma Team Dip. DEA-EAS, Ospedale Niguarda Ca'Granda, Piazza Ospedale Maggiore 3, 20162, Milan, Italy

nation. Trauma registries contain detailed information, but this is offset by the limitation of including only patients treated at trauma centre and already triaged as "severe" at a dedicated trauma unit. On the contrary, population-based registries have usually been recorded for many years and are available for time periods before changes of the Healthcare system. Additionally, they contain readily available, alphanumeric-coded information and allow easy and low cost analysis. Moreover, population-based registries may be used to investigate resources consumption and evaluate costs of the system. Recently, many investigators have started to use large databases for quality assessment studies in trauma care, and these works are classified as providing "high end" Class III evidence [4-8].

The objective of this study was to perform an exhaustive analysis of severe trauma patients hospitalised in Lombardia, a mixed rural/industrial region of northern Italy. The hospital discharge registry, a population-based record of all hospitalised people of the country, has been used as source of data. All hospital admissions for injuries during a three years period have been included and severely injured patients have been extrapolated. This analysis may be a useful starting point for evaluating the need for resources and costs of regional Trauma System implementation.

Methods

Lombardia is a mixed rural/industrial region of the northern Italy, with an area of 24,000 Km [2] (9,302 square miles), with Alpi Mountains in the north and hill or flat in the south. Residents, evaluated at the end of 2010, were 9,737,074 (1,046 persons per square mile), 48.87% males, and Milano is the capital city. In this Region there are nine hospitals which function as level 1 or 2 Trauma Centre. The regional Hospital Discharge Registry (HDR), a part of the national HDR, includes the discharge forms of all hospitalised patients of the region since 2001. A common minimum data set, including demographics, place of residency, hospital length of stay (LOS), wards of admission or transit, discharge diagnoses, therapeutic procedures, and outcome, is adopted for all of the public or private hospitals partially or totally financed by the Regional Health Service (97% of existing hospitals). In HDR discharge diagnoses (one principal and up to five secondary diagnoses) and procedures are coded using the Clinical Modification of the International Classification of Diseases 9th edition (ICD-9-CM). In-hospital deaths are all recorded in HDR.

Reimbursement of public or private hospitals is calculated by Government of the Region using the disease-related group (DRG) system and the discharge form of HDR is the administrative document used to calculate the DRG: each patient is weighted on the sequence of ICD-9-CM diagnoses, therapeutic procedures, complications and associated morbidities and the value of assigned DRG is reimbursed to the hospital.

Data extraction

To conduct this study all hospital admissions in Lombardia during a period of three years, from 2008 to 2010, have been reviewed. The aim was to select from regional HDR all patients who suffered from serious injuries.

All patients with at least one principal or secondary diagnosis coded from 800.0 to 939.9 or from 950.0 to 959.9 have been considered. Burns, scalds and frostbites, chemical corrosion, poisoning, intoxication, drowning and hangman, suffocation, electrocution, radiation and medical treatment complications, have been excluded. Furthermore, femur fractures (820.0 and 821.9), as the only traumatic diagnosis, have been considered only if affecting people younger than 65, to exclude femur fractures of elderly due to osteoporotic complications. All patients have been coded with an individual number. Patients with the first admission in a rehabilitation or spinal unit, with a LOS less than two days, unless discharged dead or transferred from or to other facilities, have been excluded.

To select seriously injured any of the following criteria have been used:

- patients discharged dead
- patients admitted in intensive care unit (ICU) during the course of hospital stay
- patients which have been mechanically ventilated (ICD9 code 96.70-96.72) or received tracheotomy (31.1-31.29)
- patients which received invasive hemodynamic monitoring (89.60-89.69)

All patients with at least one of these characteristics have been classified as serious trauma and included in the analysis.

Distribution of severe trauma for specific age-sex population groups has been estimated. The modality of trauma has been identified as:

- accident at workplace
- accident in domestic pertinence
- road-related accident
- assault (violence inflicted by others)
- self-inflicted violence
- other

The Regional Health System allowed the analysis of the reimbursements, giving the investigators the value in euros of DRG assigned for each case. In order to characterise the time distribution of trauma deaths, from HDR it was possible to classify hospital deaths into acute (within two days following admission), early (from three to seven days), or late deaths (more than seven days).

Statistics

Data processing and statistical analysis were performed using SAS 9.2®. Continuous data were compared by ANOVA or Student's t-test, while categorical data were analysed using chi-square test. Differences for all tests were considered significant with a p value less than 0.05.

Incidence rates for severe trauma hospital admission in specific age-sex population groups were calculated, using the resident population estimated at the end of administrative year 2010.

Results

Selected records have been 12,036 from which 332 cases (2.76%) have been excluded because LOS <2 days, not deceased or transferred (Figure 1). Finally, the working database of in-hospital severe trauma counted 11,704 cases, 892 (7.62%) non-residents in Lombardia.

Table 1 describes general results of data extraction. The severely injured patients hospitalised in Lombardia during a three years period were the 0.80% of all hospital admissions, on average, 391 cases per million inhabitants

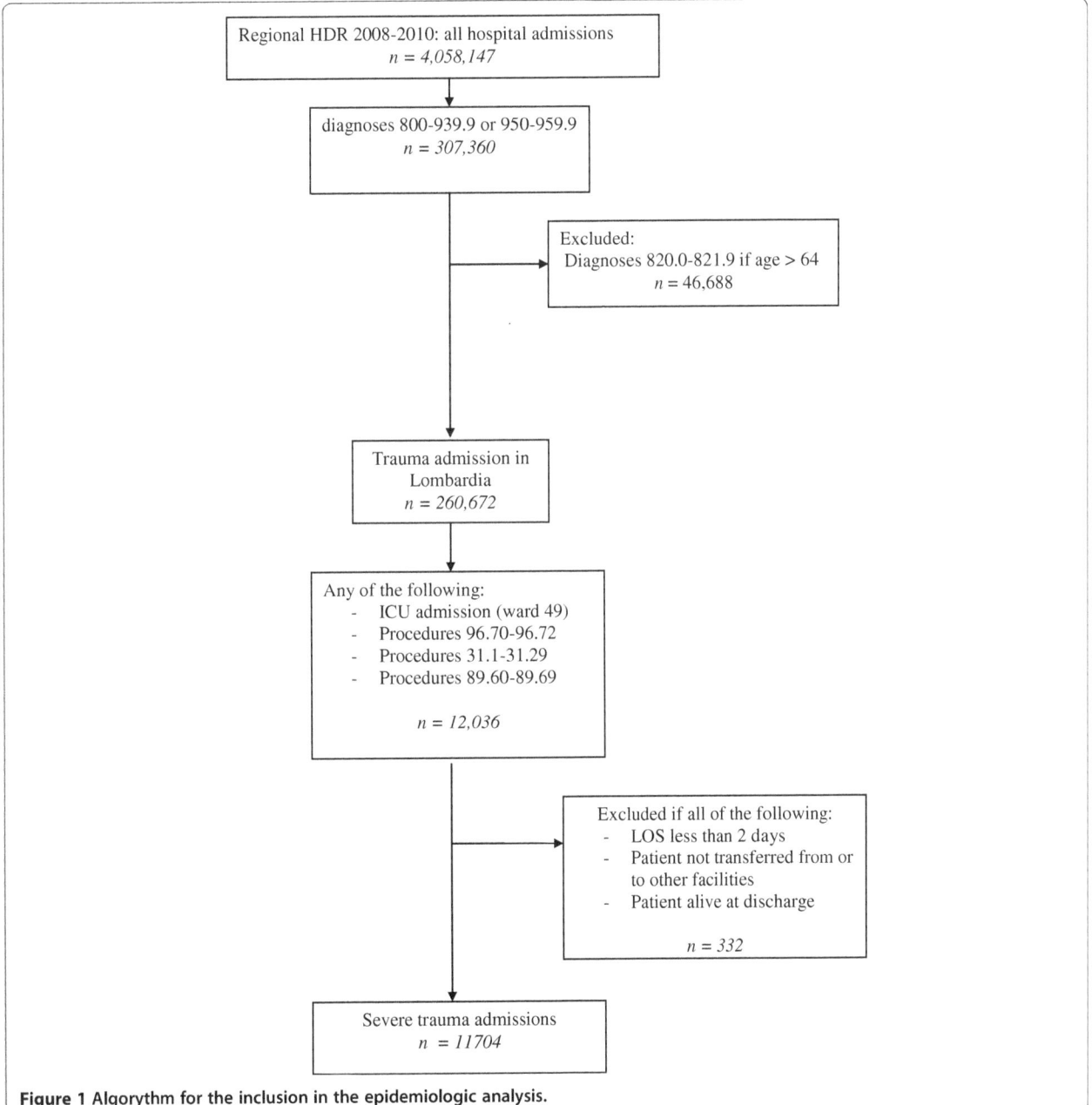

Figure 1 Algorythm for the inclusion in the epidemiologic analysis.

Table 1 Severe trauma patients hospitalized in Lombardia

	Number	Deceased	% deceased	Hosp. LOS (±SD)	% ICU adm	ICU LOS (±SD)	Avg remb (€) (±SD)
Total	11704	2829	24.17	18.53 (18.89)	74.09	6.12 (11)	13'759.82 (19347.55)
Male	7623	1588	20.83*	19.35* (20.43)	80.44*	7.02* (11.71)	15'128.02* (20464.93)
Female	4081	1241	30.41	17.00 (18.73)	62.22	4.43 (9.32)	11'204.13 (16771.51)
Year 2008	3866	954	24.68	18.77 (20.31)	74.70	6.21 (11.40)	13'684.64 (18821.89)
Year 2009	3960	961	24.27	18.48 (19.65)	73.79	6.25 (11.36)	13'757.31 (19199.84)
Year 2010	3878	914	23.57	18.34 (19.70)	73.78	5.90 (10.20)	13'837.34 (20008.15)

LOS: length of hospital stay. Avg remb: average rembursement in euros based on disease related group (DRG). ICU adm: admission in intensive care unit. SD: standard deviation. * p < .001 males vs females.

per year. Males constituted 65.13% of these cases and showed a significantly longer hospital LOS, ICU-LOS and rate of admission in ICU. Males showed also a higher value of reimbursement. Overall mortality was 24.17%, with an incidence rate of 9.68/100,000 per year. Surprisingly, mortality of males was lower than in females. Significant differences of these variables during the three years of the survey were not appreciated. The calculated incidence rate of hospital admissions for severe trauma was 40.06/100,000 inhabitants per year (27.33 for females and 53.38 for males). The highest rate was observed in the over 74 years age group (129.21/100,000), while the lowest for children between 7 and 12 years (11.73/100,000).

In Table 2 patients have been analysed according to age groups. Overall, severe trauma affected adults: 4206 cases in age 0–45, 7495 cases after 45 years. Mortality increased with age, reaching nearly 50% in trauma victims older than 75 years. Similarly, hospital and ICU-LOS, rate of admission to ICU and reimbursed DRG, all increased with age, with the higher levels in ages between 13 and 74 years. On the contrary, pediatric cases (age group 0–12) were only 482 in three years, with shorter ICU LOS, decreased mortality and lower levels of reimbursement. All of these differences were statistically significant (p < .0001, ANOVA).

The cause of accident has been indicated in 72.98% of cases (Tables 3 and 4) and "other mechanism", road-related trauma, injured in domestic pertinences and at

workplace were the principal conditions. As expected, accidents on the road and at the workplace were the principal causes of trauma for males aging from 18 to 64 years. On the contrary, accidents in domestic pertinences increased with age, being the principal cause of trauma after 64 years, and old women were affected the most. Violence inflicted by others (assault) or self-inflicted violence was rare in Lombardia and affected people 18 to 64 years old. In pediatric age most of cases were domestic or road-related. Statistic analysis demonstrated a significant association at chi-square test between gender and modality of trauma: males had more occupational injuries, trauma on the road and injuries caused by violence by others, while females were more subjected to domestic injuries and self inflicted violence.

Furthermore, the age of exposure to injuries changed with gender. The mean age of females involved in domestic, road-related trauma and in the category of other modalities was significantly higher (Table 5). Age between gender was not different in accidents during working activities and injuries derived from violence. Same differences of age between gender were evident also in deceased patients (Table 6). Women who died after trauma were significantly older when the cause of death was an accident at work, on the road, violence by others or self-inflicted, other mechanisms.

Time distribution of deaths changed with cause of trauma (Table 7). Late deaths were more often represented

Table 2 Severe trauma hospitalized in Lombardia according age groups

Age groups	Number	Deceased	Modality of trauma: absolute values			
			%_ deceased	LOS (±SD)	% ICU adm	ICU LOS (±SD)	Avg remb (€) (±SD)
00-06	322	15	4.65	10.65 (15.22)	79.165	3.36 (7.49)	6'588.98 (11828.14)
07-12	160	4	2.50	12.50 (12.74)	88.75	3.88 (7.81)	7'492.89 (10229.22)
13-17	411	19	4.62	17.20 (15.94)	95.38	6.39 (9.20)	12'908.43 (16509.47)
18-45	3313	334	10.08	20.88 (21.35)	93.96	7.66 (11.25)	16'144.73 (19550.47)
46-64	2148	356	16.57	21.01 (22.31)	85.52	7.57 (12.74)	16'207.54 (21784.13)
65-74	1657	407	24.56	20.39 (21.06)	74.83	7.13 (11.93)	16'224.24 (21679.17)
>74	3690	1693	45.88	15.21 (16.34)	45.85	3.74 (9.20)	10'067.29 (16701.65)

All differences significant (p < .0001) at ANOVA.
In three cases age informations have been missed.

Table 3 Distribution of patients according to age groups, gender and modality of trauma

| Age groups | Gender | Missing | Modality of trauma: absolute values | | | | | |
			Work	Domestic	Road	Assault	Self inflicted violence	Other mechanisms
00-06	m	32		48	44	1		82
	f	30		24	14			47
07-12	m	3	1	3	49			53
	f	3		1	21	2		24
13-17	m	16	2	7	200	2	2	92
	f	9		3	48		8	22
18-45	m	173	301	49	1479	122	70	525
	f	75	13	15	307	18	35	131
46-64	m	255	202	93	518	20	28	456
	f	137	2	67	145	11	31	183
65-74	m	311	21	141	174	5	13	392
	f	191	1	96	113	1	8	190
75-	m	538	3	289	193	3	7	602
	f	717	2	494	122	3	4	713
Total(1)		2490	548	1330	3427	190	207	3512

in domestic trauma and in the category other mechanisms. On the contrary, deaths at work, on the road and after violence were acute in the majority of cases. Females and older age people showed a tendency to increase in late deaths, although not significantly. In late deaths of patients older than 64 years a systemic complication was the principal diagnosis in 51.4% (pulmonary or cardiovascular failure, mainly), while it was only 17.6% in victims younger than 64. The overall rate of patients admission to one of the nine level 1 or 2 hospitals was 41.58%, but this percentage decreased to 29% in patients older than 64. The mortality was 17.75% in level one or two hospitals, while it was increased to 27.95% in local – non trauma center hospitals.

Figure 2 shows trends of causes of trauma during the three years of the survey. A significant increase in domestic trauma (from 422 in 2008 to 465 in 2010, +10.18%), with a concomitant decrease in road-related crashes (from 1233 to 1014, -17.76%) were observed.

Discussion
Methods of selection
The aim of this study was to perform an exhaustive analysis encompassing the whole population in Lombardia

and to identify the number of seriously injured people who need hospital admission. It is the first time in Italy that a population-based registry has been used to investigate hospitalisation of major trauma in order to design a regionalised Trauma System. A previous study [8] in our country used national HDR to investigate epidemiology of trauma deaths.

A non-integrated Trauma System, such as in Lombardia, implies that many trauma patients are treated in non-trauma hospitals and the use of specialised trauma registries for epidemiologic studies in these conditions excludes patients who receive definitive treatment in non-Trauma Centre hospitals. In our survey less than fifty percent of cases were admitted in one of the nine hospitals which function as level one or level two Trauma Centres and this observation confirms the choice of an administrative database to obtain population-based data.

The methodological approach of cases selection in the present study may be debated. Hospital databases contain ICD diagnoses which lack information about injury severity. On the other hand, specialised trauma registries, in line with international conventions, use the Abbreviated Injury Scale (AIS), an anatomically-based injury description system which allows computation of

Table 4 Differences between male and female for modalities of trauma were significant at chi square (p < .0001)

Chi square	Work	Domestic	Road	Assault	Self inflicted	Other	Total
Male	530	630	2657	155	121	2202	**6295**
Female	18	700	770	35	86	1310	**2919**
Total	548	1330	3427	190	207	3512	9214

(1) In three patients (2 assault and 1 self inflicted violence) age was not available.

Table 5 Differences between age, gender and cause of trauma (SD, standard deviation)

Trauma modality	Male			Female		
	#	Mean age	SD	#	Mean age	SD
Work	530	42.51	13.00	18	41	21.09
Domestic	630	65.30	24.17	700	75.67*	18.95
Road	2657	39.31	19.63	770	46.51*	23.60
Assault	155	35.61	14.27	35	41.49	18.67
Self inflicted violence	121	44.61	17.89	86	45.01	16.41
Other	2202	55.12	24.65	1310	67.43*	23.86

* p < .0001.

ISS, or New Injury Severity Score (NISS) the most reliable and extensively used measure of injury severity [9]. In the middle of 1990s Osler et al. introduced the ICD9 based ISS (ICISS) that allows severity to be classified based on the ICD9 classification of injuries [10]. There is limited evidence of the validation and performance of ICISS in epidemiologic studies [11,12]. ICISS is a product of survival risk ratio from each injury sustained, based on the values of the survival rates of prior patients with similar diagnoses as classified by ICD9. Validity of ICISS derives from accuracy in compilation of list of diagnoses. In Italy hospital discharge forms mainly fulfil an administrative purpose and the sequence and choice of listed diagnoses may be determined in combination in order to generate the DRG that provides maximal payment. As a result of these limitations we considered inappropriate a retrospective analysis of regional HDR for an epidemiologic study on serious injury. We preferred to consider all hospitalised trauma patients of Lombardia with an "ex-post" selection of severity based on procedures unequivocally used in critically injured (ICU admission, mechanical ventilation, tracheotomy, invasive monitoring), or based on the fatal outcome during hospital stay. Unfortunately, vital signs, number of transfusions, laboratory values were not available in HDR. A possible selection bias is the inclusion of

patients with minor trauma and severity due to complications or associated illnesses. However our focus was the use of hospital resources and a patient with minor trauma and concomitant severe illness needs in any case to be triaged to a level one Trauma Centre.

Epidemiology of serious injury

Severe trauma patients hospitalised in Lombardia have been on average 391 per million inhabitants: because in the trauma deaths study [8] we observed a proportion of out-of-hospital deaths (on site and in emergency department) of 38% in the capital Milano during 2007. This suggest that in the regional area the Emergency System, pre-hospital and in-hospital, has to manage about 5258 major trauma patients per year, 540 per million inhabitants. This datum may be overestimated because it considers as the denominator only the resident population and the 7.62% of seriously injured patients at the numerator were non-residents in Lombardia. However, it is not possible to calculate transients or tourists of the Region. The resulting number of 540 major trauma patients per million is analogous to that described by Di Bartolomeo et al. in a study, based on specialised trauma registry, in a north-east region of Italy [13] with 1,200,000 inhabitants, an established Trauma System and only two Trauma Centres receiving major trauma. The Italian data of both these studies are higher than those showed in other European countries, as Mersey-Wales [14] and Ireland [15] but lower than United States reports [16,17]. The selection criteria used in this study seem to be appropriate: all trauma patients who needed ICU treatment or who died during hospital stay have been included. A possible explanation of differences between Italian and US data may be the lower rate in Europe of interpersonal violence. Severe trauma admissions in Italy are due to blunt trauma in 94% (in Lombardia more than 97%), with less than 17% of surgical cases for torso injuries [18]. These observations outline the need of a reduced number of Trauma Centres, to obtain local concentration of cases and surgical skill.

The hospital mortality in Lombardia of 24.17% (incidence rate of 9.68/100,000) is lower than that described

Table 6 Age of deceased patients according to cause of trauma and gender

Cause of trauma	Male		Female	
	#	Mean ± SD	#	Mean ± SD
Missing	405	72.66 16.72	383	79.83 13.28
Work	44	43.14 14.10	2	61.5* 40.31
Domestic	223	76.86 14.99	268	82.15 11.69
Road	355	50.58 22.57	140	60.53* 21.51
Assault	23	43.57 17.46	5	60.00* 14.63
Self inflicted	29	49.43 22.30	15	53.20* 14.34
Others	509	71.92 17.46	428	80.49* 12.28
Total	1588	71.48 17.80	1241	77.95* 15.57

* = p < .001.

Table 7 Time distribution of deaths in deceased patients

	Total #	%	Age (±SD)	% male	Work %	Domestic %	Road %	Assault %	Self inflict %	Other %
Acute	1111	39.27	64.13 (23.19)	60.21	63.04	35.44	67.47	64.29	75.00	33.40
Early	658	23.26	77.00 (16.00)	52.12	17.39	27.70	13.74	10.71	9.09	27.85
Late	1060	37.47	75.76 (15.17)	54.33	19.57	36.86	18.79	25.00	15.91	38.74

in overall Italy in 2002 in the national trauma death study [8] (14.5/100,000) and comparable with the data recorded by Creamer et al. in Auckland in 2004 [19].

Analysis according age groups demonstrates that the highest number of severe trauma occurs in old adults, while pediatric cases are unusual. An increasing average of the age of the victims of serious trauma is common in Western countries studies [20].

The high mortality of our study needs to be discussed. Less than half of trauma patients have been admitted to level one or two hospitals and this percentage was further reduced in patients older than 64. This is a common result in many epidemiologic studies. Ciesla et al. [21] observed that access to a designated trauma centre was dependent on proximity for severely injured elderly, while distance from trauma centre did not limit admissions for children and adults. Hsia et al. [22] demonstrated that the odds of admission to a trauma centre decreased with increasing age.

In Lombardia the percentage of hospital deaths has been higher in non level one or two hospitals: the lack of local expertise, reduced technology as well as unavailability of specialists are recognized causes of increased trauma mortality. At the time of the study a regionalized trauma system did not exist, triage protocols for centralization of severely injured were not uniformly applied and a formal hospital trauma team organization was active only in one hospital of the region. Moreover, severely injured older than 64 were the 46% of study population,

with the highest hospital death rate (from 25% to 46%). All these considerations may explain why the mortality presented in this Italian study is higher than other reports [23]. During the late 2012 a new law has formally instituted in Lombardia the regional trauma system. Now, efforts are needed to determine trauma resources and triage protocols and this study may be helpful to this project.

A special consideration is due to the severe trauma in the elderly, in terms of amount of resources expended with regard to the level of functional recovery. Recently, Grossman et al. [24] demonstrated an appreciable acute survival (66% or 69%, with or without brain injury) for geriatric trauma patients (>64) admitted to a level one trauma centre with an ISS > 29. Moreover, a good long term recovery has been observed in 67%. The prolonged life expectancy and active life style of many elderly, the increasing number of severe trauma after 64 years, together with promising results of modern trauma care, suggest the use of significant resources also in geriatric trauma, although with specific protocols to avoid futility.

Causes of trauma

Evaluating the causes of trauma, a precise definition in our study has been possible only in half of cases: in 21.27% the datum has been missed (i.e. not indicated on hospital report) while in 30% the category "other mechanism" has been assigned. Nevertheless, it is possible to

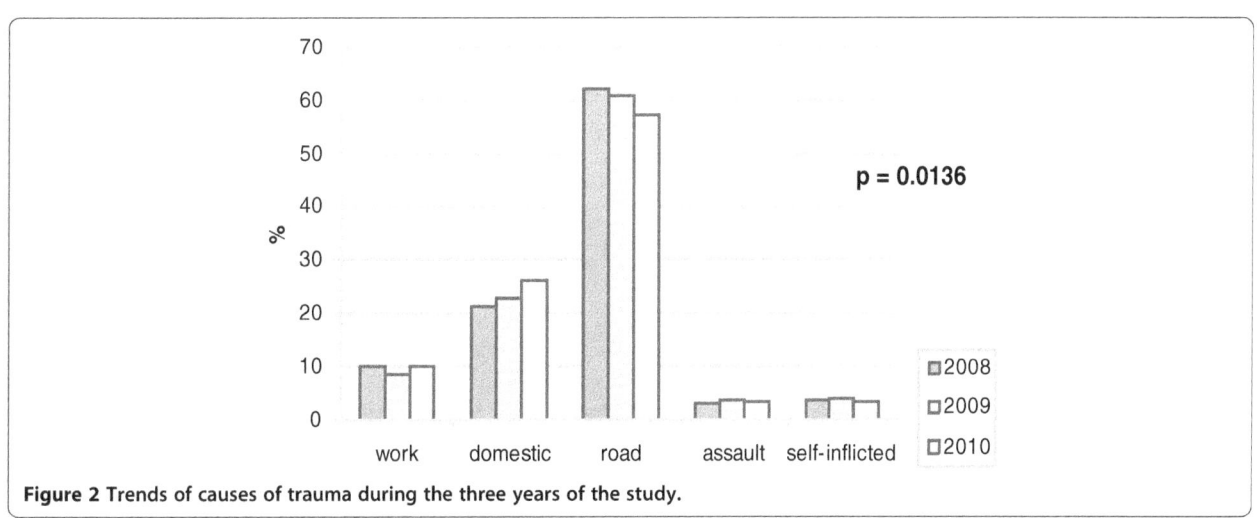

Figure 2 Trends of causes of trauma during the three years of the study.

make some observation in more than five thousands of cases for whom cause of trauma was precise and available. Young-adult males have been more exposed to road related accidents, while females in old age have been principally victims of unintentional domestic injuries. These results are consistent with other epidemiologic surveys [25-27]. Moreover, the age of injured females has been higher for all causes of injury and the same has been also observed in fatal trauma. Because trauma mortality increased with age, this might explain why in Lombardia trauma mortality in women has been globally higher than in men.

Another important observation is the trend of causes of trauma during the three years of the study. The 17.76% decrease in road-related injuries demonstrates that primary and secondary prevention programs for car, motorcycle, pedestrian, cycling accidents have obtained appreciable results. On the contrary many efforts need to be made for trauma prevention in houses, particularly of falls in old women living at home. The design of a new Trauma System must take into account these data: the new challenge will be the need to treat an increasing number of serious injuries in elderly people, with all the problems of concomitant illnesses, complications, prolonged ICU and hospital LOS, increased costs of healthcare and need of complex rehabilitation programs for the social reinstatement. On the other hand, pediatric cases are less than 200 per year in ten millions inhabitants and injured children need to be centralized in few highly specialised centres.

The low number of trauma due to violence underlines a significant difference in trauma epidemiology between Europe and overseas Countries. In Lombardia only 2.06% of serious trauma (where the cause has been formally indicated) were consequence of assaults (both penetrating or blunt) and this amount is sharply lower than North America [28]. However, media reports of stabbing and shootings and anecdotal evidence based on presentations to the emergency departments support the idea that interpersonal violence is on the rise, particularly between immigrates from Asia and Africa, as also observed in other countries [29].

Finally time distribution of hospital trauma deaths demonstrated that acute and early deaths regarded principally road-related injuries, trauma at workplace and assaults or self-inflicted violence. On the contrary, late deaths increased in victims of domestic trauma. Differences in age between victims with acute-early deaths and victims of late deaths suggest that young patients demise has been related in the acute – early phase to the severity of injuries, while elderly people died principally for related complications [30]. These observations are consistent with the results obtained also in the national trauma deaths study [8].

A late mortality close to 40%, mostly related to domestic trauma in elderly, is a substantial change and may impact significantly costs of trauma care. Notwithstanding the highest mortality, a reduced rate of ICU admission has been observed in patients older than 74. Although the datum was not available, this may suggest use of resources weighted on functional recovery possibilities. Again, this observation outlines the need of further studies to define protocols of care in this category of patients.

Funding of trauma system
In Italy, as in many other Countries, public or private hospitals are reimbursed using the DRG system. Data of Lombardia showed that the average amount paid to hospitals for seriously injured patients has been € 13,759.82 per patient. Trauma Systems in Europe demonstrate a significant country-by-country variation of costs, which is in part explained by the level of economic resources available for trauma care [31]. Iapichino et al. demonstrated [32] in a prospective Italian cohort study that variable costs of ICU for poly-trauma amounted € 4,423 per patient. In the UK [33], Sikand et al. examined hospital costs in poly-trauma patients, indicating a cost for the initial hospital LOS of € 20,408 per patient. Morris et al. [34]. In an international clinical trial about blunt trauma reported an average cost of 37,914 for initial hospital care. In general, ICU stay accounted for the majority of costs and other significant resource use included transfusion requirements and surgical procedures. Moreover, fixed costs of emergency care hospitals, rescue management and rehabilitation of trauma victims consume healthcare resources considerably. These data suggest that average reimbursement based on DRG for serious injuries which has been paid in Lombardia has been largely insufficient. Determining the cost-effectiveness of trauma interventions requires accurate data on the fixed and variable costs and outcome for trauma victims. This process is fundamental in the design of regionalized Trauma System where major trauma patients are concentrated in few specialised hospitals capable of high quality definitive care which need to be adequately budgeted for trauma capacity.

Strengths and limitations
The strength of this study was the use of a sample that is representative of all claims for a serious injury in a given Region, obtained from a population-based source at the individual level, coupled with demographics and causes of injuries. These data were used to analyse the incidence rates, mortality, type of accidents across different age groups, for men and women, with different patterns emerging for various population groups. The weakness of the study may be the quality of the sanitary data, with the limit that serious injuries number may be only indirectly

derived and not calculated from a specific anatomic score. However, the incidence rates of serious injury which have been derived in this study are comparable with those calculated in another Italian study using trauma registry and this represents a confirmation of the reliability of data extraction.

Conclusions

This study, although with an indirect evaluation of patient severity, has demonstrated that seriously injured who need hospital admission in Lombardia still represent a consistent healthcare problem. Road-related injuries in young-adult males are the principal causes of severe trauma, with a significant acute and early mortality, but there is a tendency toward the increase of elderly people, particularly females, who are exposed to serious domestic trauma, characterised by an elevated late mortality.

These results may be useful for the planning of a new regionalised Trauma System, adequately designed on epidemiologic evidences.

Competing interests
The authors declared that they have no competing interests.

Authors' contributions
OC and SC carried out the study design, CM and SL performed statistical analysis, AM retrieved the data. All authors read and approved the final manuscript.

Acknowledgements
This study was funded by the "Centro Studi Libera Orlandi", granted to one of the authors (AM). The authors are grateful to Ing. Carlo Zocchetti (General Direction of Health of the Regional Government of Lombardia) who allowed the consultation of the regional hospital discharge registry.

Author details
[1]Trauma Team Dip. DEA-EAS, Ospedale Niguarda Ca'Granda, Piazza Ospedale Maggiore 3, 20162, Milan, Italy. [2]Quality Department, Ospedale Niguarda Ca'Granda Milan, Milan, Italy. [3]Universita' di Milano, Dip, Scienze cliniche Luigi Sacco, Milan, Italy.

References
1. Celso B, Tepas J, Langland-Orban B, Pracht E, Papa L, Lottenberg L, et al: A systematic review and meta-analysis comparing outcome of severely injured patients treated in trauma centers following the establishment of trauma systems. J Trauma 2006, 60:371–378.
2. MacKenzie EJ, Rivara FP, Jurkovich GJ, Nathens AB, Frey KP, Egleston BL, et al: A national evaluation of the effect of trauma center care on mortality. N Eng J Med 2006, 354:366–378.
3. Moore EE: Trauma systems, trauma centers and trauma surgeons: opportunity in managed competition. J Trauma 1995, 39:1–11.
4. Stephenson SC, Langley JD, Civil ID: Comparing measures of injury severity for use with large databases. J Trauma 2002, 53:326–332.
5. Reilly JJ, Chin B, Berkowitz J, Weedon J, Avitable M: Use of a state-wide administrative database in assessing a national trauma system: the New York City experience. J Am Coll Surg 2004, 198:509–518.
6. Chiara O, Cimbanassi S, Pitidis A, Vesconi S: Preventable trauma deaths: from panel review to population-based studies. World J Em Surg 2006, 1:1–7.
7. Creamer GL, Civil I, Koelmeyer T, Adams D, Cacala S, Thompson J: Population-based study of age and causes of severe injury in Auckland, 2004. ANZ J Surg 2008, 78:995–998.
8. Chiara O, Pitidis A, Lispi L, Buzzone S, Ceccolini C, Cacciatore P, et al: Epidemiology of fatal trauma in Italy in 2002 using population-based registries. Eur J Trauma Emerg Surg 2010, 36:157–163.
9. Seow-Yian T, Sloan EP, Zun L, Zaret P: Comparison of the new injury severity score and the injury severity score. J Trauma 2004, 56:162–164.
10. Osler T, Rutledge R, Deis J, Bedrick E: An international classification of disease –9 based injury severity score. J Trauma 1996, 41:380–388.
11. Moore L, Clark DE: The value of trauma registries. Injury 2008, 39:686–695.
12. Stephenson S, Henley G, Harrison JE, Langley JD: Diagnosis based injury severity scaling: investigation of a method using Australian and New Zealand hospitalisations. Inj Prev 2004, 10:379–383.
13. Di Bartolomeo S, Sanson G, Michelutto V, Nardi G, Burba I, Francescutti C, et al: Epidemiology of major injury in the population of Friuli Venezia Giulia – Italy. Injury 2004, 35:391–400.
14. Gorman DF, Teanby DN, Sinha MP, et al: The epidemiology of major injuries in Mersey Region and North Wales. Injury 1995, 26:51–54.
15. McNicholl B, Cooke RS: The epidemiology of major trauma in Northern Ireland. Ulster Med J 1995, 64:142–146.
16. Newgard CD, Schmicker RH, Sopko G, Andrusiek D, Bialkowski W, Minei JP, et al: Trauma in the neighborhood: a geospatial analysis and assessment of social determinants of major injury in North America. Am J Public Health 2011, 101:669–677.
17. Cothren CC, Moore EE, Hedegaard HB, Meng K: Epidemiology of urban trauma deaths: a comprehensive reassessment 10 years later. World J Surg 2007, 31:1507–1511.
18. Chiara O, Cimbanassi S, Andreani S, Girotti P, Pizzilli G, Vesconi S: Niguarda trauma team: outcome of three years of activity. Minerva Anestesiol 2008, 74:11–15.
19. Creamer GL, Civil I, Koelmeyer T, Adams D, Cacala S, Thompson J: Ethnicity of severe trauma patients: results of a population-based study, Auckland, New Zealand. NZ Med J 2010, 123(1316):26–32.
20. Boland M, Staines A, Fizpatrick P, Scallan E: Urban–rural variation in mortality and hospital admission rates for unintentional injury in Ireland. Inj Prev 2005, 11:38–42.
21. Ciesla DJ, Tepas JJ, Pracht EE, Langland-Orban B, Cha JY, Flint LM: Fifteen year trauma system performance analysis demonstrates optimal coverage for most severely injured patients and identifies a vulnerable population. J Am Coll Surg 2013, 216:687–695.
22. Hsia RY, Wang E, Saynina O, Wise P, Perez-Stable EJ, Auerbach A: Factor associated with trauma center use for elderly patients with trauma: a statewide analysis 1999–2008. Arch Surg 2011, 146:585–592.
23. Dutton RP, Stansbury LG, Leone S, Kraimer E, Hass JR, Scalea TM: Trauma mortality in a mature system: are we doing better? An analysis of trauma mortality patterns, 1997–2008. J Trauma 2010, 69:620–626.
24. Grossman MD, Ofurum U, Stehly CD, Stoltzfus J: Long term survival after major trauma in geriatric trauma patients: the glass is half full. J Trauma Acute Care 2012, 72:1181–1185.
25. Peel NM, Kassulke DJ, McClure RJ: Population-based study of hospitalised fall related injuries in older people. Inj Prev 2002, 8:280–283.
26. Bergland A, Wyller TB: Risk factors for serious fall related injury in elderly women living at home. Inj Prev 2004, 10:248–251.
27. Stevens JA, Sogolow ED: Gender differences for non fatal unintentional fall related injuries among older adults. Inj Prev 2005, 11:115–119.
28. Demetriades D, Murray J, Sinz B, Myles D, Chan L: Epidemiology of major trauma and trauma deaths in Los Angeles county. J Am Coll Surg 1998, 187:373–383.
29. O'Mullane PA, Mikocka-Walus AA, Gabbe BJ, Cameron PA: Incidence and outcomes of major assaults: a population-based study in Victoria. MJA 2009, 190:129–132.
30. McGwin GL, McLennan PA, Fife JB, Davis GG, Rue LW: Pre-existing conditions and mortality in older trauma patients. J Trauma 2004, 56:1291–1296.
31. Pape HC, Neugebauer E, Ridley SA, Chiara O, Nielsen TG, Christensen MC: Cost-drivers in acute treatment of severe trauma in Europe: a systematic review of literature. Eur J Trauma Emerg Surg 2009, 35:61–66.
32. Iapichino G, Raddrizzani F, Simini B, Rossi C, Albicini M, Ferla L, et al: Effectiveness and efficiency of intensive care medicine: variable costs in different diagnosis groups. Acta Anaestesiol Scand 2004, 48:820–826.

8

TEG® and ROTEM® in trauma: similar test but different results?

Ajith Sankarankutty[1,2], Bartolomeu Nascimento[2], Luis Teodoro da Luz[2], Sandro Rizoli[3*]

From World Trauma Congress 2012
Rio de Janeiro, Brazil. 22-25 August 2012

Abstract

Introduction: Transfusion in trauma is often empiric or based on traditional lab tests. Viscoelastic tests such as thromboelastography (TEG®) and rotational thromboelastometry (ROTEM®) have been proposed as superior to traditional lab tests. Due to the similarities between the two tests, general opinion seems to consider them equivalent with interchangeable interpretations. However, it is not clear whether the results can be similarly interpreted. This review evaluates the comparability between TEG and ROTEM and performs a descriptive review of the parameters utilized in each test in adult trauma patients.

Methods: PUBMED database was reviewed using the keywords "thromboelastography" and "compare", between 2000 and 2011. Original studies directly comparing TEG® with ROTEM® in any area were retrieved. To verify the individual test parameter used in studies involving trauma patients, we further performed a review using the keywords "thromboelastography" and "trauma" in the PUBMED database.

Results: Only 4 studies directly compared TEG® with ROTEM®. One in liver transplantation found that transfusion practice could differ depending on the device in use. Another in cardiac surgery concluded that all measurements are not completely interchangeable. The third article using commercially available plasma detected clinically significant differences in the results from the two devices. The fourth one was a head-to-head comparison of the technical aspects. The 24 articles reporting the use of viscoelastic tests in trauma patients, presented considerable heterogeneity.

Conclusion: Both tests are potentially useful as means to rapidly diagnose coagulopathy, guide transfusion and determine outcome in trauma patients. Differences in the activators utilized in each device limit the direct comparability. Standardization and robust clinical trials comparing the two technologies are needed before these tests can be widely recommended for clinical use in trauma.

Introduction

Coagulation is a complex, dynamic, highly regulated and interwoven process involving a myriad of cells, molecules and structures. Only recently, the unique changes in coagulation caused by trauma are starting to be understood, but remain mostly unknown [1,2]. Trauma patients are among the largest consumers of blood and blood products and the decision of what, when and how much blood and blood product to transfuse is often empiric or based on traditional coagulation lab tests such as INR/PT, PTT and platelet count. However, traditional lab tests have been heavily criticized for their limitations in assisting the physicians with the clinical decision to transfuse, and alternatives are warranted.

The traditional laboratorial evaluation of coagulation evolved initially to quantify specific cellular, molecular or factor deficiencies. Numeric values (quantity) of individual elements do not necessarily indicate how well hemostasis is functioning. As an example, a cirrhotic patient with low platelet count and an abnormal INR of 2 does not necessarily bleed and probably can tolerate minor invasive procedures. In contrast, a hypothermic

* Correspondence: Sandro.Rizoli@sunnybrook.ca
[3]Departments of Surgery and Critical Care Medicine, Sunnybrook Health Sciences Centre, University of Toronto, Canada

trauma patient with normal platelet count and INR might bleed to death [3,4]. Another limitation of traditional lab tests is the prolonged time to obtain the results or turnaround time. Dealing with rapid changes as frequently occurs in massively bleeding trauma patients, is challenging. In such situations, any delay in obtaining the lab results can lead to inadequate transfusion and increased morbidity and mortality [4]. Thus in trauma, global, functional and immediately available laboratorial evaluation of hemostasis can improve both patient management and outcome.

Viscoelastic tests such as thromboelastography (TEG®) and rotational thromboelastometry (ROTEM®) have been enthusiastically proposed by some, as superior compared to traditional lab tests. Both tests can be performed as point of care, and the faster availability of results may assist clinical decisions of what, when and how much blood and products to transfuse [5-7]. Other advantages of viscoelastic tests include their ability to provide a global and functional assessment of coagulation, which may prove superior to quantitative tests that evaluate segments of the hemostasis. A recent systematic review on massive transfusions concluded that despite an apparent association with bleeding reduction, the use of TEG® or ROTEM® to guide blood transfusion remains uncertain [8].

The interest in TEG® and ROTEM® in trauma is recent and the topic lacks large numbers of studies. However, the available evidence suggests that TEG® and ROTEM® could have important roles in trauma in 3 ways: by promptly diagnosing early trauma coagulopathy (diagnostic tools); guiding blood transfusion and revealing patients' prognosis. The two tests have the same foundational principles and share many similarities, from hardware (equipment) and procedures (technique) to tracing (graph) and parameters. Figure 1 merges the tracings obtained from both tests and Table 1 shows the parameters from each test and their normal values.

The preference for which viscoelastic tests to use appears to reside primarily on geography, with centers in North America favouring TEG® while Europeans prefer ROTEM®. Overall, the prevalent opinion is that the two tests are equivalent with interchangeable results and interpretations. It is curious to note however, that treatment recommendations seem to vary according to which test it is based on. Transfusion algorithms based on ROTEM® appear to frequently recommend fibrinogen [9] while TEG®-based algorithms appear to recommend plasma [7]. It is not clear whether the results from these two apparently related tests are interchangeable and can be similarly interpreted. Considering the growing importance of TEG® and ROTEM® in trauma, attested by the growing number of viscoelastic test based algorithms and trauma centers adopting them as

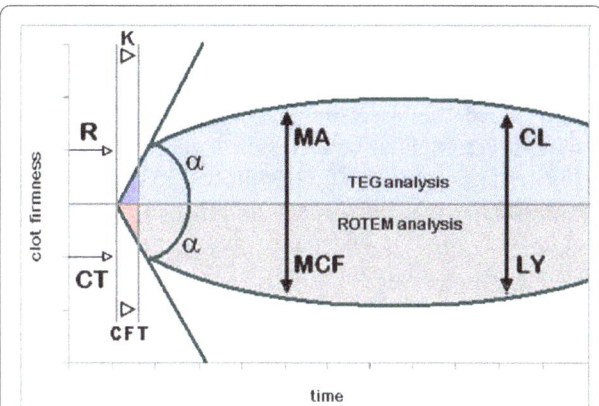

Figure 1 TEG® and ROTEM® tracing TEG® parameters: R – reaction time; k – kinetics; ∝ - alpha angle; MA – maximum amplitude; CL – clot lysis. ROTEM® parameters: CT – clotting time; CFT – clot formation time; ∝ - alpha angle; MCF – maximum clot firmness; LY – clot lysis.

standard of care, we proposed a literature review on the topic. The goal is to appraise the evidence on the comparability between TEG® and ROTEM® as well as to perform a descriptive review of the parameters used in each test, in the setting of adult trauma patients.

Table 1 TEG® and ROTEM® parameters and their reference values (adapted from Luddington 2005, and Ganter MT, Hofer CK 2008).

	TEG®	ROTEM®
Clotting time (time to 2mm amplitude)	r (reaction time) WB: 4-8min Cit, kaolin : 3-8min	CT (clotting time) Cit, EXTEM: 42-74s Cit, INTEM: 137-246s
Clot kinetics (time from 2 to 20mm)	k (kinetics) WB: 1-4min Cit, kaolin: 1-3min	CFT (clot formation time) Cit, EXTEM: 46-148s Cit, INTEM: 40-100s
Alpha angle	α (slope between r and k) WB: 47°-74° Cit, kaolin: 55°-78°	α (slope of tangent at 2mm amplitude) Cit, EXTEM: 63°-81° Cit, INTEM: 71°-82°
Amplitude (at a fixed time)	A (A30, A60)	A (A10, A15, A20, A25, A30)
Maximum strenght	MA (maximum amplitude) WB:55-73mm Cit, kaolin: 51-69	MCF (maximum clot firmness) Cit, EXTEM: 49-71mm Cit, INTEM: 52-72mm Cit, FIBTEM: 9 -25mm
Lysis (at a fixed time)	CL30, CL60	CLY30, CLY60: 94 – 100%
Maximum lysis		ML : <15%

TEG® parameters: R – reaction time; k – kinetics; ∝ - alpha angle; MA – maximum amplitude; CL – clot lysis.
ROTEM® parameters: CT – clotting time; CFT – clot formation time; ∝ - alpha angle;
MCF – maximum clot firmness; LY – clot lysis.
WB – whole blood; Cit – citrated blood.

Methods

We performed a review of the literature searching PUBMED database using the keywords "thromboelastography" and "comparison", between 2000 and 2011. Studies were eligible for inclusion if they were original and directly compared TEG® with ROTEM®. In view of the possibility that only a small number of such studies would be found, we decided to perform an additional analysis. All studies on either TEG® or ROTEM® in trauma were included and each individual test parameter was scrutinized on its role in diagnosing early coagulopathy, guiding transfusion and indicating prognosis. Then the role of similar test parameters from TEG® and ROTEM® was compared aiming to identify whether they were comparable. For this additional analysis the review used the keywords "thromboelastography" and "trauma" in the PUBMED database. Studies were excluded if they were experimental or consisted of case reports. All full-text versions of the studies were retrieved and duplicate studies were excluded.

In this review (see Table 1), the viscoelastic test parameters will be referred to as r/CT, when referring to the initiation of the clotting process of both tests or as r when specifically referring to TEG® or CT when specifically referring to ROTEM®. Similarly, k/CFT will refer to amplification of the clotting process, MA/MCF to the maximal clot firmness and CL/LI to fibrinolysis, in TEG® and ROTEM® respectively. Alpha is similar in both tests (∝).

Results

Direct comparison of TEG® and ROTEM®

The literature search identified 191 studies, of which only 4 directly compared TEG® with ROTEM® and none were done in trauma. The two clinical studies were in liver transplantation and in cardiac surgery, another was an experiment using commercially available plasma and the last was a head-to-head comparison of the technical aspects, ease of use and costs [7,10-12]. Thus no study directly comparing TEG® with ROTEM® in trauma was identified. Due to the paucity of comparisons, we considered them individually.

The first clinical study by Coakley et al. compared transfusion triggers using TEG®, ROTEM® (INTEM® and FIBTEM®) and traditional coagulation tests (PT, platelet count and Clauss fibrinogen) during liver transplantation [7]. This prospective observational study showed a good correlation between TEG® MA and ROTEM® MCF and they shared moderate agreement in guiding platelet or fibrinogen transfusion. The study concluded that transfusion could differ depending on which device is used.

The second clinical study by Venema et al. compared r/CT, k/CFT, MA/MCF and the ∝ angle during cardiac surgery [10]. This study suggested that TEG® MA and

ROTEM® ∝ angle could be used interchangeably but the other parameters are not fully interchangeable.

The third study by Nielsen compared the reaction time, ∝ angle, maximal amplitude and maximal elastic modulus between the two devices using native plasma, celite-activated normal plasma as well as celite-activated hypo and hypercoagulable plasma [11]. All TEG® ROTEM® parameters were significantly different in native plasma, while in celite-activated samples most were comparable. The study concluded that the significant differences in measurements from the two devices could be attenuated with celite activation.

The head-to-head comparison of the two devices by Jackson et al., took into consideration operational aspects including installation requirements, warm-up time, pipettes, material required, reference ranges, costs and opinion of the lab staff [12]. This study consisted of a simple subjective assessment of the advantages and disadvantages of both devices.

Additional analysis of individual parameters from TEG® and ROTEM® in trauma

The additional PUBMED search identified 24 manuscripts, of which TEG® was tested in 10, rapid-TEG in 6 and ROTEM® in 9. Two studies compared TEG® with rapid-TEG®. No randomized controlled trial was found, 16 manuscripts analyzed data prospectively collected, 6 were retrospective and 2 were "before and after" studies. The techniques used to perform TEG® and ROTEM® in these 24 studies were noticeably heterogeneous. Different activators were used and different parameters evaluated making general comparisons difficult. Table 2 summarizes the main findings of the 24 manuscripts reviewed according to the test parameters evaluated and whether TEG® or ROTEM® were used to diagnose early coagulopathy, guide transfusion or indicate prognosis.

Results of 12 studies on the use of TEG® or ROTEM® as diagnostics tools

Among the studies on TEG® Schreiber et al reported a correlation between r and PTT, and between MA and platelet count [13]. While Plotkin et al found a similar correlation between MA and platelet [14], Jeger et al found that k, ∝ angle and MA correlated with platelet levels and INR [15]. Park et al found no correlation between either ∝ angle or MA to PT and PTT [16] while Cotton et al (using Rapid TEG) reported a correlation between ∝ angle and MA with platelet, PT and PTT. In this study G was failed to correlate with any traditional lab tests [17].

Johansson et al reported that all the TEG® parameters improved after the administration of predefined transfusion packages [18]. Watters et al reported that MA parameters were higher in patients after splenectomy

Table 2 The results and correlation of TEG® and ROTEM® parameters in each study for diagnosis, transfusion guidance and prognosis

Diagnosis

TEG®	Test	Study	r /ACT	k	α	A	MA	CL	G	Comments
	TEG®	Schreiber (2005)	PTT				Platelet			
		Johansson (2008b)								r, k, α, MA and G improved after Tx packages
		Plotkin (2008)					Platelet			
		Park (2009)			NO correlation to PT/PTT		NO correlation to PT/PTT			
		Watters (2010)								MA significantly higher post-splenectomy
	TEG®-PM	Nekludov (2007)								Reduced platelet response to AA in bleeders
	Rapid-TEG®	Jeger (2009)	Platelet/INR		Platelet/INR		Platelet/INR			
		Cotton (2011)	PT/PTT	PT/PTT	PT/PTT/ platelet		PT/PTT/ platelet		No correlation	

ROTEM®	Test	Study	CT	CFT	α	CA	MCF	CLI	ML	
	EXTEM®	Rugeri (2006)				PT (CA15)				
		Levrat (2008)				ELT (CA10)	ELT	ELT (CLI60)		
		Davenport (2011a)								CT, CA, MCF improves after Tx
		Davenport (2011b)								CA5 diagnosis coagulopathy
	INTEM®	Rugeri (2006)		PTT		PTT / Platelet (CA15)				
	FIBTEM®	Rugeri (2006)				Fibrinogen (CA10)				

Transfusion Guidance

TEG®	Test	Study	r / ACT	k	α	A	MA	CL	G	Comments
	Rapid-TEG®	Kashuk (2009)	Could reduces FFP Tx							

ROTEM®	Test	Study	CT	CFT	α	CA	MCF	CLI	ML	
	EXTEM®	Schochl (2011)								ROTEM guided FC/PCC reduces RBC and platelet Tx
	FIBTEM®	Schochl (2011)								ROTEM guided FC/PCC reduces RBC and platelet Tx

TEG®	Test	Study	r / ACT	k	α	A	MA	CL	G	Comments
	TEG®	Plotkin (2008)					Increased Tx			
		Park (2008)					Mortality			
		Johansson (2008a)								TEG guided Tx reduced mortality
		Carroll (2009)	Mortality				Mortality			
	TEG®-PM	Carroll (2009)								Significantly correlated to Tx

Table 2 The results and correlation of TEG®?®? and ROTEM®?®? parameters in each study for diagnosis, transfusion guidance and prognosis *(Continued)*

			CT	CFT	α	CA	MCF	CLI	ML
Rapid-TEG®	Kashuk (2010)							Mortality	
	Kashuk (2012)						Mortality	Mortality	
	Pezold (2012)								Massive Tx; Mortality
ROTEM®	Test	Study	CT	CFT	α	CA	MCF	CLI	ML
	EXTEM®	Schochl (2009)							Mortality
		Doran (2010)					Increased Tx		
		Schochl (2010)							ROTEM guided Tx reduces mortality
	INTEM®	Leemann (2010)					Increased Tx		

Abbreviations: r, k, α and MA – TEG® parameters; CT,CFT, α, MCF, CA₁₀, CA₁₅, CL₃₀-CL₆₀ – ROTEM® parameters; ACT – activated clotting time; ELT – euglobulin lysis time; FFP – fresh frozen plasma; G – maximal elastic modulus (d/sc); PC – platelet concentrate; PCC – prothrombin complex concentrate; Tx – transfusion

[19]. Using the platelet mapping sequence in the TEG®, Nekludov found that bleeding patients have reduced platelet response to arachdonic acid [20].

In ROTEM® studies Rugeri found that CA15-EXTEM® correlated with PT, CA15-INTEM® with platelets and PTT, and CA10-FIBTEM® with fibrinogen [21]. Levrat *et al* noted that in EXTEM® CA10, MCF and CLI60 correlated well with the euglobulin lysis time, which they used as the gold standard to detect fibrinolysis [22]. Davenport *et al* reported that CA5 could be an early indicator of coagulopathy in trauma and CT, CA and MCF improved after transfusion [23,24].

In summary, the single apparent similarity between TEG® and ROTEM® parameters when used to diagnose coagulopathy in trauma is between TEG® MA and ROTEM® MCF and their similar association to platelet count and PTT.

Results of the 2 studies on the use of TEG® and ROTEM® in guiding transfusion in trauma

In a retrospective study, Kashuk *et al* suggested that using TEG® parameters such as r to guide transfusion may lead to a reduction in plasma transfusion [25]. Schochl *et al* reported that ROTEM®-based protocols are useful to guide transfusion of fibrinogen concentrates and prothrombin complex that in turn reduce the need for transfusion of red blood cells and platelets [26]. As summarized in Table 2, no similarity between TEG® and ROTEM® can be made from these studies.

Results of the 11 studies on the use of TEG® and ROTEM® and outcome in trauma

Plotkin *et al* in a retrospective study on TEG® reported that low MA correlated with increased transfusion requirement [14]. For ROTEM®, 2 studies by Leeman *et al and* Doran *et al* reported the same finding with MCF (INTEM®), the later study also showed that reduced MCF (EXTEM®) is useful to guide transfusion [27,28].

Park developed a prognostic scoring system for trauma patients using inflammatory and coagulation parameters, in which of all TEG® parameters only MA was an independent predictor of mortality [29]. Carroll also detected a significant correlation between TEG® platelet mapping and transfusion requirements, and a correlation between r and MA values with mortality [30]. Kashuk in both a "before and after" and a prospective observational study found that TEG® G values were associated with survival [31]. Similarly Pezold in a retrospective TEG® study found that low G values were associated with both increased transfusion requirements and mortality [32]. Both, Johansson ("before and after" TEG® study) and Schochl (ROTEM® retrospective study) suggested that viscoelastic tests guided transfusion reduced mortality [5,9]. Schochl also reported that hyperfibrinolysis, detected by ROTEM® ML correlated with higher mortality and this parameter could be used to classify the degree of severity of the fibrinolysis [33]. In 2010 Kashuk et al found that abnormal primary lysis detected by elevated CL (similar to ROTEM® ML) is also associated with mortality [31].

As summarized on Table 2, these 11 studies showed that some TEG® and ROTEM® parameters are similarly associated with outcomes in trauma. TEG® MA and ROTEM® MCF are associated with both the need for blood transfusion and mortality, while excessive fibrinolysis diagnosed by either TEG® CL or ROTEM® ML are independent predictors of mortality.

Discussion

A few deductions can be promptly reached from reviewing the literature on these two viscoelastic tests. First that there is a lot of enthusiasm supporting their clinical application in trauma. The literature suggests that both tests are already being used in many institutions, which could be in a wider scale than suggested by the limited number of publications. The wide clinical application of any technology without supporting evidence and scientific validation is worrisome and more investigations on these tests are urgently needed and warranted.

Another plausible conclusion from this review is that the prevalent notion that the two tests are equivalent with interchangeable results and interpretations may be unfounded. While there are insufficient studies to support any conclusions on the topic, the current evidence indicates only a small number of similarities between the tests. Concerning their diagnostic capacity, the similarities found were limited to TEG® MA and ROTEM® MCF and their similar association with platelet count and PTT. Another apparent similarity was of TEG® CL and ROTEM® ML in diagnosing excessive fibrinolysis and mortality (prognosis). Prognostication was where these tests showed more similarities. TEG® MA and ROTEM MCF® were also linked to the need for blood transfusion and mortality. The few studies on TEG®- or ROTEM®-based transfusion algorithms suggested that while both tests can be used to construct transfusion guidelines, the blood products transfused differ according to the algorithm selected.

Even tough no study could be found directly comparing TEG® and ROTEM® in trauma; two studies have compared the 2 tests in transplant and cardiac surgery. Coakley *et al.*, in the liver transplant study concluded that transfusion practice could differ depending on the viscoelastic coagulation-monitoring device in use. Venema *et al.*, verified that kaolin-activated TEG® measurements correlated with those of EXTEM®, but not all the measurements of the two devices are interchangeable. These findings seem to support the concept that despite similarities, interchangeable interpretation is not recommended without further studies and standardizations.

Despite being used for a number of years, the recent wider adoption and transfer of the technology to the hemostasis laboratory has raised some concerns regarding these techniques. Among the concerns pointed out in the literature are the effect of age [34-37], gender [38], use of citrated blood sample [39], sampling site, stability and repeated sampling [40-43] on the results observed. A number of activators and inhibitors are commonly used resulting in varied specificity of the assay [44]. Different methods of data analysis have also been suggested [45]. In an interesting article Jackson *et al* "road tested" both

TEG® and ROTEM® and summarized their finding regarding technical features, costs and pooled the opinion of the direct users [12]. The reproducibility of both TEG® and ROTEM® measurements has been reported as acceptable [46].

A recent systematic review of randomized clinical trials comparing TEG®- or ROTEM®-based algorithms with standard treatment in non-trauma bleeding patients found that the current evidence supporting viscoelastic tests is weak [4]. This systematic review found only 9 randomized controlled trials, 8 in cardiac surgery and 1 in liver transplantation. Possibly the greatest contribution of the viscoelastic tests is in the detection of hyperfibrinolysis, which no other test can diagnose as expeditiously.

Interestingly, Nielsen pointed out in his study that TEG® and ROTEM® could potentially generate similar data, provided similar activators were utilized in both devices. This observation highlights the need for standardization if the tests are to be comparable. Meanwhile, caution must be exercised in utilizing treatment algorithms based on one system while analyzing patient samples from the other, or even the same system but using different activators.

In conclusion, TEG® and ROTEM® have many of the characteristics of ideal tests for use in trauma including global evaluation of coagulation, both quantitative and functional assessment, *in vitro* assays performed under conditions of "no flow". Their potential clinical utility must be balanced against limitations particularly the considerable heterogeneity in methods, reagents and parameters evaluated. The present literature review suggests that in trauma TEG® and ROTEM® are not fully equivalent tests with interchangeable results and interpretations but as pointed out by Nielsen, this could be the results of using different activators (methods). The similarities identified were limited to TEG® MA and ROTEM® MCF measurements and their association with platelet counts and PTT. Other similarities were between TEG® CL and ROTEM® ML in diagnosing excessive fibrinolysis and mortality and TEG® MA and ROTEM® MCF association with blood transfusion and mortality.

Despite their limitations, both tests are attractive and potentially useful as means to rapidly diagnose coagulopathy, guide transfusion and determine outcome of adult trauma patients. However, standardization and robust clinical trials comparing the two technologies are needed before these promising tests can be widely recommended for clinical use in trauma.

Acknowledgements

This article has been published as part of *World Journal of Emergency Surgery* Volume 7 Supplement 1, 2012: Proceedings of the World Trauma Congress

2012. The full contents of the supplement are available online at http://www.wjes.org/supplements/7/S1.

Author details
[1]Faculdade de Medicina de Ribeirão Preto, Universidade de São Paulo, Brazil. [2]Trauma Program, Sunnybrook Health Sciences Centre, University of Toronto, Canada. [3]Departments of Surgery and Critical Care Medicine, Sunnybrook Health Sciences Centre, University of Toronto, Canada.

Authors' contributions
Literature review and drafting the manuscript : AS, LTdL, BN
Drafting the manuscript and critical review: SR

Competing interests
SR had a Canadian Institutes of Health Research (CIHR) award in partnership with NovoNordisk the manufacturer of recombinant factor VIIa.
The other authors declare that they have no competing interests.

References
1. Brohi K, Singh J, Heron M, et al: Acute traumatic coagulopathy. J Trauma 2003, 54(6):1127-1130.
2. Rizoli SB, Scarpelini S, Callum J, et al: Clotting factor deficiency in early trauma-associated coagulopathy. J Trauma 2011, 71(5 Suppl 1):S427-434.
3. O'Connor SD, Taylor AJ, Williams EC, et al: Coagulation concepts update. AJR Am J Roentgenol 2009, 193(6):1656-1664.
4. Wikkelsoe AJ, Afshari A, Wetterslev J, et al: Monitoring patients at risk of massive transfusion with Thrombelastography or Thromboelastometry: a systematic review. Acta Anaesthesiol Scand 2011, 55(10):1174-1189.
5. Johansson PI, Stensballe J: Effect of Haemostatic Control Resuscitation on mortality in massively bleeding patients: a before and after study. Vox Sang 2009, 96(2):111-118.
6. Kang YG, Martin DJ, Marquez J, et al: Intraoperative changes in blood coagulation and thrombelastographic monitoring in liver transplantation. Anesth Analg 1985, 64(9):888-896.
7. Coakley M, Reddy K, Mackie I, et al: Transfusion triggers in orthotopic liver transplantation: a comparison of the thromboelastometry analyzer, the thromboelastogram, and conventional coagulation tests. J Cardiothorac Vasc Anesth 2006, 20(4):548-553.
8. Afshari A, Wikkelsø A, Brok J, et al: Thrombelastography (TEG) or thromboelastometry (ROTEM) to monitor haemotherapy versus usual care in patients with massive transfusion. Cochrane Database Syst Rev 2011, , 3: CD007871.
9. Schöchl H, Nienaber U, Hofer G, et al: Goal-directed coagulation management of major trauma patients using thromboelastometry (ROTEM)-guided administration of fibrinogen concentrate and prothrombin complex concentrate. Crit Care 2010, 14(2):R55.
10. Venema LF, Post WJ, Hendriks HG, et al: An assessment of clinical interchangeability of TEG and RoTEM thromboelastographic variables in cardiac surgical patients. Anesth Analg 2010, 111(2):339-344.
11. Nielsen VG: A comparison of the Thrombelastograph and the ROTEM. Blood Coagul Fibrinolysis 2007, 18(3):247-252.
12. Jackson GN, Ashpole KJ, Yentis SM: The TEG vs the ROTEM thromboelastography/thromboelastometry systems. Anaesthesia 2009, 64(2):212-215.
13. Schreiber MA, Differding J, Thorborg P, et al: Hypercoagulability is most prevalent early after injury and in female patients. J Trauma 2005, 58(3):475-480, discussion 480-471.
14. Plotkin AJ, Wade CE, Jenkins DH, et al: A reduction in clot formation rate and strength assessed by thrombelastography is indicative of transfusion requirements in patients with penetrating injuries. J Trauma 2008, 64(2 Suppl):S64-68.
15. Jeger V, Zimmermann H, Exadaktylos AK: Can RapidTEG accelerate the search for coagulopathies in the patient with multiple injuries? J Trauma 2009, 66(4):1253-1257.
16. Park MS, Martini WZ, Dubick MA, et al: Thromboelastography as a better indicator of hypercoagulable state after injury than prothrombin time or activated partial thromboplastin time. J Trauma 2009, 67(2):266-275, discussion 275-266.

17. Cotton BA, Faz G, Hatch QM, et al: Rapid thrombelastography delivers real-time results that predict transfusion within 1 hour of admission. J Trauma 2011, 71(2):407-414, discussion 414-407.
18. Johansson PI, Bochsen L, Stensballe J, et al: Transfusion packages for massively bleeding patients: the effect on clot formation and stability as evaluated by Thrombelastograph (TEG). Transfus Apher Sci 2008, 39(1):3-8.
19. Watters JM, Sambasivan CN, Zink K, et al: Splenectomy leads to a persistent hypercoagulable state after trauma. Am J Surg 2010, 199(5):646-651.
20. Nekludov M, Bellander BM, Blombäck M, et al: Platelet dysfunction in patients with severe traumatic brain injury. J Neurotrauma 2007, 24(11):1699-1706.
21. Rugeri L, Levrat A, David JS, et al: Diagnosis of early coagulation abnormalities in trauma patients by rotation thrombelastography. J Thromb Haemost 2007, 5(2):289-295.
22. Levrat A, Gros A, Rugeri L, et al: Evaluation of rotation thrombelastography for the diagnosis of hyperfibrinolysis in trauma patients. Br J Anaesth 2008, 100(6):792-797.
23. Davenport R, Manson J, De'ath H, et al: Functional definition and characterization of acute traumatic coagulopathy. Crit Care Med 2011, 39:2652-2658.
24. Davenport R, Curry N, Manson J, et al: Hemostatic effects of fresh frozen plasma may be maximal at red cell ratios of 1:2. J Trauma 2011, 70(1):90-95, discussion 95-96.
25. Kashuk JL, Moore EE, Le T, et al: Noncitrated whole blood is optimal for evaluation of postinjury coagulopathy with point-of-care rapid thrombelastography. J Surg Res 2009, 156(1):133-138.
26. Schöchl H, Nienaber U, Maegele M, et al: Transfusion in trauma: thromboelastometry-guided coagulation factor concentrate-based therapy versus standard fresh frozen plasma-based therapy. Crit Care 2011, 15(2):R83.
27. Leemann H, Lustenberger T, Talving P, et al: The role of rotation thromboelastometry in early prediction of massive transfusion. J Trauma 2010, 69(6):1403-1408, discussion 1408-1409.
28. Doran CM, Woolley T, Midwinter MJ: Feasibility of using rotational thromboelastometry to assess coagulation status of combat casualties in a deployed setting. J Trauma 2010, 69(Suppl 1):S40-48.
29. Park MS, Salinas J, Wade CE, et al: Combining early coagulation and inflammatory status improves prediction of mortality in burned and nonburned trauma patients. J Trauma 2008, 64(2 Suppl):S188-194.
30. Carroll RC, Craft RM, Langdon RJ, et al: Early evaluation of acute traumatic coagulopathy by thrombelastography. Transl Res 2009, 154(1):34-39.
31. Kashuk JL, Moore EE, Sawyer M, et al: Primary fibrinolysis is integral in the pathogenesis of the acute coagulopathy of trauma. Ann Surg 2010, 252(3):434-442, discussion 443-434.
32. Pezold M, Moore EE, Wohlauer M, et al: Viscoelastic clot strength predicts coagulation-related mortality within 15 minutes. Surgery 2012, 151(1):48-54.
33. Schöchl H, Frietsch T, Pavelka M, et al: Hyperfibrinolysis after major trauma: differential diagnosis of lysis patterns and prognostic value of thrombelastometry. J Trauma 2009, 67(1):125-131.
34. Pivalizza EG, Pivalizza PJ, Gottschalk LI, et al: Celite-activated thrombelastography in children. J Clin Anesth 2001, 13(1):20-23.
35. Boldt J, Haisch G, Kumle B, et al: Does coagulation differ between elderly and younger patients undergoing cardiac surgery? Intensive Care Med 2002, 28(4):466-471.
36. Ng KF: Changes in thrombelastograph variables associated with aging. Anesth Analg 2004, 99(2):449-454, table of contents.
37. Scarpelini S, Rhind SG, Nascimento B, et al: Normal range values for thromboelastography in healthy adult volunteers. Braz J Med Biol Res 2009, 42(12):1210-1217.
38. Gorton HJ, Warren ER, Simpson NA, et al: Thromboelastography identifies sex-related differences in coagulation. Anesth Analg 2000, 91(5):1279-1281.
39. Zambruni A, Thalheimer U, Leandro G, et al: Thromboelastography with citrated blood: comparability with native blood, stability of citrate storage and effect of repeated sampling. Blood Coagul Fibrinolysis 2004, 15(1):103-107.
40. Manspeizer HE, Imai M, Frumento RJ, et al: Arterial and venous Thrombelastograph variables differ during cardiac surgery. Anesth Analg 2001, 93(2):277-281, 271st contents page.

41. Camenzind V, Bombeli T, Seifert B, et al: Citrate storage affects Thrombelastograph analysis. Anesthesiology 2000, 92(5):1242-1249.
42. Vig S, Chitolie A, Bevan DH, et al: Thromboelastography: a reliable test? Blood Coagul Fibrinolysis 2001, 12(7):555-561.
43. Rajwal S, Richards M, O'Meara M: The use of recalcified citrated whole blood – a pragmatic approach for thromboelastography in children. Paediatr Anaesth 2004, 14(8):656-660.
44. Luddington RJ: Thrombelastography/thromboelastometry. Clin Lab Haematol 2005, 27(2):81-90.
45. Sørensen B, Johansen P, Christiansen K, et al: Whole blood coagulation thrombelastographic profiles employing minimal tissue factor activation. J Thromb Haemost 2003, 1(3):551-558.
46. Ganter MT, Hofer CK: Coagulation monitoring: current techniques and clinical use of viscoelastic point-of-care coagulation devices. Anesth Analg 2008, 106(5):1366-1375.

9

Cocaine-associated hemoperitoneum following atraumatic splenic rupture

Faris Azar, Elisha Brownson and Tracey Dechert*

Abstract

Introduction: Splenic hematoma or rupture of the spleen is rare in the absence of trauma. This case report with a brief review of the literature is intended to raise awareness of splenic bleeding as an etiology of abdominal pain; it highlights the importance of a detailed social history.

Presentation of case: This report of an otherwise healthy 42-year old man details hemoperitoneum with splenic rupture as a cause for hemorrhage following cocaine use. The patient was managed non-operatively in the surgical intensive care unit. He did not require transfusion and was discharged home on hospital day four with close follow-up.

Discussion: While splenic pathology associated with cocaine use has been described, this case illustrates a novel report of cocaine-associated splenic hemorrhage. A plausible mechanism is transient vasospasm with subsequent bleeding into the infarcted area.

Conclusion: Although uncommon, atraumatic splenic rupture should be recognized early because it is potentially fatal. This case is the first to describe hemoperitoneum of splenic etiology following cocaine use.

Keywords: Cocaine, Atraumatic splenic rupture, Hemoperitoneum

Background

Hematoma or rupture of the spleen is an uncommon finding in the absence of blunt abdominal trauma [1]. Splenic hemorrhage without trauma has been described in pathologic cases, such as infection, but remains exceeding rare in healthy individuals with a normal spleen. Cocaine-associated splenic pathology, ranging from infarction to hematoma, has been previously described in reports in the literature [1-3]. This report of a healthy 42-year old man is the first to describe splenic rupture as a cause for hemorrhage following use of intranasal cocaine. Although uncommon, atraumatic splenic rupture needs to be recognized because it is potentially fatal. This case report with a brief review of the literature is intended to raise awareness of splenic bleeding as an etiology to be included in the differential diagnosis of acute abdominal pain and underlines the importance of a detailed social history.

* Correspondence: Tracey.Dechert@bmc.org
Department of Surgery, Boston University Medical Center, 850 Harrison Avenue Dowling 2 South, Boston, MA 02118, USA

Presentation of case

The patient is a 42-year-old man with no significant past medical history, aside from habitual cocaine use, who presented with excruciating left-sided abdominal pain after he consumed intranasal cocaine. The pain was constant, sharp, and nonradiating. Two days prior to presentation, he felt an acute onset of left upper quadrant pain immediately following a cough. The pain then became diffuse and more severe, prompting him to seek treatment in the emergency department (ED). He endorsed a similar left upper quadrant pain a few weeks prior, but that episode was less severe and resolved on its own. He denied any history of trauma, sick contacts, or recent travel.

On arrival to the ED, the patient's vital signs were as follows: temperature of 36.7 degrees centigrade, blood pressure of 103/68 mm Hg, pulse rate of 100 beats per minute, respiratory rate of 16 breaths per minute, and an oxygen saturation of 97% on room air. On physical examination, a subtle swelling of the left upper quadrant was noted. The abdomen was soft but markedly tender to palpation diffusely with mild guarding.

Laboratory studies revealed an initial hematocrit of 42.8%, and urine toxicology was positive for cocaine. Computed tomography (CT) scan of the abdomen and pelvis with oral and intravenous contrast showed no evidence of free peritoneal air or injury to any solid organs or bones including the ribs, but did reveal fluid around the spleen, in the left paracolic gutter, and layering in the pelvis (Figures 1, 2 and 3). There was no evidence of active contrast extravasation, no vascular blushes or aneurysms, no findings of portal hypertension, and no suspicion for malignancy. These radiographic findings pointed to a splenic source for hemoperitoneum. Six hours after presenting to the ED, the patient's hematocrit had dropped to 36.6%, and repeat CT scan revealed a focal collection of fluid surrounding the spleen. Given that the patient remained hemodynamically stable, he was admitted for non-operative management in the surgical intensive care unit, where he had serial abdominal examinations and blood count monitoring.

The patient did not require transfusion as his hematocrit remained stable between 36% and 38% throughout his hospital course. During that time, infectious etiologies including Epstein-Barr virus and cytomegalovirus were ruled out as possible causes. A human immunodeficiency virus test performed two weeks prior to this admission was negative. Additionally, hematologic malignancy was excluded with a peripheral blood smear. The patient's symptoms significantly improved and he was discharged on hospital day four.

On follow-up ten days after initial presentation, the patient's symptoms had resolved and his vital signs were stable. An abdominal ultrasound revealed a subcapsular

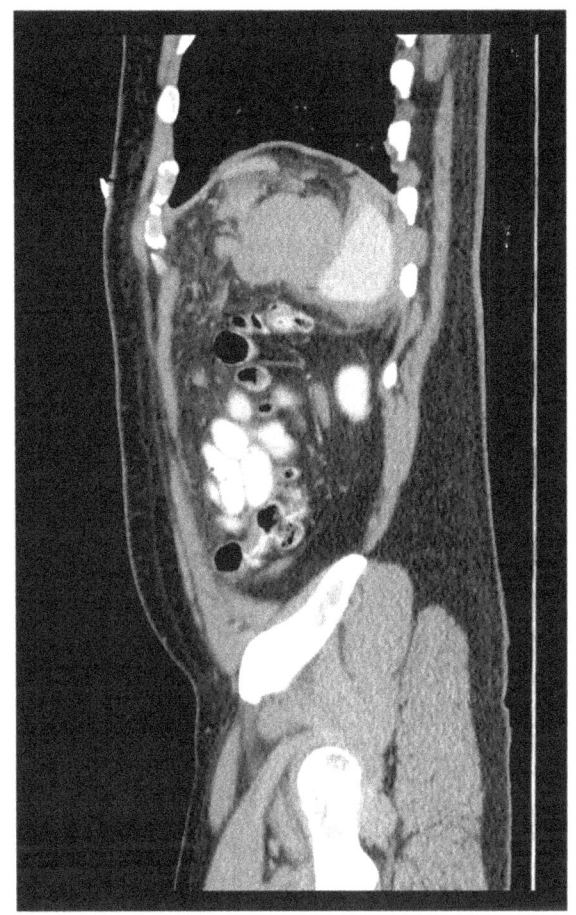

Figure 2 Sagittal, contrast-enhanced CT image demonstrates perisplenic hematoma.

splenic hematoma at the tip of the spleen tracking anteriorly with interim resolution of free fluid in the pelvis, confirming a splenic etiology for hemoperitoneum (Figure 4). Although the patient's CT scan did not show a blush suggestive of a pseudoaneurysm, the diagnosis

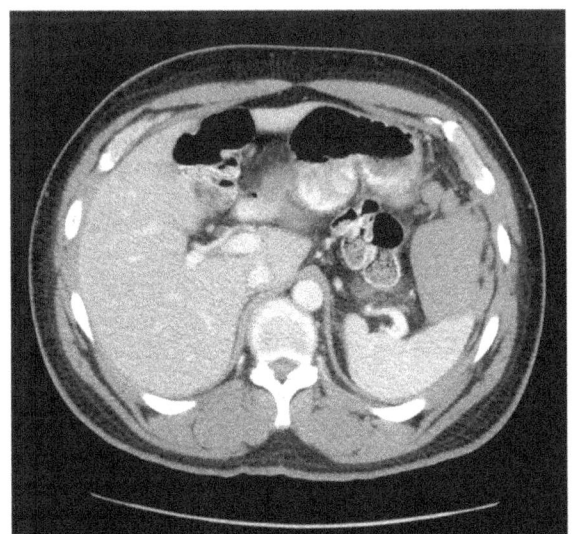

Figure 1 Axial, contrast-enhanced CT image demonstrates moderate hemoperitoneum in left upper quadrant centered around the spleen.

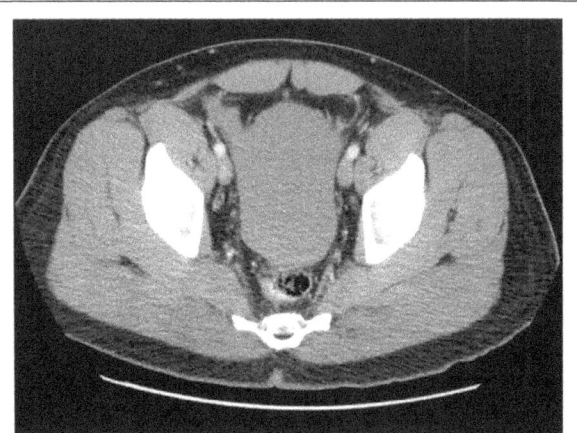

Figure 3 Axial, contrast-enhanced CT image of the pelvis demonstrates large hemoperitoneum.

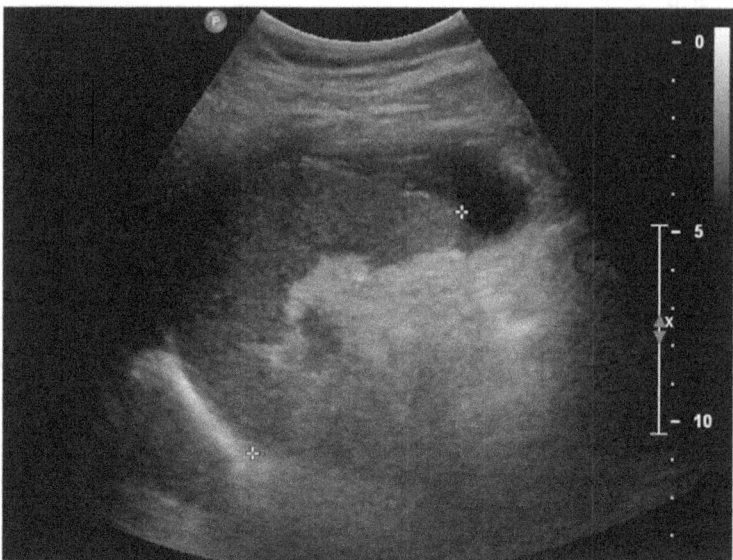

Figure 4 2D gray scale ultrasound image demonstrates small degree of subcapsular splenic hematoma.

of a splenic artery pseudoaneurysm could have been investigated further with a splenic angiogram.

Conclusions

Splenic rupture in the absence of trauma is exceedingly rare. Although atraumatic splenic rupture (ASR) is uncommon, it warrants early recognition due to the potentially fatal consequences and thus should be included in the differential diagnosis of patients with left upper quadrant abdominal pain [2]. A recent systematic review of atraumatic splenic rupture found there to be six major etiological groups: neoplastic processes (30.3%), infectious (27.3%), inflammatory (20.0%), iatrogenic (9.2%), mechanical (6.8%), and normal spleen (6.4%) [1]. ASR of the normal spleen is defined by four criteria: no history of trauma, no evidence of extrasplenic disease known to affect the spleen, no perisplenic adhesions to suggest previous trauma, and normal spleen on gross and histologic exam [3].

Clinical presentation of ASR mimics traumatic splenic rupture. Abdominal pain, especially in the left upper quadrant, or chest pain with radiation to the left shoulder, caused by subdiaphragmatic irritation, are classic symptoms of splenic pathology. There is often little or no clinical history to suggest splenic pathology, and the diagnosis is often made after imaging, which often includes ultrasonography or CT scan [4].

There are no definitive guidelines on management of ASR, although it is often modeled after that of traumatic splenic rupture. Treatment may include operative or non-operative therapy, depending upon the patient's hemodynamic stability and degree of splenic injury. The large amount of fluid within the abdomen could support operative evaluation with exploratory laparotomy. Factors favoring non-operative management in this case included total clinical stability, a soft abdomen, and duration of greater than 24 hours from the inciting event. The American Association for the Surgery of Trauma criteria for degree of splenic injury correlates with failure of conservative treatment. Given that a splenic etiology was not confirmed until the ultrasound after discharge, his injury could not be graded. At the time of follow-up, the subcapsular hematoma measured less than 10% of the surface area, consistent with a grade 1 injury [5]. Even in the setting of non-operative management, surgical teams are often involved or are the primary team managing inpatient surveillance. Work-up in patients with ASR should include studies to rule out the common causes, including neoplastic, infectious, and inflammatory processes. As this patient's work-up was negative, we conclude that the patient had a normal spleen with ASR and associate the splenic rupture with cocaine use.

Cocaine use remains epidemic and is associated with a wide range of medical complications. The well-studied physiologic effects of cocaine include increased norepinephrine reuptake with sustained alpha-adrenergic receptor stimulation and resultant vasoconstriction. Cocaine-associated vasoconstriction was shown to transiently reduce splenic volume on average by 20% [6]. This vasoconstriction transiently elevates blood pressure. In addition, increased abdominal venous pressure due to cough could suggest an inciting event for splenic hemorrhage in this patient. This has been previously described in a case report of a patient with hemoperitoneum after ingestion of cocaine and associated acute emesis; however, no etiologic source or evidence of underlying pathology was found [7].

Splenic infarction following cocaine use is rare but has been described, particularly in patients with sickle hemoglobinopathies [8]. It is plausible that cocaine-associated splenic hematoma or rupture results from transient vasospasm with subsequent bleeding into the infarcted area. Secondary infection of the infarcted spleen with resultant sepsis and death has also been detailed [9].

While the use of cocaine causing hematoma of the spleen has been described [10], this case is the first report of a case that details hemoperitoneum caused by ASR following cocaine use. Although uncommon, the potential for death due to splenic rupture warrants awareness and highlights the importance of a social history in patients presenting with acute abdominal pain.

Consent
Written informed consent was obtained from the patient for publication of this Case report and any accompanying images. A copy of the written consent is available for review by the Editor-in-Chief of this journal.

Abbreviations
ED: Emergency department; CT: Computed tomography; ASR: Atraumatic splenic rupture.

Competing interests
The authors declare that they have no competing interests.

Authors' contributions
FA and EB conducted the literature search and completed the chart review. FA authored the manuscript. EB edited the manuscript. EB provided patient care. TD was the attending physician who cared for the patient, instigated the study, edited the manuscript, and oversaw the project. All authors read and approved the final manuscript.

Acknowledgements
We would like to thank Dr. Stephan Anderson for providing the representative images and captions.

References
1. Renzulli P, Hostettler A, Schoepfer AM, Gloor B, Candinas D: Systematic review of atraumatic splenic rupture. *Br J Surg* 2009, **96**(10):1114–1121.
2. Wehbe E, Raffi S, Osborne D: Spontaneous splenic rupture precipitated by cough: a case report and a review of the literature. *Scand J Gastroenterol* 2008, **43**(5):634–637.
3. Debnath D, Valerio D: Atraumatic rupture of the spleen in adults. *J R Coll Surg Edinb* 2002, **47**:437–445.
4. Amonkar SJ, Kumar EN: Spontaneous rupture of the spleen: three case reports and causative processes for the radiologist to consider. *Br J Radiol* 2009, **82**:e111–e113.
5. Tinkoff G, Esposito TJ, Reed J, Kilgo P, Fildes J, Pasquale M, Meredith JW: American Association for the Surgery of Trauma Organ Injury Scale I: spleen, liver, and kidney, validation based on the National Trauma Data Bank. *J Am Coll Surg* 2008, **207**(5):646.
6. Kaufman MJ, Siegel AJ, Mendelson JH, Rose SL, Kukes TJ, Sholar MB: Cocaine administration induces human splenic constriction and altered hematologic parameters. *J Appl Physiol* 1998, **85**(5):1877–1883.
7. Bellows CF, Raafat AM: The surgical abdomen associated with cocaine abuse. *J Emerg Med* 2002, **23**(4):383–386.
8. Vaghjimal A: Splenic infarction related to cocaine use. *Postgrad Med J* 1996, **72**(854):768.
9. Dettmeyer R, Schlamann M, Madea B: Cocaine-associated abscesses with lethal sepsis after splenic infarction in an 17-year-old woman. *Forensic Sci Int* 2004, **140**(1):21–23.
10. Homler HJ: Nontraumatic splenic hematoma related to cocaine abuse. *West J Med* 1995, **163**(2):160–162.

Traumatic subclavian arterial rupture

Marco Assenza[1,3,4*], Leonardo Centonze[1,3], Lorenzo Valesini[1,3], Gabriele Campana[1,3], Mario Corona[2,3] and Claudio Modini[1,3]

Abstract

Subclavian artery injuries represent an uncommon complication of blunt chest trauma, this structure being protected by subclavius muscle, the clavicle, the first rib, and the deep cervical fascia as well as the costo-coracoid ligament, a clavi-coraco-axillary fascia portion. Subclavian artery injury appears early after trauma, and arterial rupture may cause life-treatening haemorrages, pseudo-aneurysm formation and compression of brachial plexus. These clinical eveniences must be carefully worked out by accurate physical examination of the upper limb: skin color, temperature, sensation as well as radial pulse and hand motility represent the key points of physical examination in this setting. The presence of large hematomas and pulsatile palpable mass in supraclavicular region should raise the suspicion of serious vascular injury. Since the first reports of endovascular treatment for traumatic vascular injuries in the 90's, an increasing number of vascular lesions have been treated this way. We report a case of traumatic subclavian arterial rupture after blunt chest trauma due to a 4 meters fall, treated by endovascular stent grafting, providing a complete review of the past twenty years' literature.

Keywords: Subclavian arterial rupture, Blunt chest trauma, Endovascular stent grafting

Introduction

Traumatic subclavian arterial rupture represents an uncommon complication of blunt chest trauma. The subclavian artery is protected by subclavius muscle, the clavicle, the first rib, and the deep cervical fascia, as well as the costo-coracoid ligament, a clavi-coraco-axillary fascia portion. Clavicular Fractures were cited as the cause of 50% of traumatic subclavian artery injuries [1]. Arterial rupture usually causes life-threatening haemorragies, and must be carefully ruled out by physical examination as well as diagnostic imaging. Physical examination of the upper limb must focus on skin color, temperature, sensation, hand motility well as radial pulse [2]. Contrast-CT represents a key diagnostic exam, while arteriography offers both a diagnostic a therapeutic approach.

Open surgery represents the classical management of subclavian rupture, but it is associated with high morbidity mostly because the need of extensive incisions, which require lengthy healing and rehabilitation.

In recent years endovascular stent grafting, thank to technical evolution and growing operators' experience, has become an attractive therapeutic approach to such kind of injuries, provided with less invasiveness and morbidity [3].

We report a case of traumatic subclavian arterial rupture after blunt chest trauma and clavicular fracture due to a 4 meters fall, treated by endovascular stent grafting.

Case report

A previously healthy 70-year old man had a fall from a 4 meters high scaffold: he reported a blunt chest trauma and a cranial trauma with temporary loss of consciousness. Immediately after trauma he was brought to our hospital.

On admittance to our hospital the patient was conscious and well oriented, and physical examination revealed patient airways, no *cornage* nor *triage* were present, he was breathing normally, not complaining about dyspnoea, his respiratory rate was 20 per minute, the trachea was lying on the midline, there were no

* Correspondence: marco.assenza@uniroma1.it
[1]Emergency Department, Division of Emergency Surgery and Trauma, Policlinico "Umberto I", Rome, Italy
[3]Umberto I General Hospital, University of Rome "Sapienza", Rome, Italy
Full list of author information is available at the end of the article

jugular veins turgor, vescicular murmur was bilaterally present and symmetric; a chest plain radiography was performed, there were no sign of pneumothorax but a left midishaft clavicular fracture was highlighted (Figure 1). The patient was hemodynamically stable, the skin was warm and dry, blood pressure was 120/90 mmHg with a 100 bpm heart rate, and he was resuscitated with 2000 ml of isotonic physiologic solution. He underwent a *Focused Assessment with Sonography for Trauma* (ECO-FAST), which showed no sign of active abdominal bleeding. There were no evidence of any neurological signs, his Glasgow Coma Scale (GCS) was 15, pupils were bilaterally isochoric, isocyclic, and reactive to light, and he was able to move the four limbs. The patient presented left parietal and periorbital ecchymotic excoriated contusion, as well as a vast hematoma with multiple excoriation in the left clavicular region and the left upper limb. The left hemithorax presented with multiple ecchymosis and was tender to palpation, while the right one was normal. There was no subcutaneous crepitation. The abdomen was flat, with physiologic respiration-associated mobility, there was no rebound tenderness, and peristalsis was present. The pelvis was stable. Palpable distal pulses were present in all extremities, and motor function of the lower limbs was preserved. Radial pulse of the left arm was slightly reduced and the limb presented with no evidence of neurological deficits (sensation, finger motility).

Urinary catheterization was performed, with an outcome of 100 ml of limpid urine. Laboratory tests showed an increase in myocytolysis enzymes with no evidence of cardiac failure (CPK = 569 UI/l; MB = 645.3 ng/ml; LDH = 338 UI/l). The haemoglobin value was initially 10.6 g/dl.

The patient underwent to a total body CT scan. The CT showed left parietal bone fracture with no signs of intracranial haemorrhage, confirmed the left clavicualr fracture viewed at RX, and revealed active bleeding from left subclavian artery; a L1 vertebral soma fracture determining medulla compression was also detected, while the abdominal scans did not show any sign of visceral trauma (Figure 2).

Because of the subclavian active bleeding the patient was sent to interventional radiology operatory theatre.

The right femoral artery was accessed using a standard Seldinger technique and a standard short 5F sheath was placed; a guidewire and a selective catheter were then used to cannulate the target vessel, and the left subclavian artery selective arteriography showed active bleeding from its 3rd segment, 3 cm after the vertebral artery's origin, due to a subtotal lesion of the arterial wall (Figure 3). A 8 × 50 mm Viabahn stent graft was advanced in anterograde fashion, then it was deployed under fluoroscopic visualization. An angioplasty balloon of appropriate size is used to iron out the proximal and distal edges of the stent and bring it up to profile (Figure 4). Next angiograms showed no active bleeding (Figure 5).

After surgical procedure, haemoglobin was checked again, and its value was 8.5 g/dl.

During the next days the patient underwent 2 blood transfusions, and its haemoglobin values returned between normal ranges (10.8 g/dl on the 6th day after trauma).

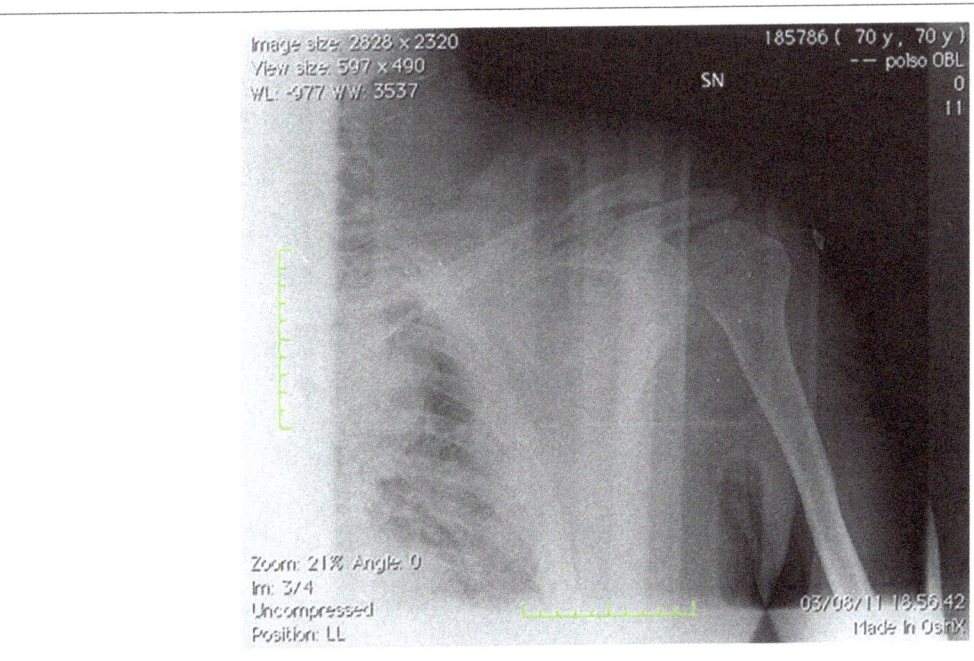

Figure 1 Plain radiography showing left midshaft clavicular fracture.

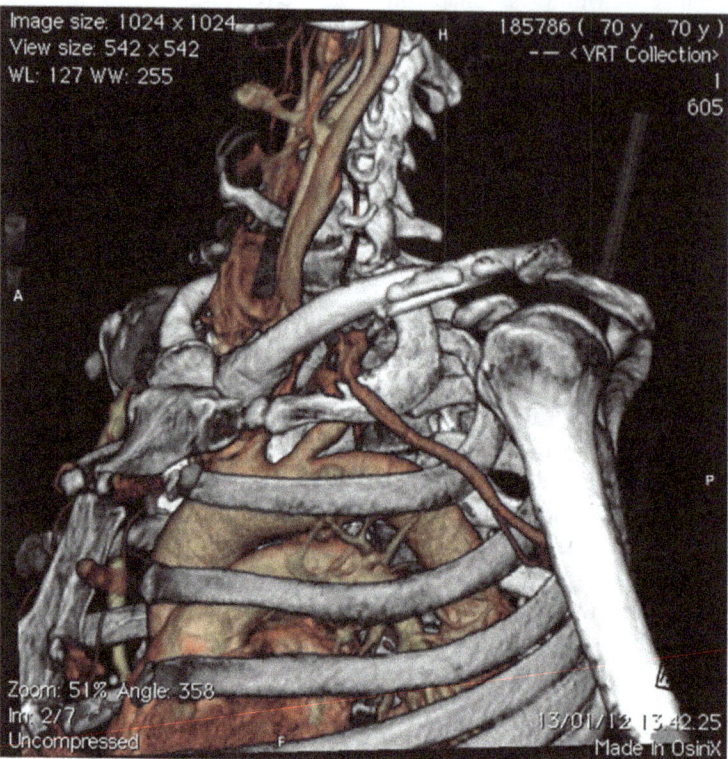

Figure 2 CT 3D reconstruction showing active left subclavian arterial bleeding and the left midshaft clavicular fracture.

The L1 vertebral soma fracture was treated on the 9th day after trauma.

The patient was discharged on the 15th day after trauma.

Discussion and review of literature

The association of subclavian arterial rupture and blunt thoracic trauma has been analyzed in many reports: in an article by Rulliat and coll. the incidence of subclavian

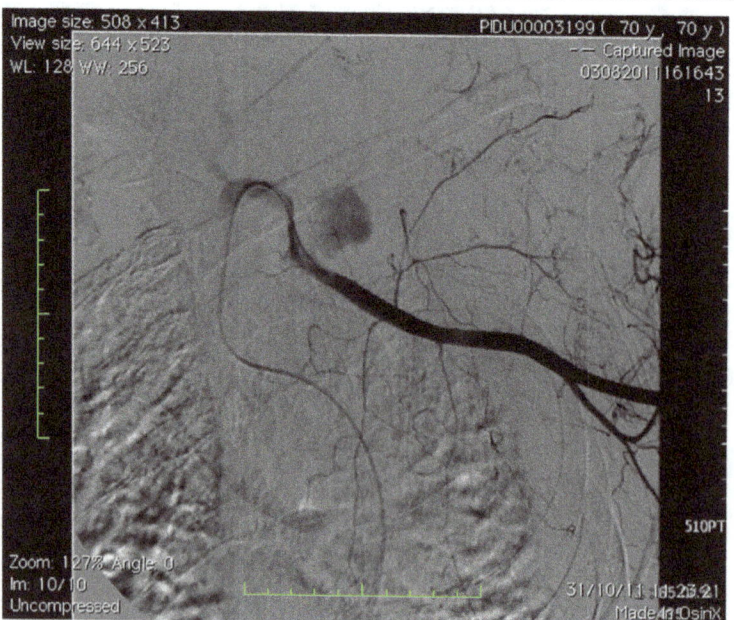

Figure 3 Arteriogram highlighting active left subclavian arterial bleeding, 3 cm after homolateral vertebral artery.

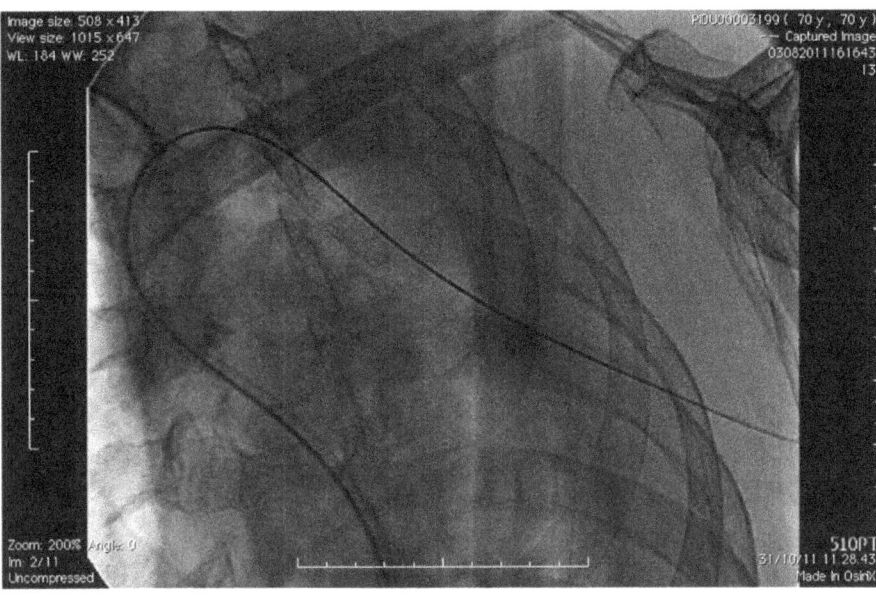

Figure 4 Covered Stent position.

arterial rupture among 1181 thoracic traumatic injuries was 0.4% [4]; a recent study by Shalhub and coll. reported a 47% incidence of subclavian arterial rupture above all the blunt thoracic outlet arterial injuries (BTOAI) [5]; furthermore, clavicular fractures were cited as the cause of 50% of traumatic subclavian artery injuries in another article by Kendall and coll. [1].

Subclavian artery injuries occurs from either elongation (stretching) or laceration mechanisms. Elongation is characteristically associated with a blunt force applied to the anterior shoulder or clavicle, as in motor vehicle crashes. This force is transmitted to fixed points along the vessel, typically the origin of the vertebral and internal thoracic artery where the vessel is then pulled apart. Laceration to the subclavian artery ensues from bony fragments produced by a fractured first rib or clavicle. The fracture is displaced into the vessel by the traction of associated chest wall muscles. Fractured clavicle has been cited as the cause of 50% of traumatic subclavian arterial injuries [1].

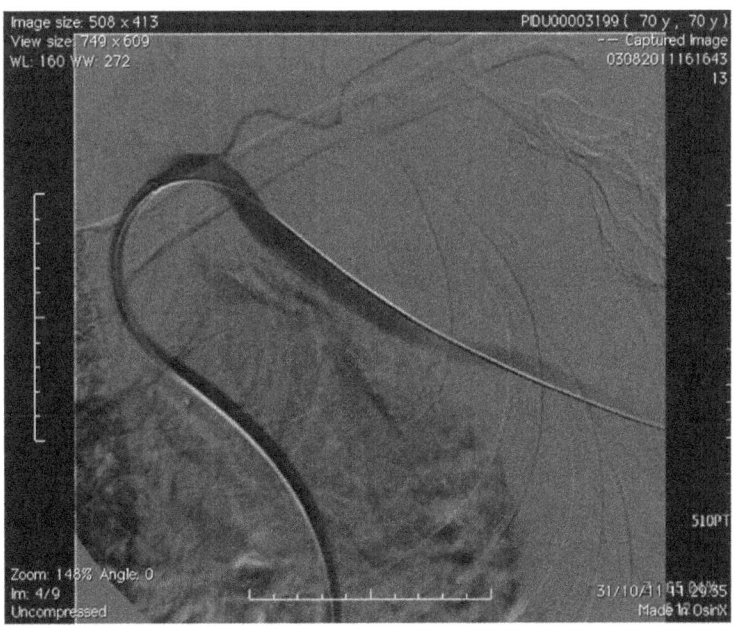

Figure 5 Arteriogram showing bleeding stop.

Subclavian arterial rupture is an uncommon complication of blunt thoracic trauma, and must be carefully ruled out because of its poor prognosis; in 1983 Sturm and Cicero have devised five criteria that should lead the examining physician to confirm the suspicion of arterial injury with arch aortography. These criteria include first rib fracture, diminished or absent radial pulses, palpable supraclavicular hematoma, chest roentgenogram demonstrating a widened mediastinum or hematoma over the area of the subclavian artery, and brachial plexus palsy [6]. Physical examination of the upper limb must focus on skin color, temperature, sensation, hand motility as well as radial pulse.

CT represents a key diagnostic exam, while selective arteriography offers both diagnostic accuracy and an operative approach.

Once identified, these injuries have historically been managed with a conventional surgical approach, associated with its own morbidity. Open repair is technically challenging and associated with significant morbidity and mortality for a variety of reasons. Exposure to obtain proximal control requires either a median sternotomy for the innominate and proximal right subclavian artery or a high anterolateral thoracotomy with potential clavicular resection for the proximal left subclavian artery. Such extensive incisions require lengthy healing and rehabilitation and carry significant morbidities.

Endovascular treatment represents a less invasive approach to these vascular injuries; furthermore, it offers less blood loss and a lesser invasive approach to an anatomically challenging problem [5]. Foremost is the benefit of approaching the lesion from a remote access site, which avoids major operative dissection in the traumatised area,

and decrease the risk of injuring important surrounding structures, such as the subclavian vein or brachial plexus, which may be difficult to identify because of haemorrhage or involvement in the original injury [7]. High success rates can be achieved if the lesion is focal and can be traversed safely with a guidewire. Complete vessel transection has been reported as a common cause for failure of an endovascular approach, primarily due to difficulty with crossing the complete transection and its associated hematoma [8]. As such, vessel transection has traditionally been approached with open vascular reconstruction. It seems convenient to perform a femoral artery access in a trauma setting, for the possibility to perform selective arteriographies of abdominal viscera. Even though rare tortuosity of supra-aortic vessels could be an obstacle for catheterization, the femoral access offers the possibility to use devices of different dimensions (until 7 F), representing the standard access for this procedure. The brachial access still offers a valid alternative in case of difficult subclavian catheterization and provides the opportunity to perform a combined brachial and femoral access to create a through-and-through brachial-femoral wire and repair of transected mid-to-distal subclavian or axillary artery with covered stent, as described by Shalhub and coll. in their recent work [9].

Analyzing the past 24 years literature [Table 1], we found out 750 subclavian arterial lesions, reported in 12 different works (associated axillo-subclavian lesions where not included in our review). Among these series, 79 patients underwent endovascular repair (10.5%). Arterial injuries were caused by blunt trauma in 56 cases (7.5%), and endovascular repair was performed in 5 of these cases (8.9%).

Table 1 Past 24 years subclavian arterial injuries' reports

Year	Authors	Number of cases	Blut trauma	Penetrating trauma	Endovascular repair	
					Blunt	Penetreting
1988	Costa et al.	167	15	152	0	0
1996	Patel et al.	6[a]	-	6	-	6
1999	Cox et al.	56	25	31	0	0
1999	Demetriades et al.	79[a]	-	79	-	1
1999	Janne d'Othée et al.	1[b,c]	1	-	1	-
2000	McKinley et al.	260	11	249	0	0
2003	Lin et al.	54[a]	-	54	-	0
2005	Castelli et al.	4[c]	1	3	1	3
2005	Bukhari et al.	1[b,c]	1	-	1	-
2008	du Toit et al.	57[a,c]	-	57	-	57
2009	Sobnach et al.	50[a]	-	50	-	1
2010	Carrick et al.	15	2	13	2	6

a - This report enrolls only Penetrating Arterial Injuries.
b - This is a Case Report.
c - This report analyses only Endovascular Treatments.

This review highlights the rarity of endovascular approach to subclavian arterial injuries: on the overall 569 cases reported from 1988 to 2000, only 8 (1.4%) underwent endovascular treatment; on the other hand, in the past 12 years 71 (39.2%) of 181 cases reported in literature were treated by endovascular approach [7,10-20].

Our analysis points out how the technical progresses and growing experience of vascular surgeons has improved the feasibility of endovascular treatment, creating a valid alternative to challenging 'classic' surgical approaches.

Conclusions

Our analysis reveals a continuous growth in the application of endovascular stent grafting vs. open repair for subclavian arterial injuries, thanks to the growing experience of endovascular surgeons coupled to rapid technologies' development. Furthermore, the indications for endovascular stent grafting were stretched: in 2005, hemodynamical instability status was still pointed out as a contraindication to endovascular approach, as well as complete vessel transaction [21]; 6 years later, the series by Shalhub and coll. [5] extended the indication to hemodynamically unstable patients as well as to patients reporting complete vessel transaction thanks to the application of a new endovascular technique based on the use of a combined brachial and femoral arterial access to create a brachial-femoral wire and repair of transected mid-to-distal subclavian or axillary artery [9]. In our opinion, according to the observation by Danetz [21] and Shalhub [5], the creation of an OR environment with full endovascular capability, where open and endovascular techniques can be used as well as other necessary procedures such as exploratory laparotomy and orthopedic fixation, without the need to transport the unstable patient, is crucial for a fast and multidisciplinary management of trauma patients.

Consent

Written informed consent was obtained from the patient for publication of this case report and any accompanying images. A copy of the written consent is available for review by the editor-in-chief of this journal.

Competing interests

The authors declare that they have no competing interests.

Author details

[1]Emergency Department, Division of Emergency Surgery and Trauma, Policlinico "Umberto I", Rome, Italy. [2]Department of Radiological Sciences, Vascular and Interventional Radiology Unit, Policlinico "Umberto I", Rome, Italy. [3]Umberto I General Hospital, University of Rome "Sapienza", Rome, Italy. [4]Surgical Research Fellow, Via Demetriade 58, Rome 00178, Italy.

Authors' contributions

MA coordinated the whole team work. LC, GC, LV cared about bibliographical research, images' collection and first draft writing. MC reviewed the radiological aspects of the article. CM carried out the final internal review. All authors read and approved the final manuscript.

References

1. Kendall KM, Burton JH, Cushing B: Fatal subclavian artery transection from isolated clavicle fracture. *J Trauma* 2000, **48**:316–318.
2. Stokkeland PJ, Soreide K, Fjetland L: Acute endovascular repair of right subclavian arterial perforation from clavicular fracture after blunt trauma. *J Vasc Interv Radiol* 2007, **18**:689–690.
3. Brandt MM, Kazanjian S, Wahl W: The utility of endovascular stents in the treatment of blunt arterial injuries. *J Trauma* 2001, **51**:901–905.
4. Rulliat E, Ndiaye A, David J-S, Voiglio EJ, Lieutaud T: Subclavian artery rupture after road crash: many similitaries. *Ann Fr Anesth Reanim* 2011, **30**(12):909–913.
5. Sherene Shalhub, Starnes Benjamin W, Hatsukami Thomas S, Riyad Karmy-Jones, Tran Nam T: Repair of blunt thoracic outlet arterial injuries: an evolution from open to endovascular approach. *J Trauma* 2011, **71**:E114–E121.
6. Sturm JT, Cicero JJ: The clinical diagnosis of ruptured subclavian artery following blunt thoracic trauma. *Ann Emerg Med* 1983, **12**:17–19.
7. Castelli P, Caronno R, Piffaretti G, Tozzi M, Lagana D, Carrafiello G: Endovascular repair of traumatic injuries of the subclavian and axillary arteries. *Injury* 2005, **36**:778–782.
8. Xenos ES, Freeman M, Stevens S, Cassada D, Pacanowski J, Goldman M: Covered stents for injuries of subclavian and axillary arteries. *J Vasc Surg* 2003, **38**:451–454.
9. Shalhub S, Starnes BW, Tran NT: Endovascular treatment of axillosubclavian arterial transection in patients with blunt traumatic injury. *J Vasc Surg* 2011, **53**(4):1141–1144. Epub 2011 Jan 26.
10. Costa MC, Robbs JV: Nonpenetrating subclavian artery trauma. *J Vasc Surg* 1988, **8**(1):71–75.
11. Patel AV, Marin ML, Veith FJ, Kerr A, Sanchez LA: Endovascular graft repair of penetrating subclavian artery injuries. *J Endovasc Surg* 1996, **3**(4):382–388.
12. Cox CS Jr, Allen GS, Fischer RP, Conklin LD, Duke JH, Cocanour CS, Moore FA: Blunt versus penetrating subclavian artery injury: presentation, injury pattern, and outcome. *J Trauma* 1999, **46**(3):445–449.
13. Demetriades D, Chahwan S, Gomez H, Peng R, Velmahos G, Murray J, Asensio J, Bongard F: Penetrating injuries to the subclavian and axillary vessels. *J Am Coll Surg* 1999, **188**(3):290–295.
14. Janne d'Othée B, Rousseau H, Otal P, Joffre F: Noncovered stent placement in a blunt traumatic injury of the right subclavian artery. *Cardiovasc Intervent Radiol* 1999, **22**(5):424–427.
15. McKinley AG, Carrim AT, Robbs JV: Management of proximal axillary and subclavian artery injuries. *Br J Surg* 2000, **87**(1):79–85.
16. Lin PH, Koffron AJ, Guske PJ, Lujan HJ, Heilizer TJ, Yario RF, Tatooles CJ: Penetrating injuries of the subclavian artery. *Am J Surg* 2003, **185**(6):580–584.
17. Bukhari HA, Saadia R, Hardy BW: Urgent endovascular stenting of subclavian artery pseudoaneurysm caused by seatbelt injury. *Can J Surg* 2007, **50**(4):303–304.
18. du Toit DF, Lambrechts AV, Stark H, Warren BL: Long-term results of stent graft treatment of subclavian artery injuries: management of choice for stable patients? *J Vasc Surg* 2008, **47**(4):739–743. Epub 2008 Feb 1.
19. Sobnach S, Nicol AJ, Nathire H, Edu S, Kahn D, Navsaria PH: An analysis of 50 surgically managed penetrating subclavian artery injuries. *Eur J Vasc Endovasc Surg* 2010, **39**(2):155–159. Epub 2009 Nov 11.
20. Carrick MM, Morrison CA, Pham HQ, Norman MA, Marvin B, Lee J, Wall MJ Jr, Mattox KL: Modern management of traumatic subclavian artery injuries: a single institution's experience in the evolution of endovascular repair. *Am J Surg* 2010, **199**(1):28–34. Epub 2009 Jun 11.
21. Danetz JS, Cassano AD, Stoner MC, Ivatury RR, Levy MM: Feasibility of endovascular repair in penetrating axillosubclavian injuries: a retrospective review. *J Vasc Surg* 2005, **41**(2):246–254.

11

Surgeon-performed sonographic findings in a traumatic trans-anal rectal perforation

Fikri M Abu-Zidan[1*], Mohamed I Abusharia[2] and Katharina Kessler[3]

Abstract

Early diagnosis and active management of trans-anal rectal injuries is essential for a favorable outcome. Intraperitoneal free air (IFA) is usually diagnosed by an erect Chest X-ray. Point-of-care ultrasound has been recently used to detect IFA. We report a 45-year-old male who presented to the Emergency Department with lower abdominal peritonitis. Surgeon-performed portable point-of-care ultrasound as an extension of the abdominal examination revealed an inflamed omentum with hypoechoic stranding, thickened non compressible small bowel, and free fluid in the pelvis. A transverse abdominal section of the right upper quadrant showed free intraperitoneal air. Rectal examination revealed a longitudinal rectal tear. Laparotomy has confirmed the sonographic findings. There was a 12 cm intraperitoneal tear of the anterior wall of the rectum which was necrotic. This case clearly demonstrates that portable point-of-care ultrasound gives very useful detailed information even when performed by a non radiologist. Surgeons should be encouraged to use point-of-care ultrasound after appropriate training.

Keywords: Rectal trauma, ultrasound, free intraperitoneal air

Introduction

Rectal injuries are uncommon. They are mainly caused by penetrating trauma. Early diagnosis and active management of trans-anal rectal injuries is essential for a favorable outcome [1,2]. Intraperitoneal rectal injuries will cause peritonitis, sepsis and even death if not detected early. Intraperitoneal free air (IFA) is usually diagnosed by an erect Chest X-ray [2]. If the erect chest X-ray was normal, then an abdominal CT scan is recommended. Point-of-care ultrasound has been recently used to detect IFA [3,4]. Hereby, we report an unusual case of trans-anal rectal injury in which point-of-care ultrasound was of a great help for an early diagnosis.

Case presentation

A 45-year-old male presented to the Emergency Department complaining of lower abdominal pain and dysuria of two days duration. His blood pressure was 120/80 mmHg, his pulse was 107 beat per minute and his temperature was 36.8°C. Abdominal examination revealed

tenderness and guarding in the lower abdomen. Surgeon-performed portable point-of-care ultrasound as an extension of the abdominal examination was done immediately and revealed an inflamed omentum with hypoechoic stranding in the right upper quadrant (Figure 1A), thickened non compressible small bowel (Figure 1B), and free fluid in the pelvis. A transverse abdominal section of the right upper quadrant showed free intraperitoneal air (Figure 2). Rectal examination revealed a large longitudinal rectal tear 8 cm from the anal verge with an inflamed floppy mucosa. The patient admitted that he has inserted a glass bottle through his anus two days before, which was associated with sudden lower abdominal pain and a small amount of rectal bleeding. Erect chest X-ray confirmed the presence of air under the diaphragm (Figure 3). C-reactive protein was 418 mg/L (Normal less than 0.7 mg/L), serum creatinine was 139 micromol/L (normal less than 107 micromol/l) and white blood cell count was 13.8×10^9/L. Arterial blood gas has shown an arterial oxygen tension of 50 mmHg on normal air. Laparotomy has confirmed the sonographic findings with thickened omentum, an edematous small bowel, pelvic abscess, and a 12 cm intraperitoneal tear of the anterior wall of the rectum which was necrotic (Figure 4). The rectum was dissected

---
* Correspondence: fabuzidan@uaeu.ac.ae
[1]Head Trauma Group, Faculty of Medicine and Health Sciences, UAE University, Al-Ain, UAE

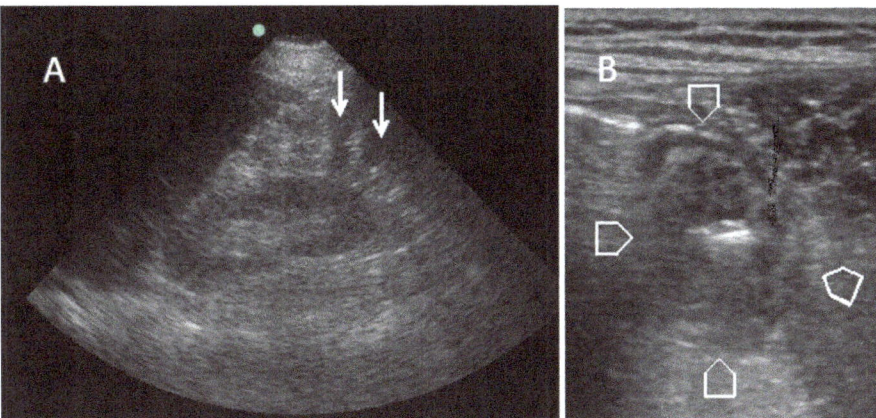

Figure 1 Surgeon-performed bedside ultrasound showing (A) an edematous omentum with hypoechoic stranding in the right upper quadrant of the abdomen (arrows) and (B) a thickened non compressible small bowel in the right lower quadrant of the abdomen (arrow heads).

and transected 8 cm from the anus. Low mesorectal excision of the necrotic rectum and a Hartman's procedure was performed. Two surgical drains without suction were left in the pelvis. Postoperatively, the patient was ventilated in the ICU. His arterial oxygen tension was 80 mmHg using an oxygen concentration of 50%. The patient received Tazocine intravenously 4.5 gms 8 hourly and Clexane 40 mg subcutaneously daily for one week. His respiratory and renal functions became normal within 4 days. The patient was discharged home on day 10 with good general condition and he is planned for reconnection of the colon after 3 months.

Discussion

The diagnosis of trans-anal rectal injuries is usually delayed because of patient's denial and late presentation.

Some of these injuries are self inflicted or caused by criminal assault [1,2]. High index of suspicion is essential for diagnosis.

In the present patient, portable surgeon-performed point-of-care ultrasound gave very useful information. Point-of-care ultrasound is an extension of the clinical examination. It is a goal-directed study that can be used for rapid diagnosis. It is accurate, non-invasive, cost effective, repeatable, without risk of radiation, and can be done in unstable patients parallel to physical examination and resuscitation [5,6].

It may be argued that ultrasound did not change the clinical management of our present patient. Bedside ultrasound is much quicker when performed by the treating surgeon as an extension of the abdominal examination than doing a formal chest X-ray in the

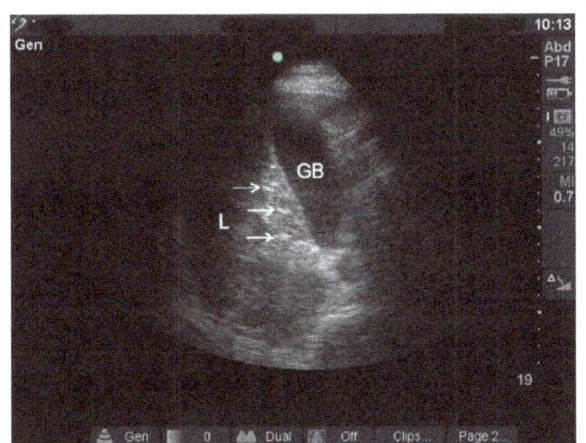

Figure 2 Transverse sonographic section of the right upper quadrant using a curvilinear probe showing hyperdence echogenic small areas (arrows) between the gall bladder (GB) and the liver (L) indicating free air.

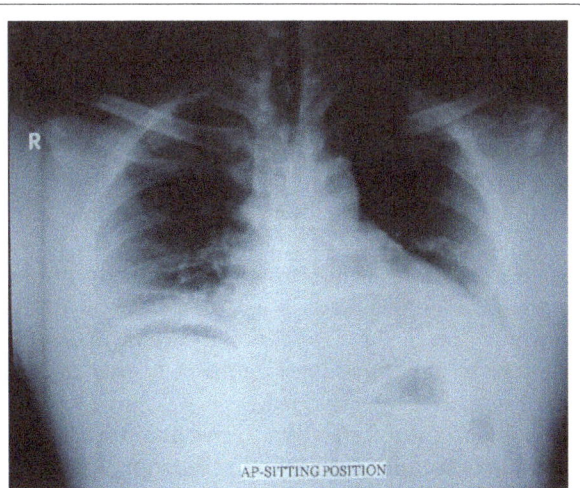

Figure 3 Erect chest X-ray showing free air under the right diaphragm.

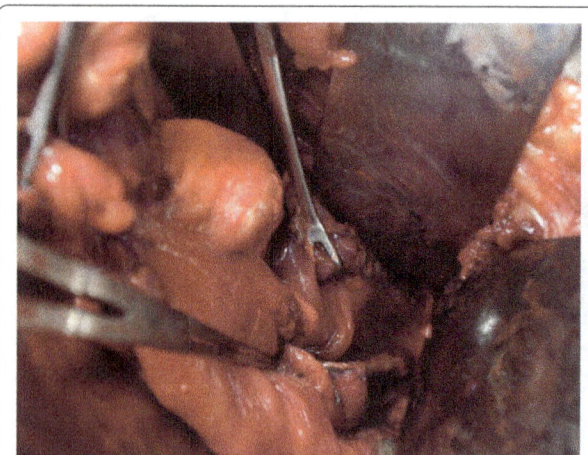

Figure 4 Laparotomy showing a 12 cm necrotic wound of the anterior wall of the rectum.

Radiology Department. Furthermore, ultrasound can be done while the patient is in the supine position, and may detect small amount of free intraperitoneal air compared with an erect chest X-ray which may be negative in up to 10% of patients with perforated bowel. Small amount of free intraperitoneal air can be detected under the anterior abdominal wall and in Morison's pouch [7]. This would be useful even in early bowel perforation without peritonitis. Furthermore, ultrasound is useful in disaster and austere situations when formal X-rays cannot be performed [8].

The ultrasound image of IFA results from the reverberation artefact of the ultrasound waves which swings between the ultrasound transducer and the highly reflective air. An increased echogenicity of a peritoneal stripe behind the anterior abdominal wall may be present [3,7,9]. The position of the stripe will change when changing the patient's position. Similar to our patient, trapped free intraperitoneal air bubbles in a localized fluid collection will give rise to echogenic foci [4,7]. The associated findings of thickened omentum and bowel, and free pelvic fluid pointed towards peritonitis in our patient [3,10].

We have performed bedside ultrasound as an extension of the abdominal examination in our patient before performing the rectal examination. Initially the patient denied the history of inserting a foreign body through his anus and he was diagnosed as having lower urinary tract infection in the Emergency Department. He was suspected to have bowel perforation only after the bedside ultrasound was performed.

It is important to stress that ultrasound usually rules in and does not rule out a bowel perforation which indicates that a negative study does not exclude a bowel perforation. FIA detection is operator dependable and

can be difficult even for an experienced ultrasound operator [11,12]. The ultrasound findings should be correlated with the clinical picture as a whole and used within defined diagnostic algorithms. If needed, and if the patient was haemodynamically stable, then an abdominal CT scan may give more information than ultrasound [13,14].

It may also be argued that laparotomy would have reached the diagnosis in our patient any way. There are different decisions to be made in cases of peritonitis including the indication for laparotomy and its timing. It would be also useful to collect information about the cause and site of perforation if possible as this may help to decide on what incision to use. Ultrasound may occasionally diagnose the cause of peritonitis, like a perforated duodenal ulcer [4,15].

Early diagnosis and active treatment results in a good prognosis. The good outcome of our patient, despite his multi-organ failure, occurred possibly because of his young age, and active surgical critical care management.

Consent
Written informed consent was obtained from the patient for publication of his clinical details and accompanying images.

Author details
[1] Head Trauma Group, Faculty of Medicine and Health Sciences, UAE University, Al-Ain, UAE. [2] General Surgeon, Al-Ain Hospital, Al-Ain, UAE. [3] Visceral, and Proctology Surgeon, Al-Ain Hospital, Al-Ain, UAE.

Authors' contributions
FA operated on the patient, had the idea, and assured the quality of data collected, drafted the paper, repeatedly edited it, and approved its final version. MA assisted in the operation and follow-up of the patient, helped in the idea, and approved the final version of the manuscript. KK operated on the patient, helped in the idea and drafting of the paper, and approved the final version of the manuscript.

Competing interests
The authors declare that they have no competing interests.

References
1. Orr CJ, Clark MA, Hawley DA, et al: Fatal anorectal injuries: A series of four cases. *Journal of Forensic Sciences* 1995, **40**:219-22.
2. El-Ashaal YI, Al-Olama A-K, Abu-Zidan FM: Trans-anal rectal injuries. *Singapore Med J* 2008, **49**:54-6.
3. Blaivas M, Kirkpatrick AW, Rodriguez-Galvez M, Ball CG: Sonographic depiction of intraperitoneal free air. *J Trauma* 2009, **67**:675.
4. Patel SV, Gopichandran TD: Ultrasound evidence of gas in the fissure for ligamentum teres: a sign of perforated duodenal ulcer. *Br J Radiol* 1999, **72**:901-2.
5. Abu-Zidan FM, al-Zayat I, Sheikh M, Mousa I, Behbehani A: Role of ultrasonography in blunt abdominal trauma, a prospective study. *Eur J Surg* 1996, **162**:361-365.
6. Abu-Zidan FM, Freeman P, Diku Mandivia: The first Australasian workshop on bedside ultrasound in the Emergency Department. *NZ Med J* 1999, **112**:322-324.

7. Hefny AF, Abu-Zidan FM: **Sonographic diagnosis of intraperitoneal free air.** *J Emerg Trauma Shock* .

8. Dittrich K, Abu-Zidan FM: **Role of Ultrasound in Mass-Casualty Situations.** *International Journal of Disaster Medicine* 2004, **2**:18-23.

9. Pattison P, Jeffrey RB Jr, Mindelzun RE, Sommer FG: **Sonography of intraabdominal gas collections.** *AJR Am J Roentgenol* 1997, **169**:1559-64.

10. Lee DH, Lim JH, Ko YT, Yoon Y: **Sonographic detection of pneumoperitoneum in patients with acute abdomen.** *AJR Am J Roentgenol* 1990, **154**:107-9.

11. Chen SC, Wang HP, Chen WJ, Lin FY, Hsu CY, Chang KJ, *et al*: **Selective use of ultrasonography for the detection of pneumoperitoneum.** *Acad Emerg Med* 2002, **9**:643-5.

12. Chadha D, Kedar RP, Malde HM: **Sonographic detection of pneumoperitoneum: An experimental and clinical study.** *Australas Radiol* 1993, **37**:182-5.

13. Radwan MM, Abu-Zidan FM: **Focussed Assessment Sonography for Trauma (FAST) and CT scan in blunt abdominal trauma: surgeon's perspective.** *Afr Health Sci* 2006, **6**:187-90.

14. Abu-Zidan FM, Sheikh M, Jaddallah F, Windsor JA: **Blunt abdominal trauma: Comparison of ultrasonography and computed tomography.** *Austral Radiol* 1999, **43**:440-3.

15. García Santos JM: **Direct sonographic signs of acute duodenal ulcer.** *Abdom Imaging* 1999, **24**:226-7.

12

Demographics of the injury pattern in severely injured patients with an associated clavicle fracture

Jacqueline JEM van Laarhoven[1*], Steven Ferree[1], R Marijn Houwert[2], Falco Hietbrink[1], EgbertJan MM Verleisdonk[2] and Luke PH Leenen[1]

Abstract

Background: Despite an increasing interest in the treatment of clavicle fractures, this is still a not yet defined area in severely injured patients as most studies exclude these patients. Analyzing fracture type and evaluate accompanying injuries can provide valuable information in an early stage of trauma care.

Objective: To identify prevalence, fracture type and accompanying injuries of clavicle fractures in the severely injured patient.

Methods: We included all severely injured patients (ISS ≥ 16) with a clavicle fracture from January 2007 - December 2011. We prospectively collected data about demographics, injuries, trauma mechanism and mortality. Fractures were classified using the Robinson classification.

Results: A total of 1534 patients had an ISS ≥16, of which 164 (10.7%) patients had a clavicle fracture. Traffic related accidents were the main cause of injury (65%). Most fractures were midshaft fractures (66.5%) of which 56% were displaced. Seven patients were treated operatively. There was no significant difference in ISS between the three fracture types. 83% of the patients sustained additional injury to the head and neck; the most prevalent injuries were skull or skull base fractures (41.5%) and maxillofacial fractures (29%). Furthermore 77% of the patients had additional thoracic injury; the most prevalent injuries were rib fractures (59%) and a pneumothorax (38%). The mortality rate was 21.4%.

Conclusion: A clavicle fracture was present in more than 10% of the severely injured patients. Displaced midshaft clavicle fractures were the most common type of fracture. Additional injuries to the head and neck region occurred in 83% of the patients and thoracic injuries occurred in 77% of the patients.

Keywords: Clavicle fracture, Trauma care, ISS, Severely injured, Associated injury pattern

Introduction

Clavicle fractures account for approximately 5% of all fractures. Most often it concerns a midshaft clavicle fracture (80%) of which 50% is dislocated [1,2]. In the past years there has been increasing interest in the treatment of clavicle fractures, especially in the midshaft fractures. However, most studies evaluating treatment of clavicle fractures exclude severely injured trauma patients [3,4]. Therefore the clavicle fracture in the severely injured patient is a not yet defined area.

Advanced Trauma Life Support (ATLS) principles advocate that in all severely injured trauma patients a chest x-ray is made to identify potential thoracic injuries [5]. Treatment-dictating injuries are frequently missed at the chest x-ray as 50% of all rib fractures and a significant number of hemato- and pneumothorax are not identified [6,7]. Clavicle fractures, on the other hand, can almost always be diagnosed at chest x-ray. Therefore it is

* Correspondence: jlaarho2@umcutrecht.nl
[1]Department of Surgery, University Medical Center Utrecht, Heidelberglaan 100, 3584, CX Utrecht, The Netherlands

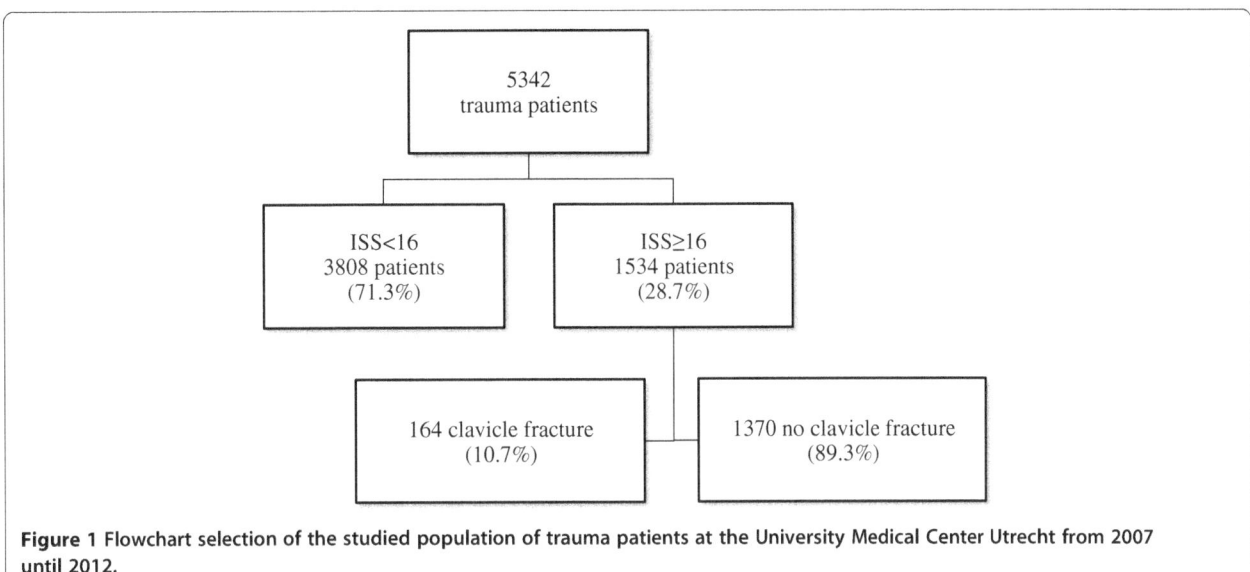

Figure 1 Flowchart selection of the studied population of trauma patients at the University Medical Center Utrecht from 2007 until 2012.

of great interest to analyze which accompanying injuries most frequently occur in severely injured patients with a clavicle fracture. These "expected" associated injuries can be taken into account in an early stage of trauma care for severely injured patients.

Table 1 Demographics of the studied population of severely injured patients with a clavicle fracture

			Clavicle fracture
Age overall			45.8 (± 21.9)
Age	Type I		39.1 (± 22.7)
	Type II		44.0 (± 20.8)
	Type III		56.0 (± 20.4)
Gender (M/F)			110/54
Trauma mechanism	Traffic	Car	34 (20.7%)
		Motor	36 (22.0%)
		Bike	32 (19.5%)
		Pedestrian	6 (3.7%)
	Sports		1 (0.6%)
	Fall		47 (28.6%)
	Other		8 (4.9%)
Injured side (L/R/both)			92/70/2
HET*			115 (70.1%)
ISS **			29.4 (± 10.4)
Admission at Intensive Care Unit			64 (39.0%)
Admission at Medium Care Unit			40 (24.4%)
Direct transport to OR			22 (13.4%)
Mortality	At emergency room		2 (1.2%)
	Within < 24 hours		17 (10.4%)
	During admission		16 (9.8%)

*Patients involved in an high energy trauma ** Injury of Severity Score.

The aim of this study is to identify prevalence, fracture type and accompanying injuries of clavicle fractures in the severely injured patient.

Materials and methods

Patients included in this study were those admitted in a level 1 trauma center from January 2007 until December 2011. The organisation of trauma care in the Netherlands is based on the American model of trauma regionalization. The Netherlands is divided in 11 separate trauma regions, each region contains a level one trauma center [8].

In this study prospective data from the Dutch National Trauma Database (DNTD) for the area Central Netherlands were used. The DNTD contains documentation on all trauma patients that are treated at the emergency department and subsequently admitted. Data in the DNTD were collected in a standardized manner and include detailed information on demographics, trauma event and mechanism, primary trauma survey, initial treatment and injuries. Injuries were diagnosed at

Table 2 Robinson classification of clavicle fractures in severely injured patients

Robinson classification	No. of patients (% of population)	Mean age ± SD	Mean ISS* ± SD
1A	8 (4.9%)	33.9 (± 20.6)	36.3 (± 11.2)
1B	2 (1.2%)	60.0 (± 24.0)	27.5 (± 9.1)
2A	51 (31.1%)	48.9 (± 22.7)	29.2 (± 9.5)
2B	61 (37.2%)	39.5 (± 18.3)	29.8 (± 11.8)
3A	32 (19.5%)	57.5 (± 21.0)	29.0 (± 9.7)
3B	10 (6.1%)	51.3 (± 18.3)	23.7 (± 4.8)

*Injury of Severity Score.

Table 3 Treatment of clavicle fractures in severely injured patients treated at the University Medical Center Utrecht, classified by the Robinson classification

Robinson classification	Operative	Conservative
1A	0	8
1B	1	1
2A	0	50
2B	5	54
3A	0	32
3B	1	9
Total	7	154

primary survey, subsequent surgery or during admission. Thoracic and pelvic x-ray imaging were performed for all trauma patients and when indicated supplemented with ultrasound and computed tomography (CT). The database accuracy is constantly evaluated by two database managers.

All injuries were coded using Abbreviated Injury Scale (AIS) location codes allocated to one of the six body regions (head and neck, face, chest, abdomen, extremities and external) to calculate the Injury of Severity Score (ISS) [9]. Patients with a clavicle fracture were selected using AIS location codes. The ISS provides an overall score for patients with multiple injuries and is used to determine injury severity; 0 corresponds with no injury, the maximum score of 75 corresponds with injury leading to death [10]. Patients with an ISS ≥ 16, obtained from ≥2 AIS regions and physiological alterations due to the injuries are considered severely injured and were included in our analysis [11].

For these patients, age, gender, trauma mechanism, injured side, additional injuries, department of admission (Intensive care Unit, Medium Care Unit, Operation Room) and discharge facility were collected from the DNTD. In all patients trauma mechanism was analysed and determined if it was a high energy trauma. The ATLS definition for high energy trauma was used [5]. Furthermore death associated with the trauma was obtained from the electronic patient documentation (EPD).

To evaluate the clavicle fractures we used the imaging studies performed. These radiological tests allowed for clear images of the fracture and of possible dislocation in anterior-posterior or cranial-caudal direction.

Fractures were classified by the researchers (JL, SF and MH) using the Robinson classification. This classification divides the clavicle in a medial fifth (type 1), a diaphyseal part (type 2) and a lateral fifth (type 3). This is further divided by three other variables; intra-articular extent, degree of comminution, and degree of displacement [12].

Data analysis

Mean numbers were noted with standard deviation (SD), median numbers were noted with interquartile range (IQR). Statistical analysis was performed using the χ^2 test for categorical variables and t-test and one-way-ANOVA for continuous variables. Binary logistic regression was used for the calculation of the dependent variables in additional injuries. A p-value of ≤0.05 was considered significant. Data were analyzed with SPSS Version 20.0, Chicago, IL, USA.

Results

A total of 5357 trauma patients were treated at the emergency department and subsequently admitted over the 5 year period (January 2007- December 2011). Of these patients 1534 had an ISS of 16 or higher, of which 164 (10.7%) patients had a clavicle fracture (Figure 1). The mean age of the entire studied population was 45.8 (± 21.9), four patients were aged under 16 years and 160 patients were aged 16 years and older (Table 1). Patients were predominantly male (66.5%). The main part of patients (65%) were involved in traffic accidents and 112 patients sustained a high energy trauma. The mortality rate was 21.4%. The majority of patients died due to injury to the central nervous system (74.3%), other causes were organ failure (14.3%), exsanguinations (8.6%) and one patient died due to sepsis. There were no missing data in baseline characteristics (Table 1). Most of the fractures were midshaft clavicle fractures (66.5%) of which 56% were displaced (Table 2).

Patients with type III fractures were older than patients with type I (P = 0.022; 16.9 95% CI 2.43-31.37) or II fractures (P = 0.001; 12.2 95% CI 4.78-19.65). No difference in age was found between patients with type I and II fractures. Patients with a displaced fracture are significantly younger than patients with a non-displaced fracture (P = 0.006; 8.933, 95% CI 2.5-15.3). There was

Table 4 Additional injuries in severely injured patients per type of clavicle fracture

	Upper extremity	Lower extremity	Abdominal injury	Thorax injury	Face injury	Head & neck injury
	n (%)	n (%)	n (%)	n (%)	n (%)	n (%)
Type I fracture (n = 10)	3 (30.0 %)	4 (40.0%)	4 (40.0%)	9 (90.0%)	1 (10.0%)	6 (60.0%)
Type II fracture (n = 112)	33 (29.7%)	36 (32.4%)	38 (34.2%)	88 (79.3%)	43 (38.7%)	90 (82.6%)
Type III fracture (n = 42)	7 (16.7%)	13 (31.0%)	11 (26.2%)	28 (66.7%)	16 (38.1%)	37 (88.1%)
No of patients (% of population)	43 (26.4 %)	53 (32.5%)	53 (32.5%)	125 (76.7%)	60 (36.8%)	133 (82.6%)

no significant difference in ISS between the three groups and no significant difference in ISS in patients with a displaced or non-displaced fracture.

In 7 patients, the clavicle fracture was treated operatively, the mean time was admission day 5 (range 1-11 days). All patients received plate fixation. In one case it concerned a type 1B fracture, in 5 cases a type 2B fracture and in one case a type 3B fracture. One patient was directly transferred and the remaining 153 patients were treated conservatively (Table 3).

Of all patients, 83% sustained additional injuries to head and neck. The most prevalent injury was a skull or skull base fracture (41.5%) followed by maxillofacial fractures in 29%. Seventy-seven percent had additional thoracic injuries (Table 4; Figure 2), 59% of the patients had rib fractures and 38% of the patients had a pneumothorax. There was no significant difference in displaced and undisplaced fractures concerning additional injuries.

Discussion

The main findings of this study were that 10% of all severely injured patients had a clavicle fracture and 21.4% of multitrauma patients with a clavicle fracture died during trauma care or admission. Midshaft clavicle fractures were most common and 44% of all fractures were displaced. Eighty-three percent of our patients had additional head and neck injuries and 77% had additional thoracic injuries.

Two large epidemiologic studies report incidence rates of clavicle fractures in the normal population between 2,6 and 4% [1,2]. Therefore clavicle fractures seem to occur at least twice as common in severely injured patients. In comparison to the study of Robinson et al, less fractures in our population were displaced. This difference might be explained by the fact that in severely injured patients, energy forces are distributed over the body. This is different compared to the direct energy on the clavicle in case of a single fracture [13,14]. Results of this study indicate that the clavicle is the gate-keeper of the thorax in severely injured patients. This hypothesis can be supported by the high rate of additional thoracic injuries.

The overall mortality of the study population was 21.4%, which includes deaths at the emergency room. Our results are similar to an abstract published by Mc Kee et al, which showed that in multitrauma patients the presence of a clavicle fracture was found to be associated with a mortality rate of 32% (thirty-four of 105 patients), mainly due to concomitant chest and head injuries [15].

Previous studies have been performed to identify associated injury in patients with upper extremity injury. Analysis showed significantly more rib fractures (52.9%), lung injuries (47.1%) and spinal fractures (29.1%) in patients with scapula fractures [16]. Also a correlation

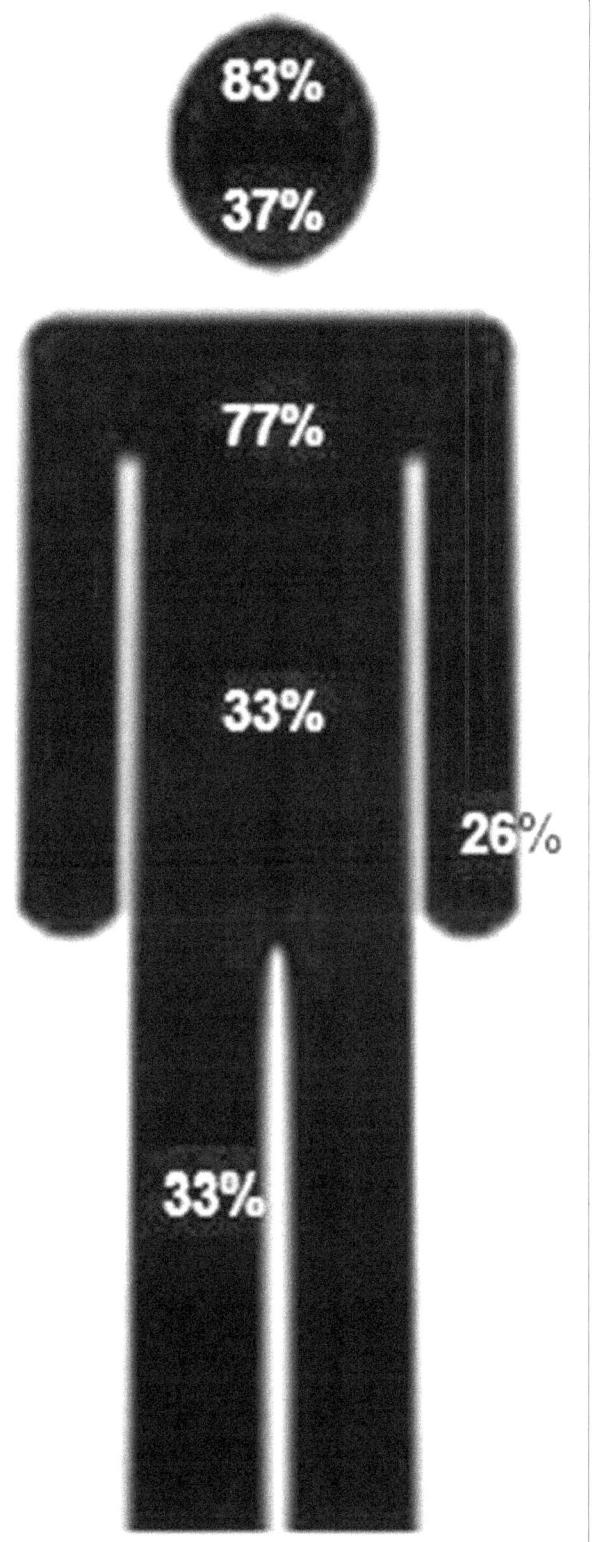

Figure 2 Additional injuries in severely injured patients with a clavicle fracture.

between shoulder girdle injuries and rates of head (31.5%), great vessel (3.9%) and thoracic injury (36.8%) has been described [17]. Compared to scapula and upper extremity injury a clavicle fracture is more likely to be identified on chest x-ray. Therefore clavicle fractures are a good predictor for additional injury and can be better identified and used in an early stage. Horst et al. found a correlation between a clavicle fracture and additional upper extremity injuries in polytrauma patients [18]. Therefore the clavicle fracture can also play an important role in the tertiary survey.

This study represents an analysis based on a prospective database, although retrospectively analyzed, and is one the first to analyze clavicle fractures in the severely injured patients. Because of the detailed description of all injuries, we were able to perform a profound analysis.

The DNTD includes patients who were treated at the Emergency Room of our hospital and subsequently admitted. Therefore patients with a clavicle fracture and an ISS ≥ 16 who were not admitted, are not included in our database. Considering the additional injuries in case of an ISS ≥ 16 we can safely assume that the number of patients we missed is small and this database provides a representative study population.

Conclusion

Clavicle fractures occur frequently (10%) in severely injured patients and 21,4% of the patients died during trauma care or admission. Midshaft clavicle fractures were most common and 44% of all fractures were displaced. Eighty-three percent of our patients had additional head and neck injuries and 77% had additional thoracic injuries.

Competing interests
The authors declare that they have no competing interests.

Authors' contributions
All authors: 1) have made substantial contributions to conception and design, or acquisition of data, or analysis and interpretation of data; 2) have been involved in drafting the manuscript or revising it critically for important intellectual content; 3) have given final approval of the version to be published. JL: Study conception and design, acquisition of data, analysis and interpretation of data, drafting of manuscript. SF: Acquisition of data, analysis and interpretation of data, drafting of manuscript. MH: Study conception and design, analysis and interpretation of data, drafting of manuscript. FH: Study conception and design, analysis and interpretation of data, critical revision. EV: Analysis and interpretation of data, critical revision of manuscript. LL: Study conception and design, critical revision of manuscript. All authors have given final approval for this manuscript to be published.

Author details
[1]Department of Surgery, University Medical Center Utrecht, Heidelberglaan 100, 3584, CX Utrecht, The Netherlands. [2]Department of Surgery, Diakonessenhuis Utrecht, Bosboomstraat 1, 3582, KE Utrecht, The Netherlands.

References
1. Postacchini F, Gumina S, De Santis P, Albo F: **Epidemiology of clavicle fractures.** *J Shoulder Elbow Surg* 2002, 11(5):452–456.
2. Nordqvist A, Petersson C: **The incidence of fractures of the clavicle.** *Clin Orthop Relat Res* 1994, 300:127–132.
3. Wijdicks FJ, Houwert RM, Dijkgraaf MG, De Lange DH, Meylaerts SAG, Verhofstad MHJ, Verleisdonk EJJM: **Rationale and design of the plate or pin (POP) study for dislocated midshaft clavicular fractures: study protocol for a randomised controlled trial.** *Trials* 2011, 15(12):177. doi: 10.1186/1745-6215-12-177.
4. Stegeman SA, de Jong M, Sier CF, Krijnen P, Duijff JW, Van Thiel TPH, De Rijcke PAR, Soesman NMR, Hagenaars T, Boekhoudt FD, De Vries MR, Roukema GR, Tanka AFK, Van Den Bremer J, Van Der Meulen HGWM, Bronkhorst MWGA, Van Dijkman BA, Van Zutphen SWAM, Vos DI, Schep NWL, Eversdijk MG, Van Olden GDJ, Van Den Brand JGH, Hillen RJ, Frölke JPM, Schipper IB: **Displaced midshaft fractures of the clavicle: non-operative treatment versus plate fixation (Sleutel-TRIAL). A multicentre randomised controlled trial.** *BMC Musculoskelet Disord* 2011, 24(12):196.
5. American College of Surgeons: *Advanced trauma life support for doctors. Student course manual.* 7th edition. Chicago, IL: American College of surgeons; 2004.
6. Aukema TS, Beenen LF, Hietbrink F, Leenen LPH: **Initial assessment of chest X-ray in thoracic trauma patients: awareness of specific injuries.** *World J Radiol* 2012, 4(2):48–52. doi: 10.4329/wjr.v4.i2.48.
7. Livingston DH, Shogan B, John P, Lavery RF: **CT diagnosis of Rib fractures and the prediction of acute respiratory failure.** *J Trauma* 2008, 64(4):905–911. United States.
8. Spijkers ATE, Meylaerts SAG, Leenen LPH: **Mortality Decreases by Implementing a Level I Trauma Center in a Dutch Hospital.** *J Trauma-Injury Infect Crit Care* 2010, 69(5):1138–1142.
9. Committee on Injury Scaling: *The Abbreviated Injury Scale, 1998 revision (AIS-98).* Des Plaines (IL): Association for the Advancement of Automotive Medicine; 1998.
10. Baker SP, O'Neill B, Haddon W, Long WB: **The injury severity score: a method for describing patients with multiple injuries and evaluating emergency care.** *J Trauma* 1974, 14(3):187–196. United States.
11. American College of Surgeons: *Resources for the Optimal Care of the Injured Patient.* Chicago, IL; 1987.
12. Robinson CM: **Fractures of the clavicle in the adult. Epidemiology and classification.** *J Bone Joint Surg Br* 1998, 80(3):476–484.
13. Nowak J, Mallmin H, Larsson S: **The aetiology and epidemiology of clavicular fractures. A prospective study during a two-year period in Uppsala, Sweden.** *Injury* 2000, 31:353–358.
14. Stanley D, Trowbridge EA, Norris SH: **The mechanism of clavicular fracture. A clinical and biomechanical analysis.** *J Bone Joint Surg Br* 1988, 70(3):461–464.
15. McKee MD, Schemitsch EH, Stephen DJ, Kreder HJ, Yoo D, Harrington J: **Functional outcome following clavicle fractures in polytrauma patients** [abstract]. *J Trauma* 1999, 47:616.
16. Baldwin KD, Ohman-Strickland P, Mehta S, Hume E: **Scapula fractures: a marker for concomitant injury? A retrospective review of data in the National Trauma Database.** *J Trauma* 2008, 65(2):430–435. United States.
17. Gottschalk HP, Browne RH, Starr AJ: **Shoulder girdle: patterns of trauma and associated injuries.** *J Orthop Trauma* 2011, 25(5):266–271. United States.
18. Horst K, Dienstknecht T, Pfeifer R, Pishnamaz M, Hildebrand F, Pape HC: **Risk stratification by injury distribution in polytrauma patients -- does the clavicular fracture play a role?.** *Patient Saf Surg* 2013, 7(1):23.

13

Strangulated intercostal liver herniation subsequent to blunt trauma

Cino Bendinelli[1*], Andrew Martin[1], Shane D Nebauer[2] and Zsolt J Balogh[2]

Abstract

Traumatic transdiaphragmatic intercostal hernia, defined as an acquired herniation of abdominal contents through disrupted intercostal muscles, is a rarely reported entity. We present the first reported case of a traumatic transdiaphragmatic intercostal hernia complicated by strangulation of the herniated visceral contents.

Following blunt trauma, a 61-year old man developed a traumatic transdiaphragmatic intercostal hernia complicated by strangulation of liver segment VI. Due to pre-existing respiratory problems and the presence of multiple other injuries (grade III kidney laceration and lung contusion) the hernia was managed non-operatively for the first 2 weeks.

The strangulated liver segment eventually underwent ischemic necrosis. Six weeks later the resulting subcutaneous abscess required surgical drainage. Nine months post injury the large symptomatic intercostal hernia was treated with laparoscopic mesh repair. Twelve months after the initial trauma, a small recurrence of the hernia required laparoscopic re-fixation of the mesh.

This paper outlines important steps in managing a rare post traumatic entity. Early liver reduction and hernia repair would have been ideal. The adopted conservative approach caused liver necrosis and required staged procedures to achieve a good outcome.

Keywords: Strangulated, Intercostal hernia, Liver herniation, Blunt trauma, Laparoscopic mesh repair

Introduction

Traumatic transdiaphragmatic intercostal hernia (TTIH) is a rare pathology with only sporadic cases published in the literature [1-21]. TTIH is defined as an acquired herniation of the abdominal contents through intercostal muscles [1-21]. The condition generally occurs following the disruption of intercostal muscles and the diaphragm as a consequence of either blunt [1-13] or penetrating trauma [5,13-15]. However, in elderly and demented patients TTIH following strenuous coughing have been reported [16-18]. To date, there are no published cases describing a TTIH complicated by strangulation of the herniated visceral contents. We report the case of a TTIH with associated strangulation and necrosis of segment VI of the liver.

* Correspondence: cino.bendinelli@hnehealth.nsw.gov.au
[1]Department of Traumatology, John Hunter Hospital, Newcastle, NSW, Australia

Statement of approval by Local Ethical Committee and patient was obtained.

Case report

Stage 1. Acute

A 61-year old man was admitted at Level 1 Trauma Centre, following a 3 metre fall from scaffolding onto a trestle stand. On arrival the patient showed normal vital signs and was complaining of pain in the right thoracoabdominal region, where a seriously injured skin mark and swelling was obvious. A right haemopneumothorax was identified on chest X-ray and treated with a 32Fr chest tube. Computer tomography (CT) with intravenous contrast demonstrated: right lung contusions, lateral 9th to 12th rib fractures with herniation of segment VI of the liver through an acquired defect in the 9th -10th intercostal space, a grade III liver laceration and a grade III laceration of right kidney without contrast extravasation. Medical history included: obesity, hypertension, and obstructive sleep apnoea requiring a continuous positive airway pressure device at night.

The initial management of these injuries was conservative. The patient required High Dependency Unit admission for non invasive ventilation, pain relief and aggressive chest physiotherapy. Follow-up CT (48 hours postinjury) demonstrated the absence of contrast enhancement suggesting strangulation of the herniated liver (Figure 1). Transaminases and all liver function test were only slightly elevated. Conservative management was successful and the patient was discharged 12 days post injury.

Stage 2. Sub Acute

At 45 days follow-up the patient presented with a large and painful collection (70 x 65 mm). This was treated with incision and drainage. About 50 ml of necrotic liver was debrided (Figure 2). Definitive repair of the TTIH was further postponed due to the risk of a prosthetic mesh infection. Intra-operative cultures taken however showed no growth.

Stage 3. Chronic

At 7 months follow-up, the patient presented with a large reducible TTIH (Figure 3). On CT, the defect measured 120 x 90 mm and the sac contained the hepatic flexure of the colon and a small part of the liver margin (Figure 4). The repair of the defect was planned in 2 months in order to allow full recovery from injury and optimization of body weight.

Definitive surgical repair was performed under general anaesthetic, with the patient on left lateral decubitus position. Laparoscopic port placement involved a 10 mm umbilical port, one 15 mm port and two 5 mm ports in

equidistant subcostal positions. After initial orientation, the hepatic flexure, the omentum and the liver margin were sharply dissected from the sac. Once the sac and its neck were clearly demonstrated, a 21.0x15.9 cm low profile polypropylene and expanded polytetrafluoroethylene (ePTFE) double mesh prosthesis (Bard® Composix® L/P Mesh, US) was used for the repair. Due to the proximity of the diaphragm to the defect, it was decided to use a combination of intracorporal suturing and endoscopic tacks. The caudal part of the mesh was secured to the abdominal wall with helical tacks (5 mm Protack® Autosuture® Tyco®, US). The cranial aspect of the mesh was sutured to the diaphragm with a continuous 1 braided polyester (CT-1 Ethibond®, US). The postoperative course was uneventful, with hospital discharge on the fourth postoperative day.

At the twelve months follow up after hernia repair the patient presented with some discomfort and features suggesting a recurrent hernia. CT confirmed the diagnosis and identified the presence of omentum in the sac.

At laparoscopic exploration the mesh appeared well embodied and completely peritonealised. There was a 2 x 2 cm defect between the abdominal wall and the lower

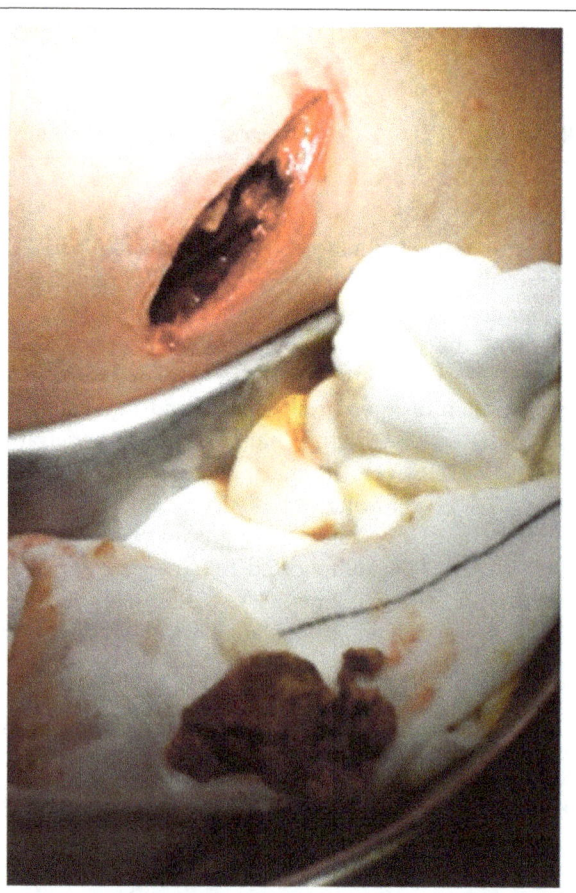

Figure 2 Incision and drainage of subcutaneous collection containing necrotic liver.

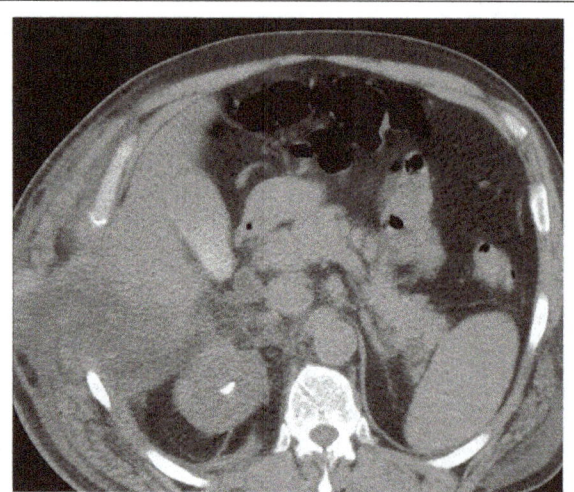

Figure 1 CT at 48 hours post injury: herniated segment VI of the liver without contrast enhancement, suggesting strangulation.

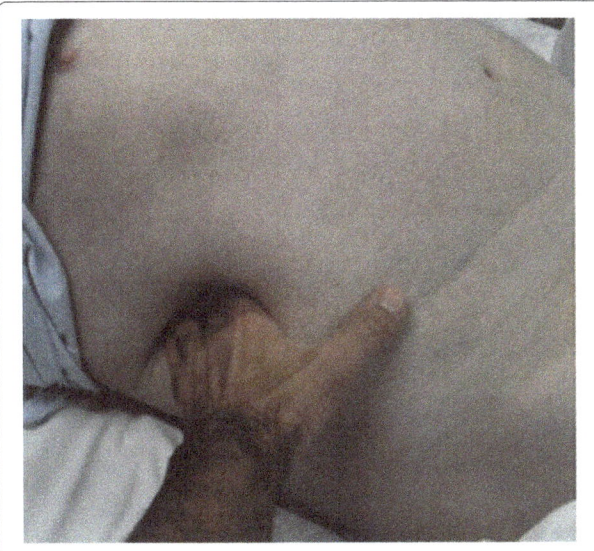

Figure 3 Easily reducible TTIH.

part of the mesh (due to failure of the endotack fixation). The omentum was reduced in the abdomen and the mesh sutured to abdominal wall by laparoscopic means. In order to increase the strength of the repair, the intercostal space was partially re-approximated with three figure of eight braided polyester stiches (CT-1 Ethibond®, US) through a 5 cm incision. The patient was discharged 48 hours post procedure with minimal discomfort. At the 12-month follow up after the second reconstructive procedure there was no evidence of recurrence.

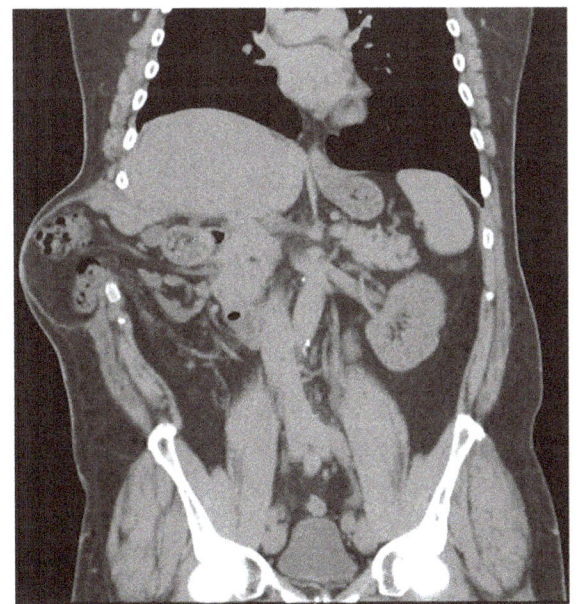

Figure 4 Coronal CT view: Hepatic colonic flexure and some liver tissue are included in the sac of TTIH.

Discussion

TTIH is rare sequelae of injury. In 1911 Gerster already challenged this concept. He reviewed 10 cases and concluded "that the occurrence of these herniae is not as rare as the few published communications on this subject would lead one to believe" [13]. TTIH are most commonly the result of penetrating injuries [5,13-15] or high energy and focused blunt strikes [1-13]. More frequently seen on the left side, TTIH may contain omentum, colon, spleen, stomach, and/or small bowel. The diagnosis of TTIH has historically been difficult to make, with delayed diagnosis to up to several years [5,13]. On initial clinical examination, intercostal hernias have been mistaken for lipomas or hematomas [3]. In these cases, it was not until a CT that the diagnosis of intercostal herniation was confirmed.

We know of no reports in the literature in which a TTIH was associated with liver strangulation. The closest, albeit clearly different, reported cases being a left TTIH due to coughing with infarcted omentum found at elective repair [16] and a patient with Chilaiditi's syndrome who required ileocecal resection during repair of a non-traumatic intercostal incisional hernia [22]. Conservative management of TTIH has been reported. Most often the patient presents with pain and increasing lump size and the repair is then considered [4].

The decision to elect the non-interventional approach despite liver strangulation was dictated by the patient's comorbidities, severe lung contusion, non-operatively managed abdominal solid organ injuries (kidney, liver), partial thickness skin necrosis and the lack of compromised liver function. More aggressive operative approach could have prevented later readmissions but also could have resulted in severe complications such as major bleeding, respiratory failure and wound/mesh infection. This dilemma cannot be addressed by case studies of this rare injury, but our example highlights what can be expected with conservative approach. Whether this is applicable to a given patient to a given time requires the informed judgement of the treating surgeon.

Several repair techniques have been described: endogenous tissue repair [8], prosthetic mesh reinforced by cable banding around the ribs [18], open transthoracic mesh repair [20] and tension free laparoscopic absorbable mesh repair [21]. We favoured the laparoscopic tension-free approach and the use of a non absorbable dual layer mesh. The choice of a running suture for mesh fixation to the diaphragm was based upon manufacturer warnings, which contraindicate helical tacks for use in tissues less than 4 mm thick. The thickness of the diaphragm has been measured by ultrasound as low as 2 mm [23]. As a matter of fact, a fatal injury of the heart has been reported during hiatus hernia repair with helical tack [24].

Conclusion

TTIH are rarely encountered and may be difficult to diagnose and treat without relevant imaging and pre-operative planning. Liver strangulation, if not treated promptly, results in liver necrosis and mandates a staged surgical management of TTIH. Laparoscopic tension-free repair with a permanent prosthetic mesh and the use of suture for fixation to diaphragm are keys for a successful outcome.

Competing interests

The authors declare that they have no competing interests.

Authors' contributions

CB and AM performed the surgical procedures and wrote the paper. SDN helped in data collection and in writing the paper. ZJB provided critical analysis and reviewed the paper. All authors read and approved the final manuscript.

Author details

[1]Department of Traumatology, John Hunter Hospital, Newcastle, NSW, Australia. [2]University of Newcastle, Newcastle, NSW, Australia.

References

1. Couso JL, Ladra MJ, Gómez AM, Pérez JA, Prim JM: Post-traumatic intercostal digestive hernia. *J Chir* 2009, **146:**189–190.
2. Bobbio A, Ampollini L, Prinzi G, Sarli L: Endoscopic repair of an abdominal intercostal hernia. *Surg Laparosc Endosc Percutan Tech* 2008, **18:**523–525.
3. Biswas S: Keddington J. Soft right chest wall swelling simulating lipoma following motor vehicle accident: transdiaphragmatic intercostal hernia. A case report and review of literature. *Hernia* 2008, **12:**539–543.
4. Smith E, Spain L, Ek E, Farrell S: Post-traumatic intercostal liver herniation. *ANZ J. Surg.* 2008, **78:**615–616.
5. Sharma OP, Duffy B: Transdiaphragmatic intercostal hernia: review of the world literature and presentation of a case. *J Trauma* 2001, **50:**1140–1143.
6. Hruska LA, Corry D, Kealey GP: Transdiaphragmatic intercostal hernia resulting from blunt trauma: case report. *J Trauma.* 1998, **45:**822–824.
7. Serpell JW, Johnson WR: Traumatic diaphragmatic hernia presenting as an intercostal hernia: case report. *J Trauma.* 1994, **36:**421–423.
8. Le Neel JC, Mousseau PA, Leborgne J, Horeau JM, Labour PE, Mousseau M: La hernie intercostale abdominale. Rapport de quatre observations. *Ann Chir* 1978, **32:**138–141 (French).
9. Guivarc'h M, Fournier F: La hernie intercostale abdominale: a propos d'un cas de hernie droite. *Chirurgie* 1978, **104:**149–158.
10. Testelin GM, Ledon F, Giordano A: A propos d'un cas de hernie intercostale abdominale. *Mem Acad Chir* 1970, **96:**569–570.
11. Herning MM, Maistre B: Hernie intercostale abdominale chez un Africain. *Mem Acad Chir* 1968, **94:**315–317.
12. Forestier MM: A propos d'un cas de hernie intercostale abdominale. *Mem Acad Chir* 1965, **91:**531–532.
13. Gerster JC: Intercostal diaphragmatic hernia: with report of a case. *Ann Surg.* 1911, **54:**538–548.
14. Balkan ME, Kara M, Oktar GL, Unlü E: Transdiaphragmatic intercostal hernia following a penetrating thoracoabdominal injury: report of a case. *Surg Today.* 2001, **31:**708–711.
15. Francis D, Barnsky WC: Intercostal herniation of abdominal contents following a penetrating chest injury. *Aust N Z J Surg.* 1979, **49:**357–358.
16. Rogers FB, Leavitt BJ, Jensen PE: Traumatic transdiaphragmatic intercostal hernia secondary to coughing: case report and review of the literature. *J Trauma.* 1996, **41:**902–903.
17. Kallay N, Crim L, Dunagan DP, Kavanagh PV, Meredith W, Haponik EF: Massive left diaphragmatic separation and rupture due to coughing during an asthma exacerbation. *South Med J.* 2000, **93:**729–731.
18. Losanoff JE, Richman BW, Jones JW: Recurrent intercostal herniation of the liver. *Ann Thorac Surg* 2004, **77:**699–701.
19. Losanoff JE, Richman BW, Jones JW: Transdiaphragmatic intercostal hernia: review of the world literature. *J Trauma* 2001, **51:**1218–1219.
20. Wu YS, Lin YY, Hsu CW, Chu SJ, Tsai SH: Massive ipsilateral pleural effusion caused by transdiaphragmatic intercostal hernia. *Am J Emerg Med.* 2008, **26:**252.
21. Kurer MA, Bradford IMJ: Laparoscopic repair of abdominal intercostal hernia: a case report and review of the literature. *Surg Laparosc Endosc Percutan Tech* 2006, **16:**270–271.
22. Rompen JC, Zeebregts CJ, Prevo RL, Klaase JM: Incarcerated transdiaphragmatic intercostal hernia preceded by Chilaiditi's syndrome. *Hernia.* 2005, **9:**198–200.
23. Ueki J, De Bruin PF, Pride NB: In vivo assessment of diaphragm contraction by ultrasound in normal subjects. *Thorax.* 1995, **50:**1157–1161.
24. ECRI: Patient injury or death could result from improper use of U.S. surgical helical tacks. *Health Devices* 2004, **33:**293–295.

14

Evaluation of gastrointestinal injury in blunt abdominal trauma "FAST is not reliable": the role of repeated ultrasonography

Afshin Mohammadi[1*] and Mohammad Ghasemi-rad[2]

Abstract

Background: To determine the diagnostic Accuracy of Focused Assessment Sonography for Trauma (FAST) and repeated FAST in the patients with blunt abdominal trauma.

Methods: In this retrospective study we collected the data of all patients from September 2007 to July 2011 with gastrointestinal injury. The intraoperative outcome was compared with FAST technique and the repeated or delayed sonography.

Results: A total number of 1550 patients with blunt abdominal trauma underwent FAST in a period of 4 years in our hospital. Eighty-eight (5.67%) patients were found to have gastrointestinal injury after exploratory laparotomy. Fifty-five (62.5%) patients had isolated gastrointestinal injury and 33 (37.5%) patients had concomitant injury to the other solid organs. In those with isolated gastrointestinal injury, the sensitivity of FAST was 38.5%. Repeated ultrsonography was performed in 34 patients with false negative initial FAST after 12-24 hours. The sensitivity of repeated ultrasonography in negative initial FAST patients in detection of gastrointestinal injury was 85.2% (95% CI, 68.1%, and 94.4%).

Conclusion: Repeated sonography after 12 to 24 hours in patients with negative initial FAST but sustain abdominal symptom can facilitated a diagnosis of GI tract injury and can be as effective method instead of Computed tomography in developing country.

Keywords: Ultrasonography, Gastrointestinal, Trauma, FAST

Background

Trauma is the most common cause of mortality in 1-45 year's age group [1]. Currently ultrasonography (US) is the primary method of screening patients with blunt abdominal trauma (BAT) worldwide [1-3]. Focused Assessment Sonography for Trauma (FAST) has been previously described for the evaluation of blunt abdominal trauma to observe the presence of free fluid in the abdomen or pelvis [4].

Although in some of the previous published literature they believe that it is rare to see false-negative results when screening with US (1%) [5,6]. It seems that screening BAT with FAST will lead to under diagnosis in

some abdominal injuries such as; retroperitoneal (pancreatic and adrenal), vascular injuries and diaphragmatic rupture that may have a negative impact on the patients outcome [7].

Due to subtle findings FAST has been reported to be of less value in detection of bowel and mesenteric injuries [8]. Although it is uncommon to develop hollow visceral organ injury after BAT but they are very important to diagnose, because there is no conservative treatment for these types of injuries and all of the patients with such injuries even in unequivocal cases, they need to undergo operative intervention [9]. According to the previous reports the morbidity of gastrointestinal tract injury is mostly related to delays diagnosis [10].

Because of less availability of computed tomography in developing country, the purpose of our study was to determine the role of repeated abdominal US in the

* Correspondence: Mohamadi_Afshin@yahoo.com
[1]Department of Radiology, Urmia University of Medical Sciences, Urmia, West-Azerbaijan, Iran

patients with negative " FAST "to early diagnose hollow viscous organ injury in patients with BAT. To our best knowledge this is the first report evaluating the role of repeated abdominal sonography to determine and reduce missed gastrointestinal injury by FAST technique.

Methods

This retrospective study was started from September 2007 to July 2011. On thousand five hundred and fifty emergency ultrasonography with FAST technique were performed in our University hospital in order to detect free intra-abdominal fluid as an indicator of intra-abdominal organ injury in-patient with BAT (Figure 1, 2).

The outcome of FAST technique and the data regarding type of abdominal injuries were obtained by retrospectively going through patient's operation notes. After retrospectively reviewing the operation record of 1550 BAT patients, 88 were found to have gastrointestinal injury. This study was performed in Imam training University Hospital that serves as the only trauma referral center in our provenance. University review board and ethic committee approved the study.

All the injured patients were referred to our center, maximum one hour after trauma and US examination was performed during first 30 minutes of admission. Examination was performed by one radiologist in the department of radiology at the emergency room. FAST technique was performed by using Sonoline G 40 ultrasound devise (Siemens, Germany) with 3.5-5 MHZ convex transducer. Six areas of the abdomen were examined to detect free fluid; left upper quadrant (LUQ), Morrison pouch, right upper quadrant (RUQ), pelvis, right and left para-colic gutters.

Abdomen and pelvic spiral Computed Tomography (CT) Scan examinations were performed only with IV contrast (Toshiba; X-vision scanner) in 39 patients with BAT and negative FAST after 12-24 hours due to worsening of clinical problem but stable hemodynamic condition.

Spiral CT scans were performed with 10-mm collimation and a table speed of 10 mm/sec. Images were reconstructed at 7-mm intervals. In adults, a total of 120 ml of Iohexol (Omnipaque, 300 mg/50 cc) was administered intravenously at a rate of 3-4 ml/sec. Another experienced radiologist interpreted all of the abdominal CT scans.

The routine protocol in our center is that every patient with suspected abdominal trauma should undergo FAST. Except for those patients that further delaying to intervene to undergo FAST is not possible and the patients need to directly go to the operation room. Those patients with unstable hemodynamics and observable fluid in the peritoneal cavity should immediately undergo laparotomy. Patients with stable hemodynamics and positive sonography will undergo conservative management and close observation.

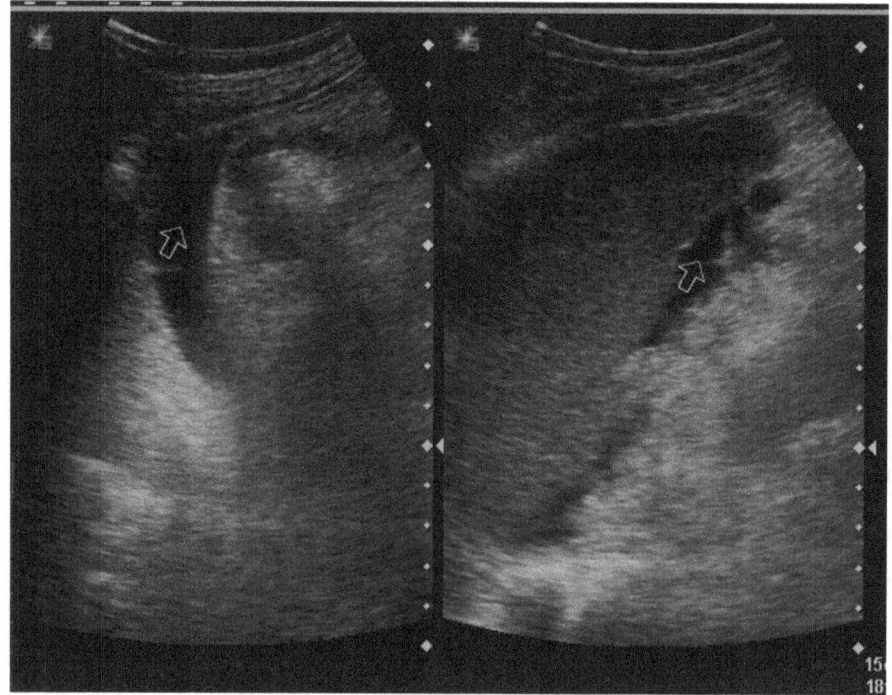

Figure 1 Longitudinal sonogram show free fluid (arrow) associated with Ileal perforation in pelvic cavity.

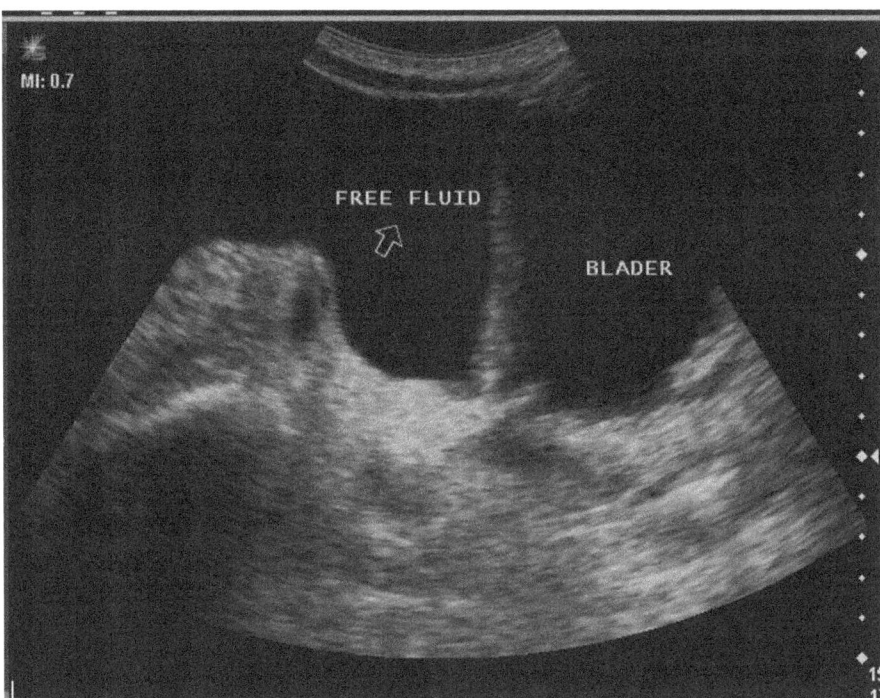

Figure 2 Ultrasonogram revealed free fluid in the paracolic gutter (right) and perisplenic (left).

Those with negative clinical signs and negative FAST are not followed by any other diagnostic methods. But in those patients with negative FAST and constant abdominal pain and stable hemodynamic due to shortage of intravenous contrast material in our center they have to undergo repeated FAST after 12 to 24 hours.

The results of FAST technique were compared with surgical results. Statistical analysis was performed to determine the sensitivity and 95% confidence interval were calculated and used for determining the diagnostic accuracy.

Results

Out of 1550 patients with BAT a total number of 352 patients (44%) underwent operation. Eighty- eight (5.67%) patients had gastrointestinal injury in exploratory laparotomy (66 (75%) were male and 22 (25%) were female).

The mean age was 28.9 ± 16.5 years (Age range: 3-80 Years). Seventy-one (80.6%) patients had abdominal tenderness during primary physical examination. Forty-seven (53%) patients had stable hemodynamic condition and 41 (46.5%) patients were hypotensive at the time of US examination.

Fifty-five (62.5%) patients had isolated gastrointestinal injury and 33 (37.5%) patients had concomitant injury to the other solid organ such as spleen (n = 14), liver

(n = 13), Diaphragm (n = 2), Pancreas (n = 2) and kidney (n = 2).

Emergency US with FAST technique was positive for free fluid in 49 (55.6%) patients (True positive) and was negative (false negative) in 39 (44.3%) patients with gastrointestinal injury.

From 49 patients with true positive FAST, 28 (57.1%) patients had solid organ injury concomitant with bowel injury and 21 (42.8%) patients had isolated gastrointestinal injury. A total of 55 (62.5%) out of 88 patients had isolated bowel injury; FAST exam was positive only in 21 (38.1%) patients (True positive) and was negative in 34 (61.8%) patients. In 34 patients with isolated gastrointestinal injury FAST was negative for free fluid (False negative).

In 39 (44.3%) patients with BAT that the result of emergency US did not show free intra peritoneal fluid in 34 patients, the underwent conservative management and after 12-24 hours serial physical examination showed abdominal tenderness and guarding and worsening of abdominal pain. Upon repeated ultrasonography there was free intra-peritoneal fluid in 29 patients and negative results in 10 patients. All those patients (39 patients) underwent abdominal and pelvic CT, which revealed hollow viscous organ injury in 24 (61.5%) patients. In 15 (38.4%) patients CT examination did not show gastrointestinal injury (false negative) all of which underwent surgical operation because of sustained guarding and unstable hemodynamic condition.

The sensitivity of FAST for detection of gastrointestinal injury in those patients with isolated gastrointestinal injury, the sensitivity was 38.5% (95% CI, 23.2%, and 53.7%).

From 34 patients with negative initial FAST the repeated ultrasonography revealed free fluid in 29 patients and was negative in 5 patients then the sensitivity of repeated ultrasonography in negative initial FAST in detection of gastrointestinal injury was 85.2% (95% CI, 68.1%, and 94.4%).

The sensitivity of CT for the detection of specific sign of gastrointestinal injury such as free air and bowel thickening in the entire study group was 61.5% (95% CI, .44.6%, 76.1%).

The distribution of gastrointestinal injury in these 88 patients is presented in table 1 and distribution of concomitant solid organ injury is presented in table 2.

Discussion

Rapid diagnosis and treatment of abdominal injury is an important step to prevent death in BAT patients [1].

Physical examination is frequently unreliable in the setting of acute trauma [11].

Many of the previous reports show that emergency ultrasound is effective in diagnosis of hemo-peritoneum [1,12-14]. Now FAST technique has gained popularity and is been accepted as a diagnostic modality for evaluation of patients with trauma [1,10-15]. Our previous experience showed that sensitivity of FAST in the diagnosis of BAT is 95.4%[1].

MacGahan et al reported free fluid in only three patients with isolated bowel and mesenteric injury in a series of 500 trauma patients [7]. There are several articles pointing that some important abdominal organ injury can be missed by ultrasonography. Dolich et al reported a large number of abdominal injuries (33%), which required operation and were missed in US examination [16].

Table 1 table shows the distribution of gastrointestinal injury in trauma

Location	Number	Total
Small bowel		71
Duodenum	7	
Jejunum	36	
Ileum	28	
Large bowel		17
Ascending colon	3	
Sigmoid colon	10	
Transverse colon	4	

Table 2 table shows the distribution of concomitant solid organ injury is trauma patients

Location	Number
Spleen	14
Liver	13
Kidney	2
Diaphragm	2
Pancreas	2

Shanmuganathan et al showed that 34%(157 patients) of 467 patients with BAT had no free fluid in emergency US [13]. He studied more than 11,000 patients with BAT and concluded that the FAST technique may frequently miss patients with surgically correctable injuries.

Previous reports are indicative of a limited value for FAST in the diagnosis of certain type of injuries such as; diaphragmatic rupture [17], pancreatic [15] and mesenteric injury [18-20].

MacGahan JP et al demonstrated a sensitivity of 44% for diagnosis of isolated gastrointestinal injury by FAST [21]. They also showed that free abdominal fluid was not detected in the majority of patients with isolated bowel and mesenteric injury. Observation, serial physical abdominal examination, Clinical suspicion for bowel and mesenteric injury and CT can all be of help to diagnose intra-abdominal organ injuries.

In our study 39 patients with negative initial US examination and persistent abdominal pain and tenderness underwent repeated ultrasonography after a period of 12-24 hours. Repeated US detected free intra-peritoneal fluid in 29 patients.

Diagnosing gastrointestinal trauma is difficult based on emergency rooms physical examination [19-21] and necessitates using other imaging modality such as CT scan [22,23].

CT has been reported to have a sensitivity ranging from 93-100% in detection of bowel and mesenteric injury. Mirvis et al prospectively detected bowel and mesenteric injury in 17 (100%) patients undergoing laparotomy [22].

Atri et al showed that sensitivity of the three observers in diagnoses of surgically important bowel or mesenteric injury by CT scan ranged from 87%-95% [23]. They concluded that multi-detector CT has high negative predictive value and can accurately show important bowel or mesenteric injuries.

Levine et al [24] reported that only bowel wall thickening and free air were specific finding in the CT scanning (Figure 3).

And other sign such as, free fluid are nonspecific not reliable to differentiate between bowel and solid organ injuries.

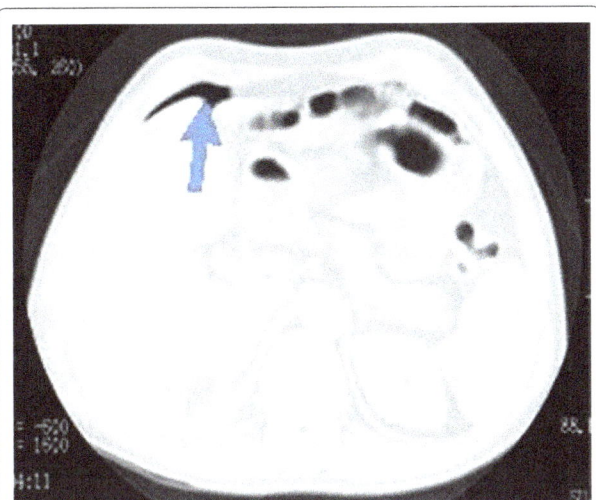

Figure 3 Abdominal CT scan with lung window shows free air adjacent to liver edge due to colon perforation.

trauma and persistent abdominal pain and tenderness, which can reduce the risk of missing major intra-abdominal injuries.

List of abbreviations
CT: Computed tomography; FAST: Focused Assessment of Sonography for Trauma.

Acknowledgements
Urmia University of Medical Sciences supported this research.

Author details
[1]Department of Radiology, Urmia University of Medical Sciences, Urmia, West-Azerbaijan, Iran. [2]Student research committee, Urmia University of medical Sciences. Urmia, Iran.

Authors' contributions
All the authors in this manuscript have read and approve the final manuscript. AM: Concept, design and the Ultrasonographic studies MG: Manuscript writing and editing and Data analysis.

Competing interests
The authors declare that they have no competing interests.

The sensitivity of CT for diagnosis of gastrointestinal trauma in our study is lower compare to other studies [22,23,25], because they used multi-detector CT that is more accurate in diagnosis of GI tract pathology.

McGahan JP et al reported that 49% of the patients with gastrointestinal injury had concomitant injury to other solid organs. The results of our study showed that 38% patients with blunt abdominal trauma had concomitant solid organ injury.

In our study jejunum and ileum were the most common sites of gastrointestinal trauma respectively. The most common solid organ injury concomitant with gastrointestinal trauma was spleen followed by the liver, which were similar to the report by Richards JL et al [18].

The limitations of our study are; single detector CT which can miss some of the intra-abdominal injuries, the retrospective part of the study which we might have missed some of the data in the records, patients with subtle injury such as mild intestinal hematoma may not show clinical symptom and could be missed because they did not underwent repeated abdominal sonography, Inability to calculate the specificity, positive predictive and negative predictive value Since the small injuries could not be seen and consequently are not going to the be operated on.

It is difficult to diagnose gastrointestinal trauma when FAST is performed immediately after admission. As is shown in our report only 38.5% of the patients with free fluid in the abdomen on initial FAST had isolated gastrointestinal trauma. We recommend performing a serial US when CT is not available in-patient suspected of GI

References
1. Mohammadi A, Daghighi MH, Poorisa M, Afrasiabi K, Pedram A: Diagnostic Accuracy of Ultrasonography in Blunt Abdominal Trauma. *Iran J Radiol* 2008, **5(3)**:135-139.
2. Brown MA, Casola G, Sirlin CB, Budorick N, Patel N, Hoyt DB: Blunt abdominal trauma: screening US in 2,693 patients. *Radiology* 2001, **218**:352-358.
3. Brown MA, Sirlin CB, Hoyt DB, Casola G: Screening ultrasound in blunt abdominal trauma. *J Intensive Care Med* 2003, **18**:253-260.
4. McGahan JP, Richards J, Gillen M: The focused abdominal sonography for trauma scan: pearls and pitfalls. *J Ultrasound Med* 2002, **21**:789-800.
5. Pinto F, Bignardi E, Pinto A, Rizzo A, Scaglione M, Romano L: Ultrasound in the triage of patients after blunt abdominal trauma: our experience in 3,500 consecutive patients. *Radiology* 2002, **225**:358.
6. Sirlin CB, Casola G, Brown MA, Patel N, Bendavid EJ, Hoyt DB: Quantification of fluid on screening ultrasonography for blunt abdominal trauma: a simple scoring system to predict severity of injury. *J Ultrasound Med* 2001, **20**:359-366.
7. McGahan JP, Rose J, Coates TL, Wisner DH, Newberry P: Use of sonography in the patient with acute abdominal trauma. *J Ultrasound Med* 1997, **16**:653-662.
8. Lee BC, Ormsby EL, McGahan JP, Melendres GM, Richards JR: The utility of sonography for the triage of blunt abdominal trauma patients to exploratory laparotomy. *AJR Am J Roentgenol* 2007, **188(2)**:415-21.
9. Hughes TM: The diagnosis of gastrointestinal tract injuries resulting from blunt abdominal trauma. *Aust NZ J Surg* 1999, **69**:770-777.
10. Wisner DH, Chun Y, Blaisdell FW: Blunt intestinal injury. *Arch Surg* 1990, **125**:1319-23.
11. Schurink GW, Bode PJ, van Luijt PA, van Vugt AB: The value of physical examination in the diagnosis of patients with blunt abdominal trauma: a retrospective study. *Injury* 1997, **28**:261-265.
12. McKenney M, Lentz K, Nunez D, *et al*: Can Ultrasound replace diagnostic peritoneal lavage in the assessment of blunt trauma? *J Trauma* 1994, **37**:439-441.
13. Shanmuganathan K, Mirvis SE, Sherbourne CD, Chiu WC, Rodriguez A: Hemoperitoneum as the sole indicator of abdominal visceral injuries: a potential limitation of screening abdominal US for trauma. *Radiology* 1999, **212**:423-430.
14. Bode PJ, Edwards MJR, Kruit MC, Van Vugt AB: Sonography in a clinical algorithm for early evaluation of 1671 patients with blunt abdominal trauma. *AJR Am J Roentgenol* 1999, **172**:905-911.

15. McGahan JP, Richards JR: **Blunt abdominal trauma: the role of emergent sonography and a review of the literature.** *AJR Am J Roentgenol* 1999, 172:897-930.

16. Dolich MO, McKenney MG, Varela JE, Compton RP, McKenney KL, Cohn SM: **2,576 ultrasounds for blunt abdominal trauma.** *J Trauma* 2001, 50:108-112.

17. Simpson J, Lobo DN, Shah AB, Rowlands BJ: **Traumatic diaphragmatic rupture: associated injuries and outcome.** *Ann R Coll Surg Engl* 2000, 82:97-100.

18. Richards JR, McGahan JP, Simpson JL, Tabar P: **Bowel and mesenteric injury: evaluation with emergency abdominal US.** *Radiology* 1999, 211:399-403.

19. Bensard DD, Beaver BL, Besner GE, Cooney DR: **Small bowel injury in children after blunt abdominal trauma: is diagnostic delay important?** *J Trauma* 1996, 41:476-483.

20. Burney RE, Mueller GL, Coon GL, *et al*: **Diagnosis of isolated small bowel injury following blunt abdominal trauma.** *Ann Emerg Med* 1983, 12:71-74.

21. Bloom AI, Rivkind A, Zamir G, *et al*: **Blunt injury of the small intestine and mesentery: the trauma surgeon's Achilles heel?** *Eur J Emerg Med* 1996, 3:85-91.

22. Mirvis SE, Gens DR, Shanmuganathan K: **Rupture of the bowel after blunt abdominal trauma: diagnosis with CT.** *AJR* 1992, 159:1217-1223.

23. Atri M, Hanson JM, Grinblat L, Brofman N, Chugtai T, Tomlinson G: **Surgically important bowel and/or mesenteric injury in blunt trauma: accuracy of multidetector CT for evaluation.** *Radiology* 2008, 249(2):524-33.

24. Levine CD, Gonzales RN, Wachsberg RH, Ghanekar D: **CT findings of bowel and mesenteric injury.** *J Comput Assist Tomogr* 1997, 21(6):974-9.

25. Breen DJ, Janzen DL, Zwirewich CV, Nagy AG: **Blunt bowel and mesenteric injury:diagnostic performance of CT sings.** *J Comput Assist Tomogr* 1997, 21:706-712.

15

Negative pressure wound therapy management of the "open abdomen" following trauma

Pradeep Navsaria[1], Andrew Nicol[1], Donald Hudson[1], John Cockwill[2] and Jennifer Smith[3*]

Abstract

Introduction: The use of Negative Pressure Wound Therapy (NPWT) for temporary abdominal closure of open abdomen (OA) wounds is widely accepted. Published outcomes vary according to the specific nature and the aetiology that resulted in an OA. The aim of this study was to evaluate the effectiveness of a new NPWT system specifically used OA resulting from abdominal trauma.

Methods: A prospective study on trauma patients requiring temporary abdominal closure (TAC) with grade 1or 2 OA was carried out. All patients were treated with NPWT (RENASYS AB Smith & Nephew) to achieve TAC. The primary outcome measure was time taken to achieve fascial closure and secondary outcomes were complications and mortality.

Results: A total of 20 patients were included. Thirteen patients (65%) achieved fascial closure following a median treatment period of 3 days. Four patients (20%) died of causes unrelated to NPWT. Complications included fistula formation in one patient (5%) with spontaneous resolution during NPWT), bowel necrosis in a single patient (5%) and three cases of infection (15%). No fistulae were present at the end of NPWT.

Conclusion: This new NPWT kit is safe and effective and results in a high rate of fascial closure and low complication rates in the severely injured trauma patient.

Keywords: Negative Pressure Wound Therapy (NPWT), Grade 1 and 2 open abdomen, Abdominal trauma, Fascial closure

Introduction

Management of the open abdomen is an area of medicine which has expanded rapidly over the last 20 years [1] and has resulted in decreased mortality rates [2]. The benefits of managing patients with open abdomens include prevention of intra-abdominal hypertension (IAH) and abdominal compartment syndrome (ACS), early identification of intra-abdominal complications (e.g. bowel ischemia) and ease of re-entry. Despite these benefits, maintenance of an open abdomen creates numerous management challenges such as development of fistula and infection. Prolonged maintenance of an open abdomen may also lead to a reduced chance of re-approximation of the fascia, as abdominal contents become 'fixed'. With increasing adoption of open abdomen techniques has come an increased

demand for Temporary Abdominal Closure (TAC) methods to protect the Open Abdomen during the phase of open treatment. Principal techniques for TAC are: Negative Pressure Wound Therapy (NPWT), Vacuum-Pac method ("Vac" Pac), artificial burr (Whitmann™ patch), absorbable mesh/sheet, zipper, "plastic silo", skin closure and dynamic retention sutures. These techniques vary in their efficacy with regard to fascial closure rates, associated morbidity and mortality rates. A number of systematic reviews have concluded that the artificial burr and NPWT have the highest fascial closure and lowest mortality rates [3,4]. Because of its relative ease of application, and preservation of fascial tissue, NPWT is becoming a dominant choice for TAC in the open abdomen patient [1].

TAC can be appropriate in the treatment of OA derived from a wide range of traumatic, post-operative and septic clinical scenarios. Together these form a complex and diverse group of wounds. Much of the published literature

* Correspondence: jennifer.smith@smith-nephew.com
[3]Smith & Nephew, 101 Hessle Road, Hull HU3 2BN, UK

describing outcomes in OA is difficult to interpret due to grouping together of these heterogeneous clinical scenarios with widely varying aetiologies, prognoses and even treatment goals. This leads to highly variable reported outcomes and complication rates. The rate of fascial closure in open abdomen patients treated with NPWT has been reported as low as 22% [5] (in pancreatitis) and as high as 92% [6] (in trauma). In order to understand how outcomes and potentially treatment protocols vary in different types of open abdomen patients, researchers must first publish results from homogenous and well-defined subgroups. The World Society of Abdominal Compartment Syndrome (WSACS) has proposed a simple clinical classification for describing the open abdomen (Bjorck et al.) [7] in order to facilitate comparison of study outcomes and clinical approach (see Table 1). The aim of the current study was to use the Bjorck classification to report outcomes of a well-defined group of patients, (with grade 1 or 2 open abdomens derived from traumatic injury) following treatment with a recently introduced NPWT system for TAC in the open abdomen. A systematic review of the literature, identifying studies with comparable homogenous study populations, was carried out as a means of comparing results from this study with results from the literature.

Methods
Temporary abdominal closure
A prospective, open labelled, non-comparative study was carried out in two centres in South Africa between August 2010 and December 2011. Consecutive patients presenting with traumatic injury and 1) requiring damage control laparotomy with staged abdominal repair; or 2) developing abdominal compartment syndrome requiring laparotomy and temporary abdominal closure; or 3) with full thickness traumatic abdominal wall defects with exposed viscera requiring temporary abdominal closure were assessed for inclusion into the study. Patients with grade 1a,1b or 2a, 2b open abdomen, as classified by Bjorck et al. [7] (Table 1) were suitable for inclusion. The following exclusion criteria were also applied: <18 years, pregnant, malignancy in wound bed, unexplored fistulas, high risk for imminent death (as determined by the treating surgeon), pre-existing large ventral hernia, significant loss of abdominal wall fascia as a result of trauma or infection,

patients with grade 4 open abdomen (Bjorck et al. classification, see Table 1), patients with a known history of poor compliance with medical treatment and any patients who had previously been withdrawn from the study. The trial was approved by local ethics boards at both institutions and was carried out in strict accordance with the Helsinki declaration. Informed consent was obtained where possible from the patient, but if the patient was incapable, the patient's legal representative was asked to provide consent on the patient's behalf. If this was not possible then independent physician consent was considered acceptable as approved by the local ethics committee. All patient information was anonymised at source.

Patients suitable for inclusion underwent initial damage control laparotomy, where initial control of haemorrhage and contamination was performed. This was followed by intra-peritoneal packing when required and TAC. Further resuscitation to near normal physiology in the intensive care unit (ICU) was continued. Re-laparotomy was performed at 48 hours or earlier if indicated. Negative pressure wound therapy (RENASYS-AB Abdominal Dressing and RENASYS EZ pump Smith & Nephew; St Petersburg, FL, USA) was applied to the wound in the following way. A fenestrated non adherent film was placed directly over the exposed viscera but under the rectus sheath. Polyurethane foam was then reduced along pre-cut perforations to the appropriate size and placed on top of the film within the open abdomen. A transparent film then covered the foam and the surrounding peri-wound skin before a suction port was connected to the NPWT pump. Negative pressure was delivered at a continuous -80 mmHg. The trial comprised a maximum of 20 days of treatment with the NPWT system with an additional 8 day post-treatment initiation follow up. Dressing changes usually took place at 48 hours during re-laparotomy for removal of packs and re-establishment of bowel continuity. Full medical and wound assessments were made. Wound closure was carried out when possible and at the discretion of the attending trauma surgeon.

The primary objective was to determine the number of days taken to achieve delayed primary fascial closure. Secondary objectives were mortality, change in OA classification, intra-abdominal pressure (IAP), length of stay (days) in ICU and hospital, incidence of complications

Table 1 Open abdomen classification

Grade 1A	Clean OA without adherence between bowel and abdominal wall or fixity of the abdominal wall (lateralization of the abdominal wall).
Grade 1B	Contaminated OA without adherence/fixity
Grade 2A	Clean OA developing adherence/fixity
Grade 2B	Contaminated OA developing adherence/fixity
Grade 3	OA complicated by fistula formation
Grade 4	Frozen OA with adherent bowel, unable to close surgically, with or without fistula

Adapted from Bjorck et al. [7].

(abdominal compartment syndrome (ACS), fistula formation, sepsis, multiple organ failure (MOF), acute respiratory distress syndrome (ARDS)). SOFA, APACHE, ISS, NISS scores were also recorded.

Statistical evaluation

Kaplan-Meier estimate of the median time to achieve primary fascial closure by treatment discontinuation was presented. McNemar's test was used to test for a reduction in the presence of infection from baseline to final assessment. All other outcomes were summarised using descriptive statistics.

Systematic review

The PRISMA guidelines were used as a guide in designing the systematic review process [8]. The following PubMed search [("open abdomen" OR "abdominal compartment syndrome" OR laparotomy) AND ("negative pressure wound therapy" OR NPWT OR "Vacuum assisted" OR VAC OR "vac pack" OR "vacuum pack") NOT review] was carried out in April 2010 and updated in April 2011 and May 2012. These studies were reviewed manually and the following types were excluded: paediatric studies, studies where greater than 33% of patients had open abdomen wounds with advanced sepsis at baseline; Grade 4 wounds at baseline; Case reviews (fewer than 6 cases). Although the majority of studies did not classify the wounds according to Bjorck et al. [7], an attempt was made to classify them retrospectively based on the patient data provided. All studies carried out on non-septic Grade 1 or 2 open abdomen wounds were included regardless of aetiology. Raw data was extracted from all the papers. Outcomes (fascial closure, mortality and fistula) were expressed as a percentage of the total numbers of patients treated in order to minimise bias based on different sample sizes. This approach also corrected inherent reporting bias in several of the studies relating to whether data took numbers of deceased patients into account (i.e. expressed outcomes as a percentage of the entire cohort and not just percentage of survivors).

Results

Patients

Twenty trauma patients undergoing damage control laparotomy were recruited (see Table 2 for demographic and baseline wound details). Injury severity was measured by the Injury Severity Score (ISS) with a median value of 25 (range 9–50). An ISS of >15 (a measure of severe trauma) was present in 17/20 patients. Four (20%) patients died during the study period; One patient achieved primary fascial closure, but died following a cardiac arrest before the end of study period. Two other patients died as a result of acute renal failure and the remaining patient died as a result of multi-organ failure. Data for all 20 patients

Table 2 Patient and wound characterisation at baseline

Age; median (range)	31.4 years (22 – 44)
Male (% patients)	90%
BMI; median (range)	26.3 kg/m^2 (17.7 – 50.8)
Injury Type (% patients)	
• Blunt trauma	50% (10/20)
• Penetrating Trauma	50% (10/20)
Injury scores (median (range)	
• SOFA	11 (0–17)
• APACHE II	14.5 (3–25)
• ISS	25 (9–50)
• NISS	33 (13–66)
IAP (# patients)	
• <12 mmHg	10
• >12 mmHg (IAH)	10

IAP = intra-abdominal pressure; IAH = intra-abdominal hypertension as defined by Cheatham et al. 2007 [9].

was included in all evaluations on an 'intention to treat' basis, unless specified.

Primary objective - fascial closure rate

Fascial closure was achieved in 13 out of 20 patients (65% of patients on an intent-to-treat basis) (see Table 3; see supplemental data for Kaplan-Meier estimate data). Fascial closure rate expressed as the percentage of survivors was 75% (12/16 patients) (data not shown). One patient died following fascial closure but the remaining 12 closed abdomens were stable at a follow up 8 days after closure although a superficial wound sepsis was present in one. The median time to achieve primary fascial closure was 3 days (CI) (n=20). Two patients were withdrawn from the study after 19 and 24 days of NPWT therapy because they developed a Grade 4 (fixed) abdomen and fascial closure was no longer an option (i.e. they could no longer contribute to the primary objective). Each open abdomen was

Table 3 Progression of open abdominal wounds from initial presentation to end of therapy

Grade	Baseline	End of therapy
Closed	0	13 (65%)
1a	14 (70.0%)	2 (10%)
1b	5 (25.0%)	1 (5%)
2	1 (5.0%)	2 (10%)
2c	0	0
3	0	0
4	0	2 (10%)
N	20 (100%)	20 (100%)*

Progress of the wounds during therapy was assessed using the Bjorck et al. classification system. *one patient died less than 24 hours after having a baseline assessment. As no other data was available, it was assumed that the wound grade at death was the same as the baseline assessment (Grade 1A).

graded according to the WSACS classification [7] (Table 1) at the initial application of NPWT and at each subsequent dressing change, including the final removal of the dressing. The grade of open abdomen for the majority of patients improved during the course of therapy.

Secondary objectives

SOFA and APACHE11 scores decreased from medians of 11 and 14.5 at baseline to 9 and 12 respectively at the end of therapy. There was no apparent relationship between IAP at baseline and achievement of fascial closure. Median time in ICU was 8 days (range 1–28 days, n=20). In the remaining patients, reasons for discontinuation of NPWT were death, (3/20; 15%), poor compliance (1/20; 5%), withdrawal for other reasons (1/20; 5% - persistent bowel hematic as a consequence of an extremely large viscera). Fluid contained in the waste canister was approximately measured and this formed part of the daily fluid management of the patient. A mean volume of 871 ml (median 700 ml) was present in the canister at dressing change. Blood loss into the canister was also an early sign of internal bleeding and allowed rapid intervention (data not shown).

A range of complications were assessed and results are shown in Table 4. One fistula (5%) was observed during the study in a single patient who had received penetrating trauma. This low output fistula was observed during the second dressing change but had resolved by the next dressing change (48 hours later). No trauma was observed on removal of any of the dressing components and was therefore unlikely that adhesion of the dressing to the bowel had contributed towards the fistula formation.

Bowel necrosis was found in two patients (10%). One instance was present at baseline and was resolved prior to application of NPWT following surgical removal of 90 cm length of bowel. This patient went on to achieve fascial closure within 3 days of injury. The second instance of bowel necrosis developed at the second dressing change during the study in a patient who had a septic abdomen at baseline with a moderate degree of oedema. This patient died as a result of multi-organ failure due to sepsis and as a result of late presentation. The development of bowel necrosis was not believed to be related to the use of the NPWT device.

At baseline assessment, 5 patients had severe contamination of the abdominal cavity due to intestinal spillage. In 3 patients the contamination was controlled and there were no sign of contamination or infection by treatment discontinuation. The remaining 2 patients developed a clinically infected wound along with a further 3 patients during the course of the study. One patient, despite fistula resolution (as described above), became persistently infected preventing wound closure. The wound degraded into a grade 4 (fixed) open abdomen and was closed with a graft. A second patient with a grade 1a abdomen was progressing well but became confused and removed the dressing resulting in wound infection and withdrawal of the patient for non-compliance. The third patient who developed infection also developed bowel oedema throughout the study and evisceration. This was in part due to unusually large viscera. Therefore, at treatment discontinuation 5 patients' abdominal wounds were clinically infected.

Case study

A 27 year old male with no significant medical history was admitted 18th October, 2010 with blunt trauma to the abdomen as a result of assault. A midline laparotomy for damage control was performed (Figure 1A). Severe contamination of the peritoneal cavity due to hollow viscous injury were apparent. Intra-abdominal pressure (IAP) was 15 mmHg and abdominal perfusion pressure (APP) was 58 mmHg. Injury scores were as follows: SOFA 11, APACHE 5, ISS 25 and NISS 48. The wound was classified as a grade 1b and was complicated by the presence of necrotic bowel. Ninety centimetres of bowel were removed surgically (Figure 1B) before the NPWT dressing was applied (Figure 1C) with the intention of performing a second look laparotomy to ensure no progression of bowel necrosis. NPWT pressure was applied at -80 mmHg continuous pressure. 800 ml of ascites was removed. Active resuscitation for 24 hours was required at which point a re-laparotomy was performed in order to view the rectal stump and rigid sigmoidoscopy. A second re-laparotomy was required at 48 hours (Figure 1D). The abdomen was closed by delayed primary fascial closure on Day 3 (Figure 1E) with no further complications.

Table 4 Number of patients developing abdominal wound related complications

Complication	Incidence		
	Baseline	End of therapy*	At any point during therapy
Fistula	0	0	1 (5%)
Bowel necrosis	1 (5%)	1 (5.3%)	2 (10%)
Bowel evisceration	4 (20%)	2 (10.5%)	5 (25%)
Infection / sepsis	5 (25%)	5 (26.3%)	8 (40%)

The incidence of complications was recorded per patient. N=20 except * (where n=19 due to one patient dying after having a baseline assessment).

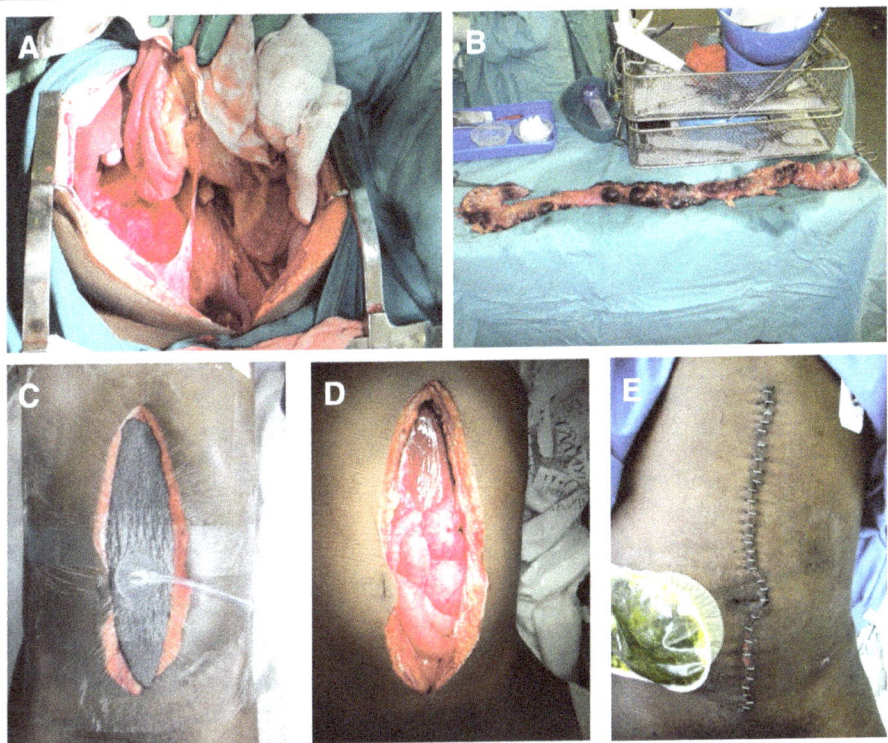

Figure 1 A 27 year old male was admitted with blunt abdominal trauma. A damage control laparotomy was performed **(A)**, 90 cm of necrotic bowel removed **(B)** and NPWT (Renasys F-AB, Smith & Nephew) applied at -80 mmHg **(C)**. Second look lapartomies were performed at 24 and 48 hours **(D)** and the fascia closed at Day 3 post injury **(E)**.

Comparison with published literature

In order to compare the results presented here with the existing literature, a systematic search was carried out. Table 5 shows the process of the systematic search. Briefly 129 papers were identified, of which 49 passed the selection criteria and were appropriate for detailed review. Of these, a further 13 did not report relevant end-points. Of the remaining 36 papers, studies where >33% of the study population was septic were excluded because the presence of sepsis has a significant effect on the prognosis and outcomes of the open abdomen patient [10]. In the present study, 25% of wounds at baseline were infected or contaminated. Studies using 'home-made' NPWT systems (i.e. vac-pack) were excluded to avoid any variability in outcomes resulting from variability in components or technique of application. Vac-pack has also been reported to have slightly less effective outcomes compared to VAC [4,11] therefore commercial NPWT provided a good

Table 5 Systematic review chart

Total number of papers identified		129
Reason for exclusion	Duplications	4
	In vivo studies	9
	Paediatric	4
	Significant modification to application technique	14
	Irrelevant clinical area	21
	Reviews/comments/letters	9
	Case series <6	18
Number of papers reviewed		**48**
Reason for exclusion	No relevant endpoints	13
	Vac-pack removed *	13
	Cohorts with >33% septic	15
Number of remaining papers		**8**

*papers describing results with a non-commercial NPWT technique known as 'vac-pack' were excluded.

benchmark. Open abdomen wounds from all aetiologies were theoretically included but in practice the majority of studies reported traumatic patients with only 2 studies reporting mixed cohorts of patients.

Results of the comparison between the present study and relevant articles identified from the systematic review are shown in Table 6. The identified studies are relatively small in size with a mean patient number of 30. Demographic variables (ISS, age, gender) were acceptably similar between this study and the reported studies (data not shown). Overall, mean fascial closure rates of 63.7% were reported; a close match with the mean value of 65% reported in the current study. These values reflect the 'intent-to-treat' population which includes all patients regardless of whether they survived their injuries. Mean mortality rate in the published studies was 22% which compares well with the values in the current study of 20%. A 3% mean percentage of patients in the published literature developed a fistula during therapy (ranging from 7 to 0%). The value in the current study of 5% compares well, especially considering that a single patient developed a fistula which was apparent at only one dressing change and was resolved by the next dressing change. In terms of the rate of other complications, the data was less reliable because not all the relevant studies reported complications (not shown). In conclusion, there is no evidence that the device used in this study is any less efficacious than the VAC^{TM} device in the treatment of Grade 1 and 2 open abdomen wounds derived from traumatic patients.

Discussion

In this study, the rate of fascial closure was 65% on an intent-to-treat basis which compares well with comparable published studies (63.7%) of patients (Table 6). All comparisons were carried out with studies using the predominant

commercially available abdominal NPWT kit, Abdominal VAC^{TM} (KCI San Antonio, Tx USA). One significant drawback of this study design was the non-comparative design. A large comparative study would be required to confirm equivalence of these two devices. The present study provides evidence that application of the alternative dressing (RENASYS^{TM} AB Smith & Nephew St Petersburg, FL USA) is likely to achieve similar outcomes. Concurrent application of fascial tension: for example through the use of 'dynamic suturing', along with NPWT may further improve the frequency of fascial closure [19,20] although, to date, no comparative studies have been carried out to support this. Achievement of fascial closure not only has significant implications for the recovery of the patients but also leads to shorter ICU and hospital length of stay, reduced need for surgical reconstruction of the abdominal wall, and shorter recovery time. These factors all have a considerable cost element so early but safe abdominal closure is the best outcome.

The most commonly cited objection to the use of NPWT TAC is a perceived increase in fistula formation. The rate of fistula formation in the current study of 5% was similar to that derived from the published studies of 3%. It is possible that these relatively low levels of fistula formation are observed in this specific population of open abdomen patients [2,21] and that higher incidence of de novo fistula formation may occur in 'high risk' subsets of patients i.e. those with more advanced grade of open abdomen (grade 3 or 4), sepsis, or in wounds where a bowel anastomosis following bowel surgery is present or where there is a delay or failure to achieve fascial closure. In fact where concern has been expressed by several commentators [22-24] the patients described tend to be 'high risk'. The potential link between NPWT and fistula formation has been disputed by others [25] including in a systematic review [26]. More evidence is needed to determine

Table 6 Comparison with published literature

Reference	Method	n	Fascial closure	Mortality	Fistula
This Study	RENASYS -AB	20	13 (65%)	4 (20%)	1 (5%)
Miller et al. 2004 [12]	VAC^{TM}	53	38	8 (15%)	1 (2%)
Garner et al. 2003 [6]		14	13	NR	0
Suliberk et al. 2003 [13]		29	25	6 (21%)	2 (8)
Stone et al. 2004 [14]		48	23	16 (33%)	2 (4%)
Weinberg et al. 2008 [15]		9*	6	NR	NR
Arigon et al. 2008† [16]		22	6	3 (14%)	0
Batacchi et al. 2010 [17]		35*	NR	8 (23%)	NR
Labler et al. 2005 [18]		18	12	5 (33%)	0
Total patients reporting relevant end-point		**228**	**193**	**205**	**5**
Weighted mean (%)			63.7	23.5	2.7

NR = Not Recorded. NA = Not Applicable. * refers to the relevant subgroup (treated with NPWT) of a wider analysis. † data extracted from abstract only (article in French). All studies described traumatic patients except Arigon et al. [16] and Batacchi et al. [17] who described a mixed group of aetiologies with the majority of reported patients being relevant to this study.

whether use of NPWT on grade 3 or 4 open abdomen is effective and whether an increased risk of fistulisation is indeed observed as a result of therapy in this sub-population. With regard to the current study, one draw-back is the relatively low sample size, which may not accurately reflect the true incidence of fistula formation in these wounds. One variable not assessed in the systematic review was the level of negative pressure used in each study. This is reported in only one study where the rela-tively high level of -175 mmHg was used [13]. Use of high levels of negative pressure is thought to a potential risk factor for increased fistula formation but the present ana-lysis is not able to clarify this assertion.

Wider adoption of the published classification system is needed when reporting outcomes on open abdomen patients in order to help clarify these and other issues.

Conclusion

Application of an alternative NPWT TAC system, when applied to trauma patients with grade 1 and 2 open abdo-mens (Bjorck et al. classification) [7] is safe and effective resulting in a high rate of fascial closure rate (65% intent-to-treat) and relatively low rate of complications. These values are similar to those presented in the published literature. Wider adoption of the published classification system is needed when reporting outcomes on open abdomen patients.

Abbreviations
NPWT: Negative Pressure Wound Therapy; IAH: Intra-abdominal Hypertension; IAP: Intra-abdominal Pressure; ACS: Abdominal Compartment Syndrome; OA: Open Abdomen; SOFA: Sequential Organ Failure Score; APACHE 11: Acute Physical and Chronic Health Evaluation Score; ISS: Injury Severity Score; NISS: New Injury Severity Score.

Competing interests
This study was funded by Smith & Nephew (S&N). Authors JS and JC are employees of S&N. DH was part of an International Expert Panel on Negative Pressure Wound Therapy funded by an unrestricted educational grant provided by Smith & Nephew.

Authors' contributions
PN, DH and AN acquired the data. JC and AN conceived and designed the study and JS interpreted the data, drafted the manuscript and carried out the systematic review. All authors provided critical revisions of the manuscript before their final approval of the manuscript.

Acknowledgements
Hussein Dharma and Alison Wraith (employees of Smith & Nephew) carried out data management and statistical analysis. S&N (the funding body) contributed to study design and provided statistical evaluation and medical writing expertise. The reporting of the study is believed to be impartial and scientific in its approach.

Author details
[1]Department of Surgery, Groote Schuur Hospital, University of Cape Town, Cape Town, South Africa. [2]Smith & Nephew, St Petersberg, Florida, USA. [3]Smith & Nephew, 101 Hessle Road, Hull HU3 2BN, UK.

References
1. MacLean AA, O'Keeffe T, Augenstein J: Management strategies for the open abdomen: survey of the American Association for the Surgery of Trauma membership. *Acta Chir Belg* 2008, **108**:212–218.
2. Cheatham ML, Safcsak K: Is the evolving management of intra-abdominal hypertension and abdominal compartment syndrome improving survival? *Crit Care Med* 2010, **38**:402–407.
3. Quyn AJ, Johnston C, Hall D, Chambers A, Arapova N, Ogston S, Amin A: *The open Abdomen and Temporary Abdominal Closure Systems - Historical Evolution and Systematic Review, Colorectal disease: the official journal of the Association of Coloproctology of Great Britain and Ireland.* 2012.
4. Boele van Hensbroek P, Wind J, Dijkgraaf MGW, Busch ORC, Goslings JC, Carel Goslings J: Temporary closure of the open abdomen: a systematic review on delayed primary fascial closure in patients with an open abdomen. *World J Surg* 2009, **33**:199–207.
5. Schmelzle M, Alldinger I, Matthaei H, Aydin F, Wallert I, Eisenberger CF, Schulte Am Esch J, Dizdar L, Topp SA, Yang Q, Knoefel WT: Long-term vacuum-assisted closure in open abdomen due to secondary peritonitis: a retrospective evaluation of a selected group of patients. *Dig Surg* 2010, **27**:272–278.
6. Garner GB DM, Ware DN, Cocanour CS, Duke JH, Mckinley BA, Ph D, Kozar RA, Moore FA: Vacuum-assisted wound closure provides early fascial reapproximation in trauma patients with open abdomens. *Am J Surg* 2002, **182**:630–638.
7. Björck M, Bruhin A, Cheatham M, Hinck D, Kaplan M, Manca G, Wild T, Windsor A: Classification–important step to improve management of patients with an open abdomen. *World J surg* 2009, **33**:1154–1157.
8. Liberati A, Altman DG, Tetzlaff J, Mulrow C, Gotzsche PC, Ioannidis JPA, Clarke M, Devereaux PJ, Kleijnen J, Moher D: The PRISMA statement for reporting systematic reviews and meta-analyses of studies that evaluate healthcare interventions: explanation and elaboration. *BMJ* 2009, **339**:b2700-b2700.
9. Cheatham ML, Malbrain MLNG, Kirkpatrick A, Sugrue M, Parr M, De Waele J, Balogh Z, Leppäniemi A, Olvera C, Ivatury R, D'Amours S, Wendon J, Hillman K, Wilmer A: Results from the International Conference of Experts on Intra-abdominal Hypertension and Abdominal Compartment Syndrome. II. Recommendations. *Intensive Care Med* 2007, **33**:951–962.
10. Mentula P: Non-traumatic causes and the management of the open abdomen. *Minerva Chir* 2011, **66**:153–163.
11. Kaplan M, Banwell P, Orgill D, Ivatury R, Demetriades D, Moore F, Miller P, Nicholas J, Henry S: Guidelines for the management of the open abdomen. *Wounds* 2005, **10**:S1–24.
12. Miller PR, Meredith JW, Johnson JC, Chang MC: Prospective Evaluation of Vacuum-Assisted Fascial Closure After Open Abdomen. *Ann Surg* 2004, **239**:608–616.
13. Suliburk JW, Ware DN, Balogh Z, McKinley BA, Cocanour CS, Kozar RA, Moore FA, Ivatury RR: Vacuum-assisted wound closure achieves early fascial closure of open abdomens after severe trauma. *J Trauma* 2003, **55**:1155–1160. discussion 1160–1.
14. Stone PA, Hass SM, Flaherty SK, DeLuca JA, Lucente FC, Kusminsky RE: Vacuum-Assisted Fascial Closure for Patients With Abdominal Trauma. *J Trauma: Inj Infect Crit Care* 2004, **57**:1082–1086.
15. Weinberg JA, George RL, Griffin RL, Stewart AH, Reiff DA, Kerby JD, Melton SM, Rue LW: Closing the open abdomen: improved success with Wittmann Patch staged abdominal closure. *J Trauma* 2008, **65**:345–348.
16. Arigon J-P, Chapuis O, Sarrazin E, Pons F, Bouix A, Jancovici R: [Managing the open abdomen with vacuum-assisted closure therapy: retrospective evaluation of 22 patients]. *J Chirurgie* 2008, **145**:252–261.
17. Batacchi S, Matano S, Nella A, Zagli G, Bonizzoli M, Pasquini A, Anichini V, Tucci V, Manca G, Ban K, Valeri A, Peris A: Vacuum-assisted closure device enhances recovery of critically ill patients following emergency surgical procedures. *Critical Care (London, England)* 2009, **13**:R194.
18. Labler L, Zwingmann J, Mayer D, Stocker R, Trentz O, Keel M: V.A.C.® Abdominal Dressing System. *Eur J Trauma* 2005, **31**:488–494.
19. Pliakos I, Papavramidis TS, Mihalopoulos N, Koulouris H, Kesisoglou I, Sapalidis K, Deligiannidis N, Papavramidis S: Vacuum-assisted closure in severe abdominal sepsis with or without retention sutured sequential fascial closure: a clinical trial. *Surgery* 2010, **148**:947–953.
20. Matthias RK-r, Nina Z: *Open Abdomen Treatment with Dynamic Sutures and Topical Negative Pressure Resulting in a High Primary Fascia Closure Rate.* 2012.

21. Mentula P, Hienonen P, Kemppainen E, Puolakkainen P, Leppäniemi A:
    Surgical decompression for abdominal compartment syndrome in
    severe acute pancreatitis. *Arch Surg (Chicago, Ill. 1960)* 2010, **145**:764–769.
22. Trevelyan SL, Carlson GL: **Is TNP in the open abdomen safe and effective?**
    J Wound Care 2009, **18**:24–25.
23. Rao M, Burke D, Finan PJ, Sagar PM: **The use of vacuum-assisted closure of
    abdominal wounds: a word of caution.** *Colorectal dis: Offic J Assoc
    Coloproctology Great Britain Ireland* 2007, **9**:266–268.
24. Fischer JE: **A cautionary note: the use of vacuum-assisted closure systems
    in the treatment of gastrointestinal cutaneous fistula may be associated
    with higher mortality from subsequent fistula development.** *Am J Surg*
    2008, **196**:1–2.
25. Shaikh IA, Ballard-Wilson A, Yalamarthi S, Amin AI: **Use of topical negative
    pressure in assisted abdominal closure does not lead to high incidence
    of enteric fistulae.** *Colorectal dis: Offic J Assoc Coloproctology Great Britain
    Ireland* 2010, **12**:931–934.
26. Stevens P: **Vacuum-assisted closure of laparostomy wounds: a critical
    review of the literature.** *Int Wound J* 2009, **6**:259–266.

16

Ex-vivo porcine organs with a circulation pump are effective for teaching hemostatic skills

Yoshimitsu Izawa[1], Shuji Hishikawa[2], Tomohiro Muronoi[1], Keisuke Yamashita[1], Masayuki Suzukawa[1] and Alan T Lefor[2*]

Abstract

Surgical residents have insufficient opportunites to learn basic hemostatic skills from clinical experience alone. We designed an ex-vivo training system using porcine organs and a circulation pump to teach hemostatic skills. Residents were surveyed before and after the training and showed significant improvement in their self-confidence (1.83 ± 1.05 vs 3.33 ± 0.87, $P < 0.01$) on a 5 point Likert scale. This training may be effective to educate residents in basic hemostatic skills.

Keywords: Ex-vivo, Trauma surgery, Education, Porcine model

Background

Simulation training for surgical skills has become essential around the world. Many methods including dry laboratories, simulators, cadavers, and live tissues have been used for basic surgical skill training, open surgery training, and laparoscopic training [1]. To improve trauma surgery education, many educational training courses have been developed. Specifically, many simulation courses such as Advanced Trauma Operative Management, Definitive Surgical Trauma Care, and Advanced Surgical Skills for Exposure in Trauma have been held around the world [2-7].

Among the various possible approaches, live animal training may be most suitable for teaching hemostatic skills [1]. However, these courses are expensive and it is difficult to provide repetitive training because they utilize live animal models necessitating general anesthesia, as well as much time and effort. Recently, the use of live animals is decreasing in surgical training. The validity of using a simulated model instead of live animals has been validated for chest tube placement and cricothyrotomy [8]. In addition, it is critically important to adopt the 3R approach to the use of animal models, including

Reduction, Refinement and Replacement, originally described in 1959 [9].

Simulation training programs may not be suitable for certain kinds of training because the bleeding encountered is not similar to live animals. Ex-vivo training as a type of simulation for surgical education is a less realistic model of hemorrhage than a live animal. However, such courses may be relatively inexpensive and allow repetitive training [1].

Recently, with fewer opportunities to participate in live animal training due to economic and ethical aspects, and limited trauma operative experience during training, residents may not be able to learn adequate hemostatic skills in clinical trauma situations alone [10]. In order to improve the competency of residents in basic hemostatic skills in the trauma setting, we created this realistic, repetitive, and ethically-advantageous ex-vivo training model to teach hemostatic procedures using a circulation motor and ex-vivo porcine organs, providing an opportunity for residents to learn hemostatic skills.

Materials and methods

This training was carried out in a humane manner after receiving approval from the Institutional Animal Experiment Committee of Jichi Medical University, and in accordance with the Institutional Regulation for Animal Experiments and Fundamental Guideline for Proper Conduct of Animal Experiment and Related Activities in Academic Research Institutions under the jurisdiction of

---

* Correspondence: alefor@jichi.ac.jp
[2]Department of Surgery, Jichi Medical University, Tochigi, Japan This manuscript was presented in part at the World Society of Emergency Surgery 1st World Congress on 2nd July 2010 in Bologna Italy

the Ministry of Education, Culture, Sports, Science and Technology. Participants were recruited from among residents (PGY 2 through PGY 5) rotating in the Emergency Department at the time of the study. Participants were informed about the nature of the program and given the option to participate.

All animals used were specific pathogen free and were tested for the absence of Hepatitis E Virus. Animals were obtained from a breeder directly, and included Mexican and Chinese mini-pigs weighing 30-45 kg each, and treated in accordance with appropriate rules and regulations for the ethical care of laboratory animals. Previous experiments included various surgical procedures that would not introduce added risks to participants. Porcine hearts, kidneys, and inferior vena cavae (IVCs) were harvested from animals used in other experiments and stored cryogenically until the training sessions. On the day of the session, the frozen organs were thawed and connected to circulation pumps. Circulating water was mixed with red ink to simulate blood. All participants received didactic training with a one hour lecture, and were were surveyed regarding their confidence to perform the procedures before the laboratory session (Table 1).

Participants then moved to the laboratory, and suture hemostasis was performed in the renal cortex (Figure 1), IVC (Figure 2) and the injured heart (Figure 3) while active bleeding was simulated by the flow of the circulating red water through native vessels. This was done under close supervision and mentorship by senior faculty in Emergency Surgery (YI, TM, KY, and SH). The dynamic nature of the bleeding simulation is easily seen in the Additional file 1: Vedio S1; Additional file 2: Vedio S2. Participants were given the opportunity to repeat the simulation, and to attempt different approaches to achieve hemostasis. The laboratory session lasted about 5 hours total, with each participant spending time with each of the three organs.

Following the training, participants were surveyed regarding their confidence and their opinion of the training. The survey used a 5-point Likert scale, with 1 indicating low confidence and 5 indicating the highest confidence. These results are shown in Tables 1 and 2.

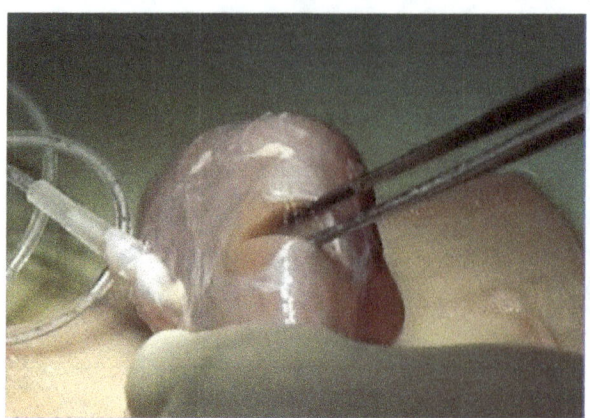

Figure 1 A Renal cortex injury is made in a kidney connected to a circulation pump with saline circulating through the renal vessels.

Statistical Analysis

Survey data was analyzed by Wilcoxson rank-sign test (Excel, Microsoft Corp, Redmond WA USA), and is reported with mean, standard deviation, and p-value comparing the scores before and after training.

Results

Twenty-four residents participated in this training program and performed hemostatic procedures. The training level of the residents included: PGY 2, 16 (67%), PGY 3, 6 (25.0%), PGY4, 1 (4%), and PGY5, 1 (4%). Their experience in trauma surgery as surgeon or assistant prior to this program included: no cases for 8 participants (33%), 1 ~ 5 cases for 13 participants (55%), 6 ~ 10 cases for 2 participants (8%), and 15 or more cases for 1 participant (4%).

Residents were divided into groups and the program for each group was conducted at a different time, to

Table 1 Self-Confidence Level of Participants Before and After Simulation Training

Time Measured	Mean	SD	P-Value
Pre-Course	1.83	1.05	< .01
Post-Course	3.33	0.87	

Self-Confidence measured on a 5-point Likert scale (1 = no confidence, 3 = Neither Confident nor lack of confidence, 5 = strong confidence)

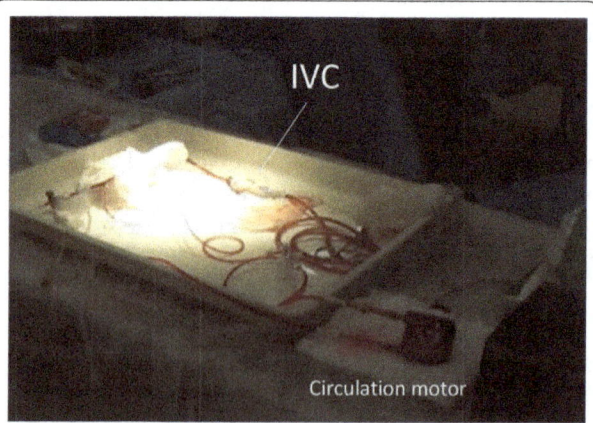

Figure 2 An ex-vivo porcine inferior vena cava (IVC) is connected to a circulation pump for teaching hemostatic techniques.

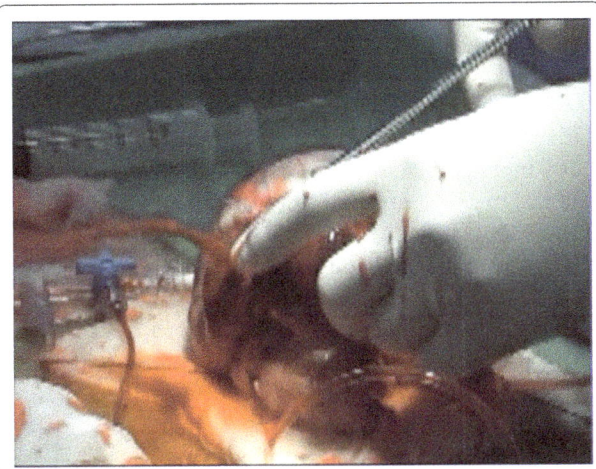

Figure 3 An ex-vivo porcine heart is connected to a circulation pump for teaching hemostatic techniques.

enable close faculty mentorship. In total, the sessions were conducted eight separate times. A questionnaire was given to all participants both before and after the program. Responses showed a significant ($p < .01$) improvement in self-confidence (Table 1) after the program compared to before the training. Each of the eight sessions utilized one porcine heart, one porcine vena cava and one or two porcine kidneys depending on the number of participants.

All participants were satisfied with the training they received, and gave very positive feedback concerning the program (Table 2).

Discussion

In Japan, nearly all trauma patients are victims of blunt traumatic injuries, particularly from automobile accidents. There is essentially no penetrating trauma at all. The number of patients undergoing surgery for blunt injuries has decreased given improvements in automotive safety and design. Hemostatic procedures are one of the most important skills in trauma surgery. Surgical residents should master the crucial hemostatic skills to deal with the hemorrhage in trauma operations. However, they have few chances to learn hemostatic skills in

actual clinical care, due to a paucity of operative cases as well as the hierarchical nature of training [10]. We sought to develop an effective simulation model to teach hemostatic skills to residents, and conducted ex-vivo training with a circulation pump to provide residents with a chance for basic hemostatic skill training.

Various types of simulation training exist in surgical education. Reznick et al described the features of the types of simulation available and concluded that live tissue is suitable for procedures requiring blood flow [1]. Live animal training may be ideal for for hemostatic skill training. Many trauma surgery courses held around the world utilize live tissue for learning hemostatic skills. However, these courses are generally expensive and do not allow repetitive experiences. Furthermore, from an ethical perspective, we must seek to reduce the use of live animals. The direct costs of this study were limited to the facility fee and the cost of consumable items such as sutures. The facility fee included the cost of storing the organs and use of instruments. There were no other associated direct costs.

Cadaver training, which demonstrates accurate anatomy, is suitable for learning complex surgical procedures [11] but cannot be used in realistic simulations for teaching hemostatic techniques because there is no bleeding. Though a virtual reality simulator is reusable and easy to prepare [12], its texture is far from realistic and its three-dimensional image is generally well simulated so that it is not a realistic model. Although some types of dry-models are useful for surgical training [13], they cannot make a realistic bleeding model.

The model used here maintains the texture of live tissue because actual organs are used. The freeze/thaw cycle did not change the tactile sensation of the tissue, nor did it destroy the large vessels with in the organs, notably the kidney in the model used here. Also, by utilizing a circulation pump, it provides a more realistic training situation than ex-vivo tissue alone, yet is much less expensive than live animal models. This study demonstrates the value of this hybrid model, which exists between using live animals and typical ex-vivo tissue models.

Table 2 Participant Evaluation of the Course

Question	Mean Score	± SD
I understood the goals and objectives for this trauma ex-vivo training program	4.63	0.647
My interest in trauma care has increased	4.75	0.442
I am satisfied with this training	4.54	0.721
I would recommend this training to my colleagues	4.75	0.531
I would like to repeat this training	4.79	0.415
Repeating this training would make me more capable in torso trauma surgery	4.75	0.442

Scores shown on a 5-point Likert scale (1 = strongly disagree, 3 = neither agree nor disagree, 5 = strongly agree). *SD*, Standard Deviation

In this study, we selected the heart, kidney and vena cava for the models. Each organ was only used for one session, but by multiple participants. The organs were not re-frozen because the multiple repairs precluded their re-use. It may be possible to use other organs, such as spleen or liver. However, cannulation of the porcine splenic vessels may be difficult because of their size. The repair of the kidney affords a similar experience to that of a spleen or liver, but was preferred because of the increased number of organs as well as the size of the kidney being conducive to easy cannulation and handling compared to the liver.

Ex-vivo training with a circulation pump model is suitable for basic hemostatic practice for residents. This training is easy to prepare and allows residents to practice hemostatic skills repeatedly, which may lead to earlier mastery some skill. Furthermore, this training is clearly advantageous from the ethical point of view compared with live tissue training. The concept of 3R is crucial regarding the ethics of using animal tissue in medical research and education. This training contributed to the Replacement and Reduction components of the 3R principle. The design of this model satisfies both reality and ethics.

There are some limitations to the sense of reality encountered in this model. This training does not use blood so that coagulation is completely absent compared to live tissue. For example, during repair of the IVC injury in this model, the oozing from the needle holes cannot be stopped.

Another limitation is the lack of a physiologic effect of bleeding. For example, the cardiac injury repair is easier in this ex-vivo model than in a live animal because it cannot offer the same motion during systole as a live heart. Donias et al made a beating heart model in an ex-vivo setting for coronary artery anastomosis training using a foot pump [14]. The cardiac muscle does not contract by itself so that the reality of ex-vivo training is not the same as that in a live animal. Precise re-creation is impossible using this model, but the practice afforded here may facilitate learning with a live animal model and requires further study.

An important aspect of this training is the close faculty participation required. Each organ used constituted a "station" and we felt it was important to have each station manned by a faculty member throughout the training, such that the time faculty time requirement is significant. Including the lecture time (1 hour) and laboratory time (5 hours), a total of 16 person-hours of faculty time are needed to conduct the session.

The effectiveness of simulation training can be defined in several ways, such as improved clinical performance following simulation training, improved patient safety following such training, or effects on the practitioner. In a study of thoracostomy tube placement by medical students, Hishikawa and colleagues found that while there was no measurable effect on performance of the task in a live porcine model with or without prior simulation training, the students who underwent simulation training felt significantly more confident when performing the task on a live animal [15]. The improved confidence observed in the present study is felt to be a valid measure of effectiveness, as was shown in the thoracostomy tube study.

This ex-vivo training level is excellent for surgical residents. This model cannot re-create hemorrhage for complex hemostatic procedures such as hemorrhage of multiple origins, so experienced trauma surgeons may not be satisfied with this training. Further studies are needed to judge the effectiveness of this training at various levels of training.

Conclusions

Ex-vivo tissue training with circulation pumps for teaching basic hemostatic skills in trauma was developed to increase residents' opportunities to learn these important skills, and serves as a hybrid model combining the realistic feel of tissue and the experience of bleeding without the need for live animals. This training improved the confidence of residents in hemostatic skills of trauma surgery, and is one of the ways to educate residents for basic hemostatic skills. The model employed is economical, effective, and respects the 3R principle of animal ethics. Continued evaluation of various teaching modalities is an important goal in surgical education. This study serves as the basis of future larger studies, which will investigate the objective benefits of simulation training for teaching hemostatic skills.

Author details
[1]Department of Emergency Medicine, Jichi Medical University, Tochigi, Japan. [2]Department of Surgery, Jichi Medical University, Tochigi, Japan This manuscript was presented in part at the World Society of Emergency Surgery 1st World Congress on 2nd July 2010 in Bologna Italy.

Authors' contributions
YI: Conceived the trial, conducted the training, collected and analyzed data, prepared the manuscript, SH: Conducted the training, collected the data, prepared the manuscript, TM: conducted the training, collected and analyzed the data, KY: conducted the training, collected and analyzed the data, MS: conceived the trial, analyzed the data, prepared the manuscript, AL: conceived the trial, Analyzed the data, preparation of manuscript, All authors read and approved the final manuscript.

Competing interests
The authors declare that they have no competing interests.

References

1. Reznick RK, MacRae H: **Teaching Surgical Skills-Changes in the wind.** *N Engl J Med* 2006, **355**:2664-2669.
2. Gaarder C, Naess PA, Buanes T, Pillgram-Larsen J: **Advanced surgical trauma care training with a live porcine model.** *Injury* 2005, **36**:718-724.
3. Jacobs LM, Burns KJ, Luk SS, Marshall WT: **Follow-Up Survey of Participants Attending the Advanced Trauma Operative Management (ATOM) Course.** *J Trauma* 2005, **58**:1140-1143.
4. Jacobs LM, Burns KJ, Luk SS, Hull S: **Advanced trauma operative management course: participant survey.** *World J Surg* 2010, **34**:164-168.
5. **Definitive Surgical Trauma Care (DSTCTM) Courses.** [http://www.iatsic.org/DSTC.html].
6. **Definitive Surgical Trauma Skills (DSTS).** [http://www.rcseng.ac.uk/education/courses/dsts.html].
7. **Advanced Surgical Skills for Exposure in Trauma (ASSET) Course.** [http://www.facs.org/trauma/education/asset.html].
8. Hall AB: **Randomized objective comparison of tissue training versus simulators for emergency procedures.** *The Am Surgeon* 2011, **77**:561-565.
9. van Zutphen LF, van der Valk JB: **Developments on the implementation of the Three Rs in research and education.** *Toxicology in Vitro* 2001, **15**:591-595.
10. Spain DA, Miller FB: **Education and training of the future surgeon in acute care surgery: trauma, critical care, and emergency surgery.** *Am J Surg* 2005, **190**:212-217.
11. Gilbody J, Prasthofer AW, Ho K, Costa ML: **The use and effectiveness of cadaveric workshops in higher surgical training: a systematic review.** *Ann R Coll Surg Engl* 2011, **93**:347-352.
12. Cherry RA, Ali J: **Current Concepts in Simulation-Based Trauma Education.** *J Trauma* 2008, **65**:1186-1193.
13. Anastakis DJ, Regehr G, Reznick RK, Cusimano M, Murnaghan J, Brown M, Hutchison C: **Assessment of Technical Skills Transfer from the Bench Training Model to the Human Model.** *Am J Surg* 1999, **177**:167-170.
14. Donias HW, Schwartz T, Tang DG, DeAnda A Jr, Tabaie HA, Boyd DW, Karamanoukian HL: **A porcine beating heart model for robotic coronary artery surgery.** *Heart Surg Forum* 2003, **6**:249-253.
15. Hishikawa S, Kawano M, Tanaka H, Konno K, Yasuda Y, Kawano R, Kobayashi E, Lefor AT: **Simulation improves operator confidence but not performance of tube thoracostomy by medical students in a porcine model: A prospective controlled trial.** *Am Surg* 2010, **76**:73-78.

17

Compliance to advanced trauma life support protocols in adult trauma patients in the acute setting

Bonnie Tsang[1*], Jessica McKee[2], Paul T Engels[3], Damian Paton-Gay[3] and Sandy L Widder[1]

Abstract

Introduction: Advanced Trauma Life Support (ATLS) protocols provide a common approach for trauma resuscitations. This was a quality review assessing compliance with ATLS protocols at a Level I trauma center; specifically whether the presence or absence of a trauma team leader (TTL) influenced adherence.

Methods: This retrospective study was conducted on adult major trauma patients with acute injuries over a one-year period in a Level I Canadian trauma center. Data were collected from the Alberta Trauma Registry, and adherence to ATLS protocols was determined by chart review.

Results: The study identified 508 patients with a mean Injury Severity Score of 24.5 (SD 10.7), mean age 39.7 (SD 17.6), 73.8% were male and 91.9% were involved in blunt trauma. The overall compliance rate was 81.8% for primary survey and 75% for secondary survey. The TTL group compared to non-TTL group was more likely to complete the primary survey (90.9% vs. 81.8%, $p = 0.003$), and the secondary survey (100% vs. 75%, $p = 0.004$). The TTL group was more likely than the non-TTL group to complete the following tasks: insertion of two large bore IVs (68.2% vs. 57.7%, $p = 0.014$), digital rectal exam (64.6% vs. 54.7%, $p = 0.023$), and head to toe exam (77% vs. 67.1%, $p = 0.013$). Mean times from emergency department arrival to diagnostic imaging were also significantly shorter in the TTL group compared to the non-TTL group, including times to pelvis xray (mean 68min vs. 107min, $p = 0.007$), CT chest (mean 133min vs. 172min, $p = 0.005$), and CT abdomen and pelvis (mean 136min vs. 173min, $p = 0.013$). Readmission rates were not significantly different between the TTL and non-TTL groups (3.5% vs. 4.5%, $p = 0.642$).

Conclusions: While many studies have demonstrated the effectiveness of trauma systems on outcomes, few have explored the direct influence of the TTL on ATLS compliance. This study demonstrated that TTL involvement during resuscitations was associated with improved adherence to ATLS protocols, and increased efficiency (compared to non TTL involvement) to diagnostic imaging. Findings from this study will guide future quality improvement and education for early trauma management.

Keywords: Advanced trauma life support, Quality improvement, Trauma team leader, Major trauma, Wounds & injuries

* Correspondence: btsang@ualberta.ca
[1]Department of Surgery, Faculty of Medicine and Dentistry, University of Alberta, 2D WMC, 8440-112 Street NW, Edmonton, AB T6G 2B7, Canada
Full list of author information is available at the end of the article

Introduction

Trauma is the most common cause of death in Canada for the age group of 44 years or less. In 2004, intentional and unintentional injuries led to 13,677 deaths, and 211,000 hospitalizations [1]. The economic burden from injuries is estimated at $10.7 billion in health care costs, and $19.8 billion in total economic costs [1].

Trauma resuscitations often involve complex decision-making and management of critical injuries in a short span of time. Errors are common; an Australian study on trauma management found 6.09 errors per fatal case in the emergency department (ED) with 3.47 errors contributing to patient death [2]. Since 1977, the Advanced Trauma Life Support (ATLS) treatment paradigm was established to improve the management of trauma patients during the initial resuscitation phase [3]. ATLS protocols provide a common framework and organized approach during these situations, and have been shown to improve outcomes [4,5]. Unfortunately, attrition rate of ATLS knowledge [6,7] and low compliance rate are issues even in major trauma centers. Deviations from ATLS protocols are common, ranging from 23% to 53% [8-11]. Compliance rate can affect patient outcome [4,5], and can serve as a surrogate marker for quality assessment of a trauma system.

Adherence to ATLS protocols is only investigated by a few studies [9-11]; specifically, whether the presence or absence of a Trauma Team Leader (TTL) affects adherence. The primary objective of this study was to determine the compliance rate with ATLS protocols in the ED in a Canadian Level I trauma centre, as well as to assess the impact on ATLS compliance with TTL involvement. Secondary objectives included assessing patient outcomes and times to diagnostic imaging.

Methods

This study was conducted in a Level I trauma center in Canada. Ethics approval for the study was obtained from the Human Research Ethics Review Board at the University of Alberta. Patients meeting inclusion criteria were identified from the Alberta Trauma Registry (ATR) from July 1, 2009 to June 30, 2010. Inclusion criteria were: age ≥17 years old, Injury Severity Score (ISS) ≥12, and patients with injuries that occurred <24 hours prior to presentation to the trauma centre. Patients with non-acute injuries (injuries sustained ≥24hrs), drowning, strangulations, missing charts and inter-hospital transfers that bypassed ED assessment were excluded.

The ATR collects data prospectively on all trauma patients with an ISS ≥12 who are admitted to one of the ten participating trauma centers in Alberta. Data obtained from the ATR included: date of injury, sex, age, mechanism of injury, discharge status, total length of stay (LOS), ICU (Intensive Care Unit) LOS, ISS, and

revised trauma score (RTS). A retrospective chart review was performed for additional data not collected in the ATR, on the completion of various actions or tasks as per ATLS protocols (see Table 2), as well as time to diagnostic tests, readmission to hospital, and presence or absence of TTL during resuscitation. Readmission rate in this study included all unplanned readmissions to a hospital in Alberta within 60 days of discharge.

Criteria for trauma team and/or TTL activation

Respiratory distress
Hemodynamic instability
Focal neurological signs or GCS ≤8
Penetrating torso trauma
Multiple casualties
Major burn
At the discretion of the ED physician or charge nurse

At the time of the study, the core trauma team was composed of the TTL, senior and junior general surgery residents, orthopedic resident, anesthesia resident, along with nursing staff, radiology technicians, and respiratory therapists. Attending surgeons were available within 30 minutes while on-call. Other surgical specialties (neurosurgery, thoracics, vascular), intensivist, as well as hemoatologist were available upon request. The decision to activate the trauma team was based on criteria listed above. In cases where the trauma team was not activated, it was at the discretion of the ED physician in charge to consult the appropriate services.

TTLs were multidisciplinary and composed of emergency physicians, general surgeons, and one neurosurgeon. All of the TTLs have ATLS certification, and a strong interest in trauma. Members of the TTL group are involved in ATLS education, quality assurance, and research. For major traumas meeting criteria (see above), the TTL on-call was activated and was expected to arrive within 30 minutes to take over the leadership role of the resuscitation. When a TTL was not available, the leadership role fell onto the ER physician in charge, a senior surgical resident, or the general surgeon on call.

Two groups were created for the analysis: the TTL group and the non-TTL group. Basic demographic analysis was completed on the two groups involving age, sex, ISS, total LOS, ICU LOS, RTS, mechanism of injury and mortality. Chi square analysis was used to compare the ATLS protocol compliance between the two groups, as well as the mortality rate and readmission rate. Independent sample T-Test was used to compare the times to diagnostic imaging and Mann–Whitney U test (2 sample) was used to compare the number of items completed in the primary and secondary survey. Statistical analysis was performed using SPSS software, version 19 (IBM Corporation, Armonk, New York).

Results

A total of 781 patients were identified from the ATR that met the inclusion criteria. Two hundred seventy three of the patients were excluded by criteria. A total of 508 patients were analyzed.

Demographics

Of the 508 patients, mean age was 39.7 (SD 17.6), 375 (73.8%) were male, and the mean ISS was 24.5 (SD 10.7) (Table 1). The majority of the patients (n = 467, 91.9%) suffered blunt trauma, whereas penetrating trauma and burns accounted for 5.7% (n = 29) and 2.4% (n = 12) of the patients respectively. Overall mortality was 4.9% (n = 25).

Approximately half of the cases (53.9%, n = 274) had a TTL present. The TTL and non-TTL groups were comparable in terms of sex, age, mechanism of injury and mortality (Table 1). The RTS was lower and ISS higher in the TTL group compared to the non-TTL group (5.81 vs. 6.55, p = 0.007 and 25.4 vs. 23.5, p = 0.045 respectively), indicating a more severely injured patient population in the TTL group.

ATLS compliance rates

The compliance rates for ATLS protocols were based on the completion of 11 items for the primary survey and 4 items for the secondary survey that were chosen a priori by a group of trauma surgeons based on ATLS guidelines (Table 2). The median rates of completion for primary and secondary survey items for all patients were 81.8% (9 out of 11 items) and 75% (3 out of 4 items) respectively (Table 3). Compliance rate for completion of the primary survey was significantly higher (p = 0.003) for the TTL group (median of 10 out of 11 items, 90.9%) compared to the non-TTL group (median of 9 out of 11 items, 81.8%). Compliance rate for completion of the secondary survey was also significantly higher (p = 0.004) for the TTL group (median of 4 of 4 items, 100%) compared to the non-TTL group (median of 3 out of 4 items, 75%). Specifically, insertion of two large bore IVs 16 gauge or larger (TTL 68.2% vs. non-TTL 57.7%, p = 0.014), performance of the digital rectal exam (DRE) (TTL 64.6% vs. non-TTL 54.7%, p = 0.023), and performance of the head to toe exam (TTL 77.0% vs. 67.1%, p = 0.013) were higher in the TTL group (Tables 2 and 3).

Time to diagnostic imaging

Mean times from arrival to the ED to performance of various diagnostic studies were obtained. Times to pelvis xray (68min vs. 107min, p = 0.007), CT of the chest (133min vs. 172min, p = 0.005), and CT of the abdomen and pelvis (136min vs. 173min, p = 0.013) were significantly faster for the TTL group compared to the non-TTL group (Table 4).

Major outcome measures and readmission rate

Patients from the TTL group required significantly longer ICU LOS compared to the non-TTL group (mean 4.5 days vs. 2.9 days, p = 0.040). Although not statistically significant, the total LOS was also higher for the TTL group compared to the non-TTL group (16.2 days vs. 12.4 days, p = 0.050). There is no difference in mortality between the two groups (TTL 5.5% vs. non-TTL 4.3%, p = 0.682). The overall rate of unplanned readmission within 60 days was 4.0% (19 out of 477 patients), and the rates were not significantly different between the TTL group (3.5%, 9 out of 257 patients) and non-TTL group (4.5%, 10 out of 220 patients; p = 0.642) (Table 1).

Table 1 Patient demographics

	All patients (n = 508)	TTL (n = 274)	Non-TTL (n = 234)	p-value
Male	375 (73.8%)	210 (76.6%)	165 (70.5%)	0.117
Mean age (years)	39.7 (SD 17.6)	39.2 (SD 17.3)	40.3 (SD 18.0)	0.457
Mean ISS	24.5 (SD 10.7)	25.4 (SD 11.0)	23.5 (SD 10.2)	0.045
Mean ICU LOS (days)	3.7 (SD 9.0)	4.5(SD 9.8)	2.9 (SD 7.8)	0.040
Mean total LOS (days)	14.5 (SD 23.0)	16.2 (SD 28.1)	12.4 (SD 14.6)	0.050
RTS	6.15 (SD 3.1)	5.81 (SD 3.30)	6.55 (SD 2.82)	0.007
Mechanism of injury				
Blunt	467 (91.9%)	248 (90.5%)	219 (93.6%)	
Penetrating	29 (5.7%)	21 (7.7%)	8 (3.4%)	
Burns	12 (2.4%)	5 (1.8%)	7 (3.0%)	
Mortality	25 (4.9%)	15 (5.5%)	10 (4.3%)	0.682
Readmission*	19 (4.0%)	9 (3.5%)	10 (4.5%)	0.642

ICU Intensive Care Unit, *ISS* Injury Severity Score, *LOS* Length of Stay, *RTS* Revised Trauma Score, *TTL* Trauma team leader.
*Unplanned readmission within 60 days of discharge.

Table 2 Compliance rates for primary survey, secondary survey and adjuncts

	All patients (%)	TTL (%)	Non-TTL (%)	p-value
Primary survey				
Airway patent	505 (99.4)	272 (99.3)	233 (99.6)	1.000
C spine immobilized	429 (84.4)	229 (83.6)	200 (85.5)	0.577
Chest auscultation	499 (98.2)	269 (98.2)	230 (98.3)	1.000
Chest palpation	295 (58.1)	163 (59.5)	132 (56.4)	0.483
Abdominal exam	499 (98.2)	270 (98.5)	229 (97.9)	0.739
Pelvis stability	333 (65.6)	183 (66.8)	150 (64.1)	0.525
Long bones exam	435 (85.6)	234 (85.4)	201 (85.9)	0.874
Two large bore IVs	322 (63.4)	187 (68.2)	135 (57.7)	0.014
Gross motor exam	439 (86.4)	243 (88.7)	196 (83.8)	0.106
Log roll	401 (78.9)	223 (81.4)	178 (76.1)	0.143
Digital rectal exam	305 (60.0)	177 (64.6)	128 (54.7)	0.023
Secondary survey and adjuncts				
Head to toe exam	368 (72.4)	211 (77.0)	157 (67.1)	0.013
AMPLE history	466 (91.7)	247 (90.1)	219 (93.6)	0.160
Trauma panel	440 (86.6)	240 (87.6)	200 (85.5)	0.484
Blood gas	357 (70.3)	197 (71.9)	160 (68.4)	0.387
Diagnostic imaging				
CXR	445 (87.6)	242 (88.3)	203 (86.8)	0.593
C spine XR	325 (64.0)	152 (55.5)	173 (73.9)	<0.001
Pelvis XR	281 (55.3)	136 (49.6)	145 (62.0)	0.005
CT head	375 (73.8)	197 (71.9)	178 (76.1)	0.287
CT chest	372 (73.2)	194 (70.8)	178 (76.1)	0.182
CT ab/pelvis	368 (72.4)	194 (70.8)	174 (74.4)	0.371
CT C spine	269 (53.0)	137 (50.0)	132 (56.4)	0.149

Ab/Pelvis Abdomen and pelvis, *AMPLE* Allergy, medication, past medical history, last meal, events, *C spine* Cervical spine, *CXR* Chest XR.

Discussion

ATLS provide a common framework and organized approach to trauma resuscitations, and has been shown to improve outcomes [4,5]. Studies have demonstrated the effectiveness of ATLS training on improving the quality of diagnostic and therapeutic procedures and decreasing mortality rate [4,5]. ATLS training and implementation, as a part of a well-organized trauma system, can improve outcomes of trauma patients [12-19].

As with any quality assessment, the results from this study demonstrated a need to improve overall ATLS compliance at our institution. However, the compliance

Table 3 Completion rates for primary and secondary surveys

	Median (%)	p-value
*Primary survey**		
All patients	9 (81.8)	
TTL	10 (90.9)	0.003
Non-TTL	9 (81.8)	
*Secondary survey^*		
All patients	3 (75)	
TTL	4 (100)	0.004
Non-TTL	3 (75)	

*Out of a total of eleven items.
^Out of a total of four items.

Table 4 Times to diagnostic imaging

Diagnostic test	TTL involved Mean time (min) (SD) (min)	Non-TTL Mean time (min) (SD) (min)	p-value
Chest X-ray	88 (172)	99 (157)	0.466
Pelvis X-ray	68 (77)	107 (160)	0.007
C spine X-ray	98 (134)	115 (146)	0.276
CT head	111 (109)	129 (82)	0.068
CT chest	133 (130)	172 (136)	0.005
CT ab/pelvis	136 (133)	173 (144)	0.013
CT C spine	131 (134)	166 (142)	0.054

Ab/Pelvis Abdomen and pelvis, *C spine* Cervical spine.

rates for primary and secondary surveys at our institution were similar or slightly higher compared to other studies [9-11]. Santora *et al.* [9] found an overall deviation rate of 23% from ATLS protocols in their study using video assessment of trauma resuscitations, while the overall compliance rate for ATLS was only 53% in the study by Spanjersberg *et al.* [10]. In our study, the presence of a TTL during trauma resuscitation led to a significantly higher compliance rate for primary and secondary surveys, and also increased efficiency of resuscitation as demonstrated by the decrease in time to diagnostic imaging compared to the absence of a TTL. Time for CT acquisition for trauma patients range widely in the literature, from 17 to 197 minutes [20-24], and there is no definition for acceptable time to completion of diagnostic imaging in trauma patients. The mean times from patient arrival to completion of CT scans in our center were within the time frame reported by other studies; however, times to completion of xrays were often delayed. Although CT acquisition time has not been directly linked to affect major outcomes such as mortality or LOS, faster CT acquisition may be associated with time reduction to live-saving interventions [25].

There were certain areas in the primary and secondary surveys where the non-TTL group seemingly outperformed the TTL group, such as the utilization of basic radiography. Although plain C spine and pelvic xrays are part of the ATLS algorithm, with the availability of CT scanners, they have a diminishing role for hemodynamically stable blunt trauma patients with a severe mechanism of injury [26-28]. Several studies have found that pelvic xray has low sensitivity compared to CT of the pelvis, and may be omitted in hemodynamically stable blunt trauma patients who will have CT of the abdomen and pelvis [26-28]. Similarly, CT C spine is superior to C spine xray (due to frequent inadequate views) [29-31], and is replacing C spine xrays in many trauma centers [32,33]. On the basis of the current evidence, a TTL may have chosen to omit C spine and pelvic xrays on patients who were receiving CT C spine, abdomen and pelvis. This may have potentially reduced redundant imaging and unnecessary delays in the trauma resuscitation area. Overall, the times to imaging, however, were longer than expected, and could be improved upon as a quality initiative.

Our study showed a significantly longer ICU stay and a trend for longer hospital stay for the TTL group compared to the non-TTL group. This may be accounted for by the lower RTS and higher ISS in the TTL group compared the non-TTL group, indicating a higher severity of injuries in the TTL group. Although we have not been able to demonstrate a direct link between ATLS compliance and mortality, the efficiency of trauma resuscitations was improved by the presence of a TTL as demonstrated by the decreased time from patient arrival to performance of various diagnostic imaging.

Studies on medical and surgical patients have shown that the rate of early readmission is associated with quality of inpatient care [34]. In addition, the American College of Surgeons' Committee on Trauma has recommended that readmissions due to complications should be an audit filter in the quality of care monitors [35]. We have therefore used readmission rate as a surrogate marker for quality of care delivered to trauma patients. Previous studies on early readmission for trauma patients showed a readmission rate ranging from 1.2 to 10.9% [36-38], which is comparable to this study. Several factors are associated with readmissions after trauma, in particular, severity of injuries [36,38]. One would expect the TTL group to have a higher readmission rate compared to the non-TTL group due to a higher severity of injuries. The fact that the readmission rates were similar between the two groups may indicate a positive effect on patient care with the presence of a TTL, since other aspects of inpatient care were standardized for both groups of patients. Further studies are required to determine the exact impact of TTL on process of care and readmission rates.

Given the findings of this study and evidence in the literature, the consistent presence of a TTL during resuscitations of major trauma patients is important for maintaining compliance with ATLS protocols. Although one can postulate that better compliance rates for performing the primary and secondary surveys in the TTL group compared to the non-TTL group were based on increased leadership abilities, it is possible that the non-TTL group had less resources and manpower available leading to lower compliance.

At the time of the study, TTLs were composed of a multidisciplinary group of ED physicians, general surgeons, and one neurosurgeon. All of the TTLs have ATLS certification, and are involved in ATLS education, quality assurance, and research. As a whole, this group is more likely to be familiar with up to date ATLS protocols and evidence-based trauma studies, and see a higher volume of major trauma patients. The TTL serves an important role in trauma resuscitations by promoting leadership, team cohesiveness, and communication within the multidisciplinary team, to ensure efficiency and efficacy of the resuscitation [19]. TTLs can also reinforce protocol-driven approaches to trauma care that improve patient care [39]. Gerardo *et al.* [19] demonstrated a reduction in mortality rate, most notably in the most severely injured patients, when a dedicated trauma team was implemented in a Level I trauma center.

During the time period examined in our institution, a TTL was present in only half of the trauma resuscitations. Reports from UK and Australia found similar rates of involvement by the trauma team and TTL [40,41].

We believe there are two contributing factors: gaps in the TTL call scheduling, and lack of TTL notification as a part of activation of the trauma team. Reviewing the TTL call schedule at the study period, an average of 31% of shifts were not covered by a TTL (data not shown). At times when a TTL was not scheduled, the leadership role fell onto the attending ED physician, the attending surgeon, or senior general surgery resident. At our institution, TTL coverage can be improved by recruitment and retention of qualified physicians interested in trauma, and by including non-surgeons such as anesthetists, emergency physicians and intensivists. Although this study was not designed to measure the appropriateness of TTL or trauma team activation, there appears to be an element of under triage regarding trauma team activation and involvement of the TTL on call. Some of the current barriers include the lack of understanding surrounding the role of a TTL, interruptions in trauma resuscitations especially when a TTL arrives late, as well as the impression of chaos and "too many people" when the trauma team is activated. Various studies have demonstrated that appropriate activation of the trauma team can improve outcomes [42,43], and under-triaged trauma patients are associated with a high risk of mortality [42]. In order to promote a culture of safety, there needs to be ongoing education on TTL activation criteria for all staff involved in trauma resuscitations. Secondly, education should also focus on the benefits of TTL activation versus harm of "under-call". Lastly, ongoing audits should target TTL activation rate and timely feedback should be provided to all players in trauma resuscitations to ensure proper and consistent TTL activation.

Attrition of ATLS knowledge may also have contributed to poor compliance. In a study by *Ali et al.* [6], significant attrition rates of cognitive knowledge and skills was evident as early as 6 months after participants completed an ATLS course. The same group showed the attrition rate was higher for participants from low-volume centers compared to high-volume centers [7]. To address this issue, continued trauma education for all members of the trauma team should be actively encouraged and supported. This can take the form of multidisciplinary trauma simulations, maintenance of ATLS certification, other advanced courses in trauma, and attendance at trauma conferences. Additional training in trauma team crisis resource management may improve team cohesiveness, and the requirement of all physicians involved in trauma resuscitations to maintain active ATLS certification should also be established.

This study has a number of limitations. Trauma resuscitations are highly dynamic and as such not all actions performed were adequately documented with certainty. The chart review revealed a lack of time entries in many areas and this has made time-dependent outcome measures hard to gather. In particular, the rate of completion of FAST exams and time to FAST exam could not be reliably obtained from the chart review due to inconsistent record keeping. The study only reviewed data from a one-year period and as a result may not have the necessary power to show differences in major outcomes between the TTL compared to the non-TTL groups. However, we have obtained important data on the performance outcomes in the form of ATLS compliance rate, readmission rate, and indirect measure of efficiency of trauma resuscitations via times to diagnostic imaging. Additionally, we have also identified areas of future improvement with this quality assessment, and hope that other institutions will use our study as a model to promote their own quality reviews.

Conclusions

We have demonstrated that TTL involvement significantly improved compliance with many aspects of ATLS, and increased the efficiency of trauma resuscitations by decreasing mean time to diagnostic imaging. There is an acute need to improve compliance with ATLS protocols at our center as well as increase TTL involvement in major traumas at our institution. The reluctance in the hospital culture to activate the trauma team and TTL should be targeted with education around the importance of trauma team activation and involvement of TTL, as well as promotion of a culture of safety. Deficiencies found in this study will guide future quality control initiatives for trauma management.

Abbreviations

ATLS: Advanced trauma life support; ATR: Alberta trauma registry; DRE: Digital rectal exam; ED: Emergency department; ICU: Intensive care unit; ISS: Injury severity score; LOS: Length of stay; RTS: Revised trauma score; TTL: Trauma team leader.

Competing interests

The authors declare that they have no competing interests.

Authors' contributions

BT and SW conceived and designed the study, and drafted the manuscript. BT was responsible for data collection. JM was responsible for statistical analysis. PE, JM and DPG helped with the drafting and editing of the manuscript. All authors read and approved the final manuscript.

Acknowledgements

We would like to thank Tala Sutherland and Liam Holliday for their help with the chart review and data entry.

Author details

[1]Department of Surgery, Faculty of Medicine and Dentistry, University of Alberta, 2D WMC, 8440-112 Street NW, Edmonton, AB T6G 2B7, Canada. [2]Alberta Centre for Injury Control and Research, School of Public Health, University of Alberta, Edmonton, AB, Canada. [3]Department of Surgery and Division of Critical Care, Faculty of Medicine and Dentistry, University of Alberta, Edmonton, AB, Canada.

References

1. SMARTRISK: *The Economic Burden of Injury in Canada*. Toronto, ON: SMARTRISK; 2009.

2. McDermott FT, Cordner SM, Tremayne AB: *A "before and after" assessment of the influence of the new Victorian trauma care system (1997–1998 vs 2001–2003) on the emergency and clinical management of road traffic fatalities in Victoria. Report of the Consulatative Committee on Road Traffic Fatalities.* Victorian Institute for Forensic Medicine: Melbourne, Australia; 2003.

3. American College of Surgeons: *Advanced Trauma Life Support Program for Doctors: 9th ed.* Chicago: American College of Surgeons; 2012.

4. van Olden GD, Meeuwis JD, Bolhuis HW, Boxma H, Goris RJ: Advanced trauma life support study: quality of diagnostic and therapeutic procedures. *J Trauma* 2004, **57:**381–384.

5. van Olden GD, Meeuwis JD, Bolhuis HW, Boxma H, Goris RJ: Clinical impact of advanced trauma life support. *Am J Emerg Med* 2004, **22:**522–525.

6. Ali J, Cohen R, Adam R, Gana TJ, Pierre I, Ali E, Bedaysie H, West U, Winn J: Attrition of cognitive and trauma management skills after the Advanced Trauma Life Support (ATLS) course. *J Trauma* 1996, **40:**860–866.

7. Ali J, Howard M, Williams J: Is attrition of advanced trauma life support acquired skills affected by trauma patient volume? *Am J Surg* 2002, **183:**142–145.

8. McCrum ML, McKee J, Lai M, Staples J, Switzer N, Widder SL: ATLS adherence in the transfer of rural trauma patients to a level I facility. *Injury* 2012. in press.

9. Santora TA, Trooskin SZ, Blank CA, Clarke JR, Schinco MA: Video assessment of trauma response: adherence to ATLS protocols. *Am J Emerg Med* 1996, **14:**564–569.

10. Spanjersberg WR, Bergs EA, Mushkudiani N, Klimek M, Schipper IB: Protocol compliance and time management in blunt trauma resuscitation. *Emerg Med J* 2009, **26:**23–27.

11. Fitzgerald M, Gocentas R, Dziukas L, Cameron P, Mackenzie C, Farrow N: Using video audit to improve trauma resuscitation–time for a new approach. *Can J Surg* 2006, **49:**208–211.

12. Shackford SR, Hollingworth-Fridlund P, Cooper GF, Eastman AB: The effect of regionalization upon the quality of trauma care as assessed by concurrent audit before and after institution of a trauma system: a preliminary report. *J Trauma* 1986, **26:**812–820.

13. McDermott F, Cordner S, Winship V: Addressing inadequacies in Victoria's trauma system: responses of the Consultative Committee on Road Traffic Fatalities and Victorian trauma services. *Emerg Med Australas* 2010, **22:**224–231.

14. Simons R, Eliopoulos V, Laflamme D, Brown DR: Impact on process of trauma care delivery 1 year after the introduction of a trauma program in a provincial trauma center. *J Trauma* 1999, **46:**811–815.

15. Alberts KA, Bellander BM, Modin G: Improved trauma care after reorganisation: a retrospective analysis. *Eur J Surg* 1999, **165:**426–430.

16. Barquist E, Pizzutiello M, Tian L, Cox C, Bessey PQ: Effect of trauma system maturation on mortality rates in patients with blunt injuries in the Finger Lakes Region of New York State. *J Trauma* 2000, **49:**63–69.

17. Nathens AB, Jurkovich GJ, Rivara FP, Maier RV: Effectiveness of state trauma systems in reducing injury-related mortality: a national evaluation. *J Trauma* 2000, **48:**25–30.

18. Abernathy JH 3rd, McGwin G Jr, Acker JE 3rd, Rue LW 3rd: Impact of a voluntary trauma system on mortality, length of stay, and cost at a level I trauma center. *Am J Surg* 2002, **68:**182–192.

19. Gerardo CJ, Glickman SW, Vaslef SN, Chandra A, Pietrobon R, Cairns CB: The rapid impact on mortality rates of a dedicated care team including trauma and emergency physicians at an academic medical center. *J Emerg Med* 2011, **40:**586–591.

20. Easton R, Sisak K, Balogh ZJ: Time to computed tomography scanning for major trauma patients: the Australian reality. *ANZ J Surg* 2012, **82:**644–647.

21. Lee KL, Graham CA, Lam JM, Yeung JH, Ahuja AT, Rainer TH: Impact on trauma patient management of installing a computed tomography scanner in the emergency department. *Injury* 2009, **40:**873–875.

22. Wurmb TE, Fruhwald P, Hopfner W, Keil T, Kredel M, Brederlau J, Roewer N, Kuhnigk H: Whole-body multislice computed tomography as the first line diagnostic tool in patients with multiple injuries: the focus on time. *J Trauma* 2009, **66:**658–665.

23. Fung Kon Jin PH, Goslings JC, Ponsen KJ, van Kuijk C, Hoogerwerf N, Luitse JS: Assessment of a new trauma workflow concept implementing a sliding CT scanner in the trauma room: the effect on workup times. *J Trauma* 2008, **64:**1320–1326.

24. Fung Kon Jin PH, van Geene AR, Linnau KF, Jurkovich GJ, Ponsen KJ, Goslings JC: Time factors associated with CT scan usage in trauma patients. *Eur J Radiol* 2009, **72:**134–138.

25. Bernhard M, Becker TK, Nowe T, Mohorovicic M, Sikinger M, Brenner T, Richter GM, Radeleff B, Meeder PJ, Buchler MW, Bottiger BW, Martin E, Gries A: Introduction of a treatment algorithm can improve the early management of emergency patients in the resuscitation room. *Resuscitation* 2007, **73:**362–373.

26. Guillamondegui OD, Pryor JP, Gracias VH, Gupta R, Reilly PM, Schwab CW: Pelvic radiography in blunt trauma resuscitation: a diminishing role. *J Trauma* 2002, **53:**1043–1047.

27. Hilty MP, Behrendt I, Benneker LM, Martinolli L, Stoupis C, Buggy DJ, Zimmermann H, Exadaktylos AK: Pelvic radiography in ATLS algorithms: A diminishing role? *World J Emerg Surg* 2008, **3:**11.

28. Kessel B, Sevi R, Jeroukhimov I, Kalganov A, Khashan T, Ashkenazi I, Bartal G, Halevi A, Alfici R: Is routine portable pelvic X-ray in stable multiple trauma patients always justified in a high technology era? *Injury* 2007, **38:**559–563.

29. Bailitz J, Starr F, Beecroft M, Bankoff J, Roberts R, Bokhari F, Joseph K, Wiley D, Dennis A, Gilkey S, Erickson P, Raksin P, Nagy K: CT should replace three-view radiographs as the initial screening test in patients at high, moderate, and low risk for blunt cervical spine injury: a prospective comparison. *J Trauma* 2009, **66:**1605–1609.

30. Holmes JF, Akkinepalli R: Computed tomography versus plain radiography to screen for cervical spine injury: a meta-analysis. *J Trauma* 2005, **58:**902–905.

31. Duane TM, Dechert T, Brown H, Wolfe LG, Malhotra AK, Aboutanos MB, Ivatury RR: Is the lateral cervical spine plain film obsolete? *J Surg Res* 2008, **147:**267–269.

32. Widder S, Doig C, Burrowes P, Larsen G, Hurlbert RJ, Kortbeek JB: Prospective evaluation of computed tomographic scanning for the spinal clearance of obtunded trauma patients: preliminary results. *J Trauma* 2004, **56:**1179–1184.

33. Hennessy D, Widder S, Zygun D, Hurlbert RJ, Burrowes P, Kortbeek JB: Cervical spine clearance in obtunded blunt trauma patients: a prospective study. *J Trauma* 2010, **68:**576–582.

34. Ashton CM, Del Junco DJ, Souchek J, Wray NP, Mansyur CL: The association between the quality of inpatient care and early readmission: a meta-analysis of the evidence. *Med Care* 1997, **35:**1044–1059.

35. American College of Surgeons: *Committee on Trauma: Resources for optimal care of the injured patient.* Chicago: American College of Surgeons; 1993.

36. Battistella FD, Torabian SZ, Siadatan KM: Hospital readmission after trauma: an analysis of outpatient complications. *J Trauma* 1997, **42:**1012–1016.

37. Moore L, Thomas Stelfox H, Turgeon AF, Nathens AB, Sage NL, Emond M, Bourgeois G, Lapointe J, Gagne M: Rates, patterns, and determinants of unplanned readmission after traumatic injury: a multicentre cohort study. *Ann Surg* 2013. in press.

38. Morris DS, Rohrbach J, Sundaram LM, Sonnad S, Sarani B, Pascual J, Reilly P, Schwab CW, Sims C: Early hospital readmission in the trauma population: Are the risk factors different? *Injury* 2013. in press.

39. Driscoll PA, Vincent CA: Variation in trauma resuscitation and its effect on patient outcome. *Injury* 1992, **23:**111–115.

40. Findlay G, Martin IC, Carter S, Smith N, Weyman D, Mason M: *Trauma: Who cares? A report of the National Confidential Enquiry into Patient Outcome and Death (2007).* London, UK: NCEPOD; 2007.

41. Wong K, Petchell J: Trauma teams in Australia: a national survey. *ANZ J Surg* 2003, **73:**819–825.

42. Rainer TH, Cheung NK, Yeung JH, Graham CA: Do trauma teams make a difference? A single centre registry study. *Resuscitation* 2007, **73:**374–381.

43. Petrie D, Lane P, Stewart TC: An evaluation of patient outcomes comparing trauma team activated versus trauma team not activated using TRISS analysis. Trauma and Injury Severity Score. *J Trauma* 1996, **41:**870–873. discussion 873–5.

18

Association between increased blood interleukin-6 levels on emergency department arrival and prolonged length of intensive care unit stay for blunt trauma

Masashi Taniguchi[1], Taka-aki Nakada[1,2]*, Koichiro Shinozaki[2], Yasuaki Mizushima[1] and Tetsuya Matsuoka[1]

Abstract

Background: Systemic immune response to injury plays a key role in the pathophysiological mechanism of blunt trauma. We tested the hypothesis that increased blood interleukin-6 (IL-6) levels of blunt trauma patients on emergency department (ED) arrival are associated with poor clinical outcomes, and investigated the utility of rapid measurement of the blood IL-6 level.

Methods: We enrolled 208 consecutive trauma patients who were transferred from the scene of an accident to a level I trauma centre in Japan and admitted to the intensive care unit (ICU). Blood IL-6 levels on ED arrival were measured by using a rapid measurement assay. The primary outcome variable was prolonged ICU stay (length of ICU stay > 7 days). The secondary outcomes were 28-day mortality, probability of survival and Abbreviated Injury Scale (AIS) scores.

Results: Patients with prolonged ICU stay had significantly higher blood IL-6 levels on ED arrival than the patients without prolonged ICU stay ($P < 0.0001$). The receiver-operating characteristic curves produced an area under the curve of 0.75 (95 % confidence interval [CI], 0.66–0.84; $P < 0.0001$) for prolonged ICU stay. The patients who had increased blood IL-6 levels on ED arrival had increased 28-day mortality ($P = 0.021$) and decreased probability of survival ($P < 0.0001$). The AIS scores for the thorax, abdomen, extremity, and external body regions independently correlated with blood IL-6 levels (unstandardized coefficients [95 % CI] for the thorax: 23.8 [12.6–35.1]; $P < 0.0001$; abdomen: 42.7 [23.8–61.7]; $P < 0.0001$; extremity: 19.0 [5.5–32.4]; $P = 0.0060$; external body regions: 62.9 [13.2–112.7]; $P = 0.030$); the standardized coefficients for the thorax (0.27) and abdomen (0.28) were larger than those for the extremity (0.18) and external body regions (0.15).

Conclusions: Increased blood IL-6 level on ED arrival was significantly associated with prolonged length of ICU stay. Blood IL-6 level on ED arrival independently correlated with the AIS scores for the abdomen and thorax, and, to a lesser extent, those for the extremity and external body regions. The rapid measurement of blood IL-6 level on ED arrival can be utilized as a fast screening tool to improve assessment of injury severity and prediction of clinical outcomes in the initial phase of trauma care.

Keywords: Blunt trauma, Interleukin-6, Abbreviated Injury Scale, Injury Severity Score, Trauma and Injury Severity Score

* Correspondence: taka.nakada@nifty.com
[1]Senshu Trauma and Critical Care Center, 2-23 Rinku Orai Kita, Osaka 598-8577, Japan
[2]Chiba University Graduate School of Medicine, 1-8-1 Inohana, Chuo, Chiba 260-8677, Japan

Background

Systemic immune response to injury plays a key role in the pathophysiological mechanism of blunt trauma [1, 2]. Inflammatory mediators such as tumour necrosis factor (TNF) alpha and interleukin-6 (IL-6) are released into the bloodstream from immune cells after recognition of damage-associated molecular patterns from injured tissues [1, 2]. The exaggerated inflammatory response after trauma potentially causes development of multiorgan dysfunctions (MODs) and prolongs length of intensive care unit (ICU) stay, which lead to increased mortality, morbidity, and medical costs [1, 3–6]. Early identification of high-risk patients is crucial to improve trauma care [7, 8].

Blood IL-6 levels in human trauma have been studied [9–14]. Gebhard et al. serially measured blood IL-6 levels in patients with major trauma during the first 24 h of trauma and were the first to report the significant correlation between blood IL-6 levels during the early phase of trauma (up to 12 h after hospital admission) and injury severity score (ISS), suggesting a potential utility of IL-6 level as an early biomarker of injury severity [9]. Subsequent IL-6 studies in patients with trauma revealed a significant association between elevated blood IL-6 levels during the early phase and development of MODs [10–13]. However, the association between blood IL-6 levels during the early phase of trauma and length of ICU stay has been rarely tested, and only a few studies demonstrated the association between blood IL-6 levels and altered mortality from injury [13, 14]. Furthermore, despite investigations on the association between blood IL-6 level and ISS [9, 12, 14], the relationship between blood IL-6 levels and Abbreviated Injury Scale (AIS) score has been rarely analysed. Moreover, rapid IL-6 measurement systems including point-of-care testing are currently available for clinical practice [15]; however the investigation on potential utility of the point-of-care testing for IL-6 in blunt trauma remains insufficient.

Thus, we tested the hypothesis that increased blood IL-6 levels of blunt trauma patients on emergency department (ED) arrival are associated with poor clinical outcomes, and investigated the potential utility of rapid measurement of the blood IL-6 level in the initial phase of trauma care. We chose length of ICU stay as the primary outcome variable, and 28-day mortality and probability of survival according to Trauma and Injury Severity Score (TRISS) [16] as secondary outcome variables. We further investigated the association between the AIS scores for the six body regions and the blood IL-6 levels. We studied 222 consecutive patients with trauma who were transferred from the scene of the accident to a level I trauma centre in Japan and measured IL-6 levels by performing rapid measurement assays of blood samples on the arrival of the patient to the ED of the trauma centre.

Methods
Patients

The current observational study was prospectively conducted. In this study, 222 consecutive trauma patients who were transferred from the scene of the accident to the Senshu Trauma and Critical Care Center (level I trauma centre, Osaka, Japan) between March 2014 and December 2014 were included. Of these patients, 2 incurred burns, 2 incurred penetrating traumas, and 10 did not require ICU admission were excluded from the study population. Thus, 208 patients with blunt trauma who were admitted to the ICU were evaluated in the study. The institutional review board approved the study.

Measurement and definition

Blood IL-6 levels were measured with a rapid measurement system (Ray-Fast, Toray, Tokyo, Japan) in the ED of the trauma centre by using 200-μL whole blood samples, which were left over after use for initial blood gas analysis on the arrival of the patient to the ED. The rapid measurement system, a compact device for point-of-care testing (width 30 cm, length 42 cm, height 22 cm; weight 15 kg) that includes a chip and all reagents. It took 19 min to provide IL-6 levels automatically after loading cartridges with the whole blood samples to the rapid measurement system through microbead-based fluorescence enzyme immunoassay.

For the present study, prolonged ICU stay was defined as an ICU stay of longer than 7 days [17, 18]. Patients discharged alive from the ICU within 7 days were assigned to the "ICU stay ≤ 7 days" group, while the remaining patients were assigned to the "ICU stay > 7 days" group. Trauma severity scores, including AIS score, ISS, Revised Trauma Score, and probability of survival according to the TRISS model, were determined [19, 20]. Prehospital time was defined as the interval from the 911-call receipt to ED arrival [21].

Statistical analysis

We primarily analysed the association between blood IL-6 levels on ED arrival and prolonged ICU stay. Blood IL-6 levels were compared by using a Mann–Whitney U or Kruskal-Wallis test. The area under the curve (AUC) of the receiver-operating characteristic (ROC) curves of the blood IL-6 levels in relation to prolonged ICU stay or 28-day mortality was analysed. Patients were categorized into tertiles of TRISS, and blood IL-6 levels among the tertiles were compared.

The relationship between AIS scores and blood IL-6 levels was analysed by using multiple linear regression by the following equation: blood IL-6 levels = b1 (Head AIS score) + b2 (Face AIS score) + b3 (Thorax AIS score) + b4 (Extremity AIS score) + b5 (External AIS score) + C.

Differences were considered significant if the two-tailed p value was 0.05. Analyses were performed by using the SPSS statistical software (SPSS, version 20, Chicago, IL).

Results

In baseline characteristics, the patients who had prolonged ICU stay (length of ICU stay > 7 days) were older and had higher severity scores than the patients who had an ICU stay of ≤7 days (Table 1). The patients with prolonged ICU stay had significantly higher blood IL-6 levels on ED arrival than the patients without prolonged ICU stay ($P < 0.0001$; Fig. 1a). The ROC curves yielded an AUC of 0.75 (95 % confidence interval [CI], 0.66–0.84; $P < 0.0001$) for prolonged ICU stay (Fig. 1b).

The patients who died within 28 days had significantly higher blood IL-6 levels than the patients who survived

($P = 0.021$; Fig. 2a). The patients who had a lower probability of survival according to the TRISS model had significantly increased blood IL-6 levels on ED arrival ($P < 0.0001$; Fig. 2b). The AUC of blood IL-6 levels on ED arrival for 28-day mortality was 0.76 (95 % CI, 0.49–1.02; $P = 0.021$; Fig. 1b).

We tested for the association between blood IL-6 levels on ED arrival and severity scores. The patients who had severe ISS had significantly increased blood IL-6 levels on ED arrival (Fig. 3). ISS or TRISS significantly correlated with the blood IL-6 levels on ED arrival ($P < 0.0001$; Pearson correlation coefficient, 0.459 [ISS], –0.453 [TRISS]).

We further tested for the association between the AIS scores for the six body regions and the blood IL-6 levels by using multiple linear regression analysis. The AIS scores for the thorax, abdomen, extremity, and external

Table 1 Baseline characteristic and clinical outcomes of the patients

	ICU stay > 7 days ($n = 48$)	ICU stay ≤ 7 days ($n = 160$)	P
Age, years	58 (43–71)	40 (20–59)	0.0002
Sex, % male	77.1	73.1	0.58
Mechanism of injury, n (%)			0.50
Road injury	32 (66.7)	110 (68.8)	
Fall	13 (27.1)	32 (20.0)	
Compression/machinery	1 (2.1)	11 (6.9)	
Other	2 (4.2)	7 (4.4)	
Prehospital time, min	43 (23–54)	39 (29–53)	0.17
AIS score ≥ 3, n (%)			
Head and neck	31 (64.6)	39 (24.4)	<0.0001
Face	3 (6.3)	1 (0.6)	0.039
Thorax	19 (39.6)	26 (16.3)	0.0006
Abdomen	9 (18.8)	4 (2.5)	0.0003
Extremity	17 (35.4)	20 (12.5)	0.0003
External	0 (0)	0 (0)	-
ISS	26 (17–35)	7 (1–14)	<0.0001
RTS	6.4 (4.1–7.8)	7.8 (7.8–7.8)	<0.0001
TRISS Ps, %	0.75 (0.32–0.90)	0.99 (0.96–0.99)	<0.0001
Intervention, n (%)	30 (62.5)	19 (11.9)	<0.0001
Surgical	19 (39.6)	13 (8.1)	
Endovascular	2 (4.2)	6 (3.8)	
Both	9 (18.8)	0 (0)	
Length of ICU stay, days	14 (8–25)	2 (2–3)	<0.0001
Length of hospital stay, days	41 (19–52)	4 (2–10)	<0.0001
28-day mortality, n (%)	7 (14.6)	0 (0)	<0.0001

Prehospital time was defined as the interval from the 911-call receipt to ED arrival

Immediate intervention was defined as surgical or endovascular intervention for haemostasis within 24 h after hospital arrival. Data are presented as median (interquartile range). P values were calculated by using the chi-square test, Fisher exact test, or Mann–Whitney U test

AIS Abbreviated Injury Scale, *ISS* Injury Severity Score, *RTS* Revised Trauma Score, *TRISS* Trauma Injury Severity Score, *Ps* probability of survival

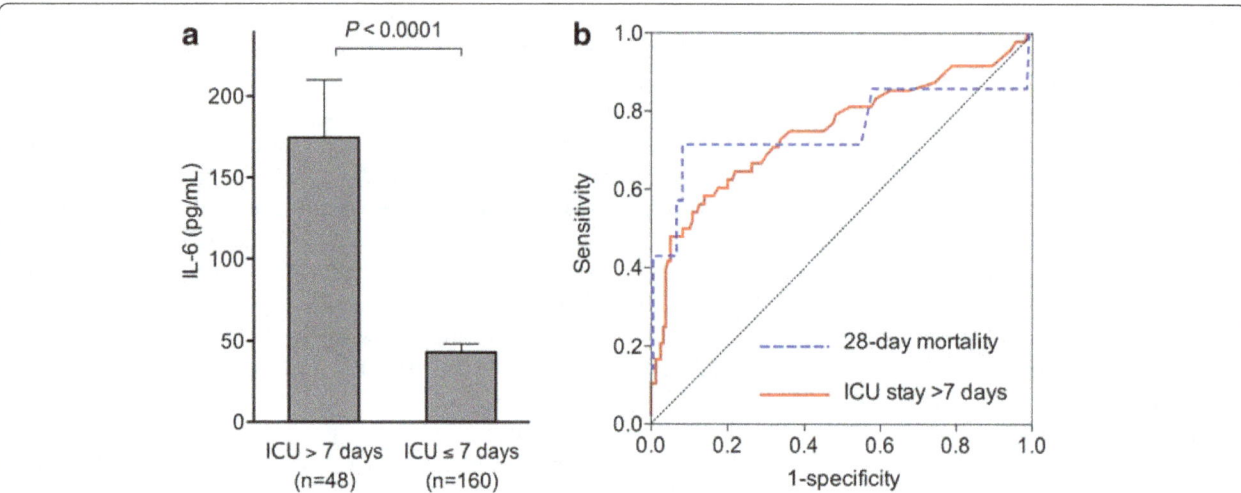

Fig. 1 Panel **a**. Blood interleukin-6 (IL-6) levels on emergency department arrival. The patients who were discharged alive from the intensive care unit within 7 days had lower blood IL-6 levels than the patients who did not survive ($P < 0.0001$). Error bars indicate the standard error of the mean. P values were calculated by using the Mann–Whitney U test. Panel **b**. Receiver-operating characteristic curve analysis. The area under the curve of the receiver-operating characteristic curves of the blood IL-6 levels was 0.76 for prolonged ICU stay (95 % confidence interval [CI], 0.67–0.84; $P < 0.0001$) and 0.76 for 28-day mortality (95 % CI, 0.50–1.02; $P = 0.021$)

body regions independently correlated with blood IL-6 levels (unstandardized coefficient [95 % CI] for the thorax: 23.8 [12.6–35.1], $P < 0.0001$; abdomen: 42.7 [23.8–61.7], $P < 0.0001$; extremity: 19.0 [5.5–32.4], $P = 0.0060$; external body regions: 62.9 [13.2–112.7], $P = 0.030$; Table 2); the standardized coefficients for the thorax and

abdomen were larger than those for the extremity and external body regions (Table 2).

Discussion

In the present study of blunt trauma, the patients who had increased blood IL-6 levels on ED arrival had prolonged

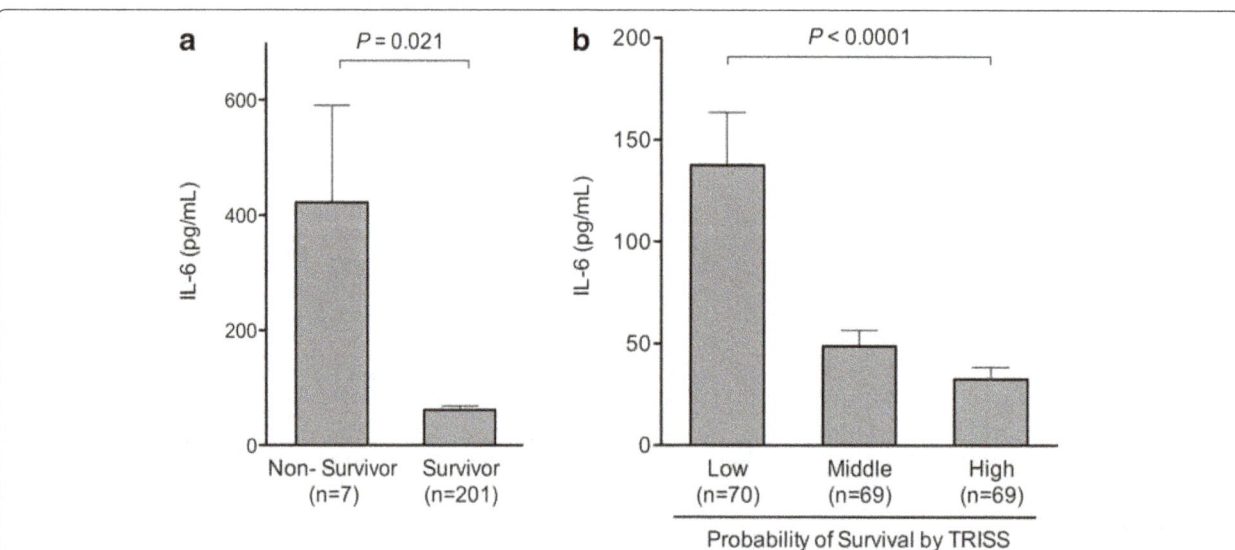

Fig. 2 Blood IL-6 levels on emergency department arrival. Panel **a**. Twenty-eight-day mortality. The patients who died within 28 days had significantly higher blood IL-6 levels than the patients who survived ($P = 0.021$). Error bars indicate the standard error of the mean. P values were calculated by using the Mann–Whitney U test. Panel **b**. Probability of survival according to trauma and injury severity score. The patients who had lower probability of survival according to Trauma and Injury Severity Score (TRISS) had higher blood IL-6 levels on emergency department arrival (low vs. middle vs. high, $P < 0.0001$; low vs. middle, $P < 0.05$; low vs. high, $P < 0.0001$; middle vs. high, $P < 0.001$). Probability of survival in tertiles (median [interquartile range]): low tertile group (0.859 [0.652–0.924]), middle tertile group (0.983 [0.969–0.991]), and high tertile group (0.997 [0.996–0.997]). Error bars indicate the standard error of the mean. P values were calculated by using the Kruskal-Wallis test with Dunn's multiple comparison test

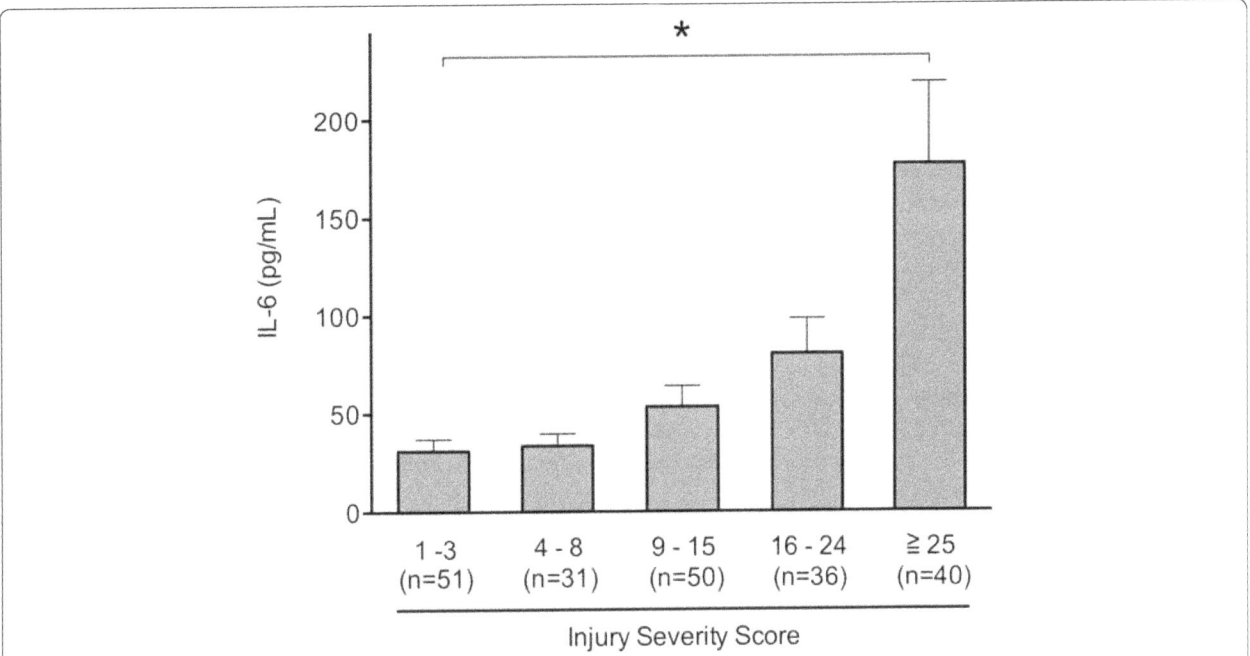

Fig. 3 Blood interleukin-6 (IL-6) levels on emergency department arrival according to injury severity score. The patients who had severe injury severity scores had significantly increased blood IL-6 levels on emergency department arrival (P < 0.0001). Error bars indicate the standard error of the mean. P values were calculated by using the Kruskal-Wallis test

ICU stay, increased 28-day mortality, and decreased probability of survival. Blood IL-6 levels independently correlated with the AIS scores for the abdomen and thorax, and, to a lesser extent, the AIS scores for the extremity and external body regions in the multivariate linear regression.

The association between blood IL-6 levels and length of ICU stay in patients with trauma has been rarely investigated, whereas the associations between increased blood IL-6 levels in early phase of trauma and the development of MODs has been reported in previous studies [10, 11, 13]. Frink et al. investigated whether blood TNF, IL-1, IL-6, IL-8, and IL-10 levels predicted the development of MODs in patients with major traumas and revealed that blood IL-6 level was the best parameter to predict MODs development among these humeral

mediators ($n = 143$; blood IL-6 levels at day 1: AUC, 0.874; 95 % CI, 0.811–0.937) [13]. Likewise, Jastrow et al. and Cuschieri et al. reported high AUC values for blood IL-6 levels in the early phase of trauma for predicting MODs (Jastrow et al.: $n = 48$; blood IL-6 levels 4–8 h after ICU admission: AUC, 0.816; Cuschieri et al.: $n = 79$; blood IL-6 levels during 12 h: AUC, 0.749, 95 % CI, 0.643–0.855) [10, 11]. Considering that the development of MODs is linked with prolonged length of ICU stay [4, 5], our study result on the association between blood IL-6 levels and prolonged ICU stay concurred with the results of the previous studies on the development of MODs.

Previous studies revealed that patients who did not survive from trauma had increased blood IL-6 levels

Table 2 Association between blood IL-6 levels on emergency department arrival and Abbreviated Injury Scale scores in the multivariate logistic regression analysis

	Unstandardized coefficient (95 % Confidence interval)	Standardized coefficient	P
AIS			
Head/neck	6.3 (−3.9 to 16.6)	0.08	0.22
Face	−1.3 (−25.7 to 23.1)	−0.07	0.91
Thorax	23.8 (12.6–35.1)	0.27	<0.0001
Abdomen	42.7 (23.8–61.7)	0.28	<0.0001
Extremity	19.0 (5.5–32.4)	0.18	0.0060
External	62.9 (13.2–112.7)	0.15	0.030

Unstandardized and standardized coefficients were calculated by using multiple linear regression analysis
AIS Abbreviated Injury Scale

during the early phase [13, 14]. Frink et al. reported a high AUC value for blood IL-6 levels at day 1 for predicting mortality in patients with multiple injuries ($n = 21/143$ [death/total]; blood IL-6 levels at day 1: AUC, 0.858; 95 % CI, 0.759–0.956) [13]. In accordance with these results, the association between blood IL-6 level on ED arrival and increased 28-day mortality or decreased probability of survival was observed in the present study of blunt trauma.

The correlations of the blood IL-6 levels in the early phase of trauma with ISSs had been well documented in the previous studies and was consistently observed in the present study (correlation coefficient, 0.46–0.61) [9, 12, 14]. As the ISS is the sum of squared AIS scores for three most severely different injured body regions, we further analysed the correlation between blood IL-6 level and AIS score in each body region. To the best of our knowledge, this is the first report on the correlation between blood IL-6 level on ED arrival and the AIS score of each body region that used multiple regression analysis. Our study showed that the AIS scores for the thorax, abdomen, extremity, and external body regions were independently correlated with blood IL-6 levels and that the AIS score for the thorax or abdomen had a greater effect on the blood IL-6 levels. The different body regions are composed of different types of cells, which may have contributed to the different effect on the blood IL-6 levels of the patients with blunt trauma.

The patients of traumatic brain injury (TBI) had increased IL-6 levels in blood and cerebrospinal fluid (CSF) during the early phase of trauma [22–24]. As the IL-6 concentrations were much higher in CSF than in blood [22, 23], IL-6 is likely to be derived from cells inside the blood–brain barrier, which restricts the movement of IL-6, resulting in the difference between blood and CFS IL-6 levels. A previous study suggested no correlation between blood IL-6 levels on hospital admission and head injury severity [25]. In accordance with this, we found no significant correlation between blood IL-6 levels on ED arrival and AIS score for the head in the present study.

The blood IL-6 levels of trauma patients peaked around 6 h after hospital arrival [9, 10]. The results of previous studies of the association between blood IL-6 levels within 4–12 h after admission and severity scores or altered clinical outcomes highlighted the potential utility of blood IL-6 measurements in clinical practice [9–11, 14]. However, the timing of 4–12 h after hospital arrival is not optimal for trauma physicians to measure blood IL-6 levels as a point-of-care testing and to utilize for predicting severity or clinical outcomes in clinical practice because detailed medical examinations, estimation of injury severity, or even immediate surgical/radiological interventions have already been completed at that time. By contrast, patient arrival to the ED may be a

more practical timing to utilize blood IL-6 level as an adjunctive clinical tool to predict outcome and improve trauma care. In our study, we measured IL-6 levels by using a rapid point-of-care testing assay in a small amount (200 µL) of whole blood samples, which were initially taken for blood gas analysis on ED arrival. It took 19 min to provide IL-6 values automatically after loading cartridges with the whole blood to the measurement system; in most cases, we obtained blood IL-6 levels within 30 min before assessing injury severity by performing detailed medical examinations. Thus blood IL-6 level on ED arrival measured by using the rapid measurement system can be utilized as a fast screening tool to improve assessment of injury severity and prediction of clinical outcomes in the initial phase of trauma care.

This study has some limitations. Although non-survivors or patients with low probability of survival according to TRISS had significantly higher blood IL-6 levels than the survivors or patients with high probability of survival, the sample size of non-survivors was small and the comparison of blood IL-6 levels on ED arrival between the survivors and non-survivors was underpowered.

Conclusions

Increased blood IL-6 levels on ED arrival was significantly associated with prolonged length of ICU stay in patients with blunt trauma. Blood IL-6 levels on ED arrival independently correlated with AIS scores for the abdomen and thorax, and, to a lesser extent, the AIS scores for the extremity and external body regions. These findings suggest the potential utility of the rapid measurement of blood IL-6 level on ED arrival as a fast screening tool to improve assessment of injury severity and prediction of clinical outcomes in the initial phase of trauma care.

Competing interests

The authors declare that they have no competing interests.

Authors' contributions

TN and KS contributed to the study conceptualization and design, acquisition of data, analysis and interpretation of data, statistical analysis, and critical revision of the manuscript for important intellectual content, and provided intellectual input to the research and manuscript. TN drafted the manuscript. MT, YM, and TM contributed to the acquisition of data and critical revision of the manuscript for important intellectual content, and provided intellectual input to the research and manuscript. All authors read and approved the final manuscript.

References

1. Lord JM, Midwinter MJ, Chen YF, Belli A, Brohi K, Kovacs EJ, et al. The systemic immune response to trauma: an overview of pathophysiology and treatment. Lancet. 2014;384:1455–65.

2. Zhang Q, Raoof M, Chen Y, Sumi Y, Sursal T, Junger W, et al. Circulating mitochondrial DAMPs cause inflammatory responses to injury. Nature. 2010;464:104–7.
3. Laupland KB, Kirkpatrick AW, Kortbeek JB, Zuege DJ. Long-term mortality outcome associated with prolonged admission to the ICU. Chest. 2006;129:954–9.
4. Ulvik A, Kvale R, Wentzel-Larsen T, Flaatten H. Multiple organ failure after trauma affects even long-term survival and functional status. Crit Care. 2007;11:R95.
5. Durham RM, Moran JJ, Mazuski JE, Shapiro MJ, Baue AE, Flint LM. Multiple organ failure in trauma patients. J Trauma. 2003;55:608–16.
6. Dewar DC, Tarrant SM, King KL, Balogh ZJ. Changes in the epidemiology and prediction of multiple-organ failure after injury. J Trauma Acute Care Surg. 2013;74:774–9.
7. Ciesla DJ, Moore EE, Johnson JL, Sauaia A, Cothren CC, Moore JB, et al. Multiple organ dysfunction during resuscitation is not postinjury multiple organ failure. Arch Surg. 2004;139:590–4. discussion 4–5.
8. Lee CC, Marill KA, Carter WA, Crupi RS. A current concept of trauma-induced multiorgan failure. Ann Emerg Med. 2001;38:170–6.
9. Gebhard F, Pfetsch H, Steinbach G, Strecker W, Kinzl L, Bruckner UB. Is interleukin 6 an early marker of injury severity following major trauma in humans? Arch Surg. 2000;135:291–5.
10. Jastrow 3rd KM, Gonzalez EA, McGuire MF, Suliburk JW, Kozar RA, Iyengar S, et al. Early cytokine production risk stratifies trauma patients for multiple organ failure. J Am Coll Surg. 2009;209:320–31.
11. Cuschieri J, Bulger E, Schaeffer V, Sakr S, Nathens AB, Hennessy L, et al. Early elevation in random plasma IL-6 after severe injury is associated with development of organ failure. Shock (Augusta, Ga). 2010;34:346–51.
12. Andruszkow H, Fischer J, Sasse M, Brunnemer U, Andruszkow JH, Gansslen A, et al. Interleukin-6 as inflammatory marker referring to multiple organ dysfunction syndrome in severely injured children. Scand J Trauma Resusc Emerg Med. 2014;22:16.
13. Frink M, van Griensven M, Kobbe P, Brin T, Zeckey C, Vaske B, et al. IL-6 predicts organ dysfunction and mortality in patients with multiple injuries. Scand J Trauma Resusc Emerg Med. 2009;17:49.
14. Stensballe J, Christiansen M, Tonnesen E, Espersen K, Lippert FK, Rasmussen LS. The early IL-6 and IL-10 response in trauma is correlated with injury severity and mortality. Acta Anaesthesiol Scand. 2009;53:515–21.
15. Pfafflin A, Schleicher E. Inflammation markers in point-of-care testing (POCT). Anal Bioanal Chem. 2009;393:1473–80.
16. Boyd CR, Tolson MA, Copes WS. Evaluating trauma care: the TRISS method. Trauma Score and the Injury Severity Score. J Trauma. 1987;27:370–8.
17. Lipsett PA, Swoboda SM, Dickerson J, Ylitalo M, Gordon T, Breslow M, et al. Survival and functional outcome after prolonged intensive care unit stay. Ann Surg. 2000;231:262–8.
18. Lin FC, Tsai SC, Li RY, Chen HC, Tung YW, Chou MC. Factors associated with intensive care unit admission in patients with traumatic thoracic injury. J Int Med Res. 2013;41:1310–7.
19. Baker SP, O'Neill B, Haddon Jr W, Long WB. The injury severity score: a method for describing patients with multiple injuries and evaluating emergency care. J Trauma. 1974;14:187–96.
20. Champion HR, Sacco WJ, Carnazzo AJ, Copes W, Fouty WJ. Trauma score. Crit Care Med. 1981;9:672–6.
21. Newgard CD, Schmicker RH, Hedges JR, Trickett JP, Davis DP, Bulger EM, et al. Emergency medical services intervals and survival in trauma: assessment of the "golden hour" in a North American prospective cohort. Ann Emerg Med. 2010;55:235–46. e4.
22. Hayakata T, Shiozaki T, Tasaki O, Ikegawa H, Inoue Y, Toshiyuki F, et al. Changes in CSF S100B and cytokine concentrations in early-phase severe traumatic brain injury. Shock (Augusta, Ga). 2004;22:102–7.
23. Maier B, Schwerdtfeger K, Mautes A, Holanda M, Muller M, Steudel WI, et al. Differential release of interleukines 6, 8, and 10 in cerebrospinal fluid and plasma after traumatic brain injury. Shock (Augusta, Ga). 2001;15:421–6.
24. Hergenroeder GW, Moore AN, McCoy Jr JP, Samsel L, Ward 3rd NH, Clifton GL, et al. Serum IL-6: a candidate biomarker for intracranial pressure elevation following isolated traumatic brain injury. J Neuroinflammation. 2010;7:19.
25. Strecker W, Gebhard F, Perl M, Rager J, Buttenschon K, Kinzl L, et al. Biochemical characterization of individual injury pattern and injury severity. Injury. 2003;34:879–87.

19

Comparison of the Canadian CT head rule and the new orleans criteria in patients with minor head injury

Cemil Kavalci[1*], Gokhan Aksel[1], Omer Salt[2], M Serkan Yilmaz[3], Ali Demir[4], Gulsüm Kavalci[5], Betul Akbuga Ozel[1], Ertugrul Altinbilek[6], Tamer Durdu[3], Cihat Yel[3], Polat Durukan[7] and Bahattin Isik[8]

Abstract

Aim: The aim of the study was to compare the New Orleans Criteria and the New Orleans Criteria according to their diagnostic performance in patients with mild head injury.

Methods: The study was designed and conducted prospectively after obtaining ethics committee approval. Data was collected prospectively for patients presenting to the ED with Minor Head Injury. After clinical assessment, a standard CT scan of the head was performed in patients having at least one of the risk factors stated in one of the two clinical decision rules.

Patients with positive traumatic head injury according to BT results defined as Group 1 and those who had no intracranial injury defined as Group 2. Statistical analysis was performed with SPSS 11.00 for Windows. ROC analyze was performed to determine the effectiveness of detecting intracranial injury with both decision rules. $p < 0.05$ was considered statistically significant.

Results: 175 patients enrolled the study. Male to female ratio was 1.5. The mean age of the patients was $45 \pm 21,3$ in group 1 and $49 \pm 20,6$ in group 2. The most common mechanism of trauma was falling. The sensitivity and specificity of CCHR were respectively 76.4% and 41.7%, whereas sensitivity and specificity of NOC were 88.2% and 6.9%.

Conclusion: The CCHR has higher specificity, PPV and NPV for important clinical outcomes than does the NOC.

Keywords: Emergency, Head injury, CT rules

Introduction

Minor head injury (MHI) is one of the most common injury type seen in the emergency departments (ED) [1]. The average incidence of MHI is reported to be 503.1/100000, with peaks among males and those <5 years of age [2]. No universally agreed definition of MHI exists. Some authors define MHI as the blunt injury of the head with alteration in consciousness, amnesia, or disorientation in a patient who has a Glasgow Coma Scale (GCS) score of 13 to 15 [3,4], although others define it as the blunt injury of the head with alteration in consciousness, amnesia, or disorientation in a patient who has a Glasgow Coma Scale (GCS) score of 14 to 15 [5]. The key to managing these patients is early diagnosis of intracranial injuries using

computed tomography (CT) [6,7]. CT is widely accepted as an effective diagnostic modality to detect rare but clinically significant intracranial injuries in patients suffering minor head injury [8]. As such, it has been increasingly utilized as a routine test for these patients [9]. Systematic evaluation by CT scan would not be a cost-effective strategy in mild head injury because potentially life-threatening complications that may require neurosurgical intervention occur in less than 1% of cases [4]. In addition, some reports warn against its harmful effects (particularly for children) due to the radiation exposure [10]. Yet, CT use is growing rapidly, potentially exposing patients to unnecessary ionizing radiation risk and costs [11].

Commonly accepted clinical decision rules for detecting life-threatening complications in patients with mild head injury are New Orleans Criteria (NOC) and the Canadian CT Head Rules (CCHR) [3,4,12]. These two rules were

---
* Correspondence: cemkavalci@yahoo.com
[1]Emergency Department, Baskent University Faculty of Medicine, Ankara, Turkey

Table 1 Canadian CT head rule and New Orleans Criteria

Canadian CT Head Rule High risk (for neurosurgical interventions)	New Orleans Criteria
• GCS score, 15 at two hours after injury	• Headache
• Suspected open or depressed skull fracture	• Vomiting
• Any sign of basal skull fracture (hemotympanum, "panda" eyes, cerebrospinal fluid otorrhoea, Battle's sign).	• Older than 60 years
• Vomiting more than once	• Drug or alcohol intoxication
• Age >65 years	• Persistent anterograde amnesia (deficits in short-term memory)
Medium risk (for brain injury on CT)	
• Persistent retrograde amnesia of greater than 30 minutes	• Visible trauma above the clavicle
• Dangerous mechanism of injury (pedestrian struck by vehicle, ejection from vehicle, fall from greater than three feet or five stairs)	• Seizure

externally validated in the previous studies but we believe that application of these decision rules may still be limited in populations with different demographic and epidemiologic features. The aim of the study was to compare the CCHR and the NOC according to their diagnostic performance in MHI patients.

Materials and methods

This study was conducted at a single tertiary care center in Turkey with an annual ED census of 70,000 visits. The study was designed and conducted prospectively after ethics committee approval. Acute MHI was defined as a patient having a blunt trauma to the head within 24 hours, with a Glasgow Coma Scale (GCS) score of 13 to 15. The patients were also required to have at least one of the risk factors stated in CCHR or NOC (Table 1).

Table 2 Characteristics of patients

	Group 1	Group 2	P value
Sex (male/female)	14/3	92/66	p>0,05
Age (mean ± sd*)	45 ± 21,3	49.57 ± 20,6	p>0,05
Trauma mechanism			
Motor vehicle accident	2	34	
Pedestrian	0	8	p>0,05
Falling	8	68	
Assault	7	48	
Symptom			
Headache	12	139	
Amnesia	1	7	
Vomiting	2	19	
Lethargy	3	6	
Loss of consciousness	1	9	
GCS			
13	3	4	
14	0	9	
15	14	145	

*Sd=standart deviation, GCS=Glasgow Coma Scale Score.

Patients with GCS score of less than 13 or instable vital signs, presentation time more than 24 hours after head trauma, patients with an obvious penetrating skull injury or obvious depressed fracture, presence of major trauma, bleeding disorder or use of oral anticoagulants (e.g., warfarin), contraindications for CT and those pregnant or fewer than 18 were excluded from the study.

All patients were assessed by an emergency physician or by supervised emergency medicine residents. Data collection was done prospectively using a data collection sheet. After clinical assessment, a standard CT scan of the head was performed in patients having at least one of the risk factors stated in one of the two clinical decision rules. The CT scans were interpreted by a radiologist who was blinded to patient data. Presence of traumatic lesions on head CT scan was the main outcome. The lesions accepted as positive CT results for the study were subarachnoid hemorrhage, epidural hemorrhage, subdural hematoma, intraparenchymal hematoma, compression fracture, cerebral edema and contusion.

Cases without a complete data sheet were excluded. Demographic characteristics, mechanism of injury, traumatic findings at CT were all evaluated. CCHR and NOC were also assessed in patients who presented with a minor head trauma. Patients with positive traumatic head injury according to BT results defined as Group 1 and those who had no intracranial injury defined as Group 2. Statistical

Table 3 Computed tomography results of the patients

BT results	N	%
Normal	156	89.1
Epidural hemorrhage	3	1.8
Depressed fracture	2	1.2
Cerebral edema	4	2.4
Subdural hematoma	3	1.8
Intraparenchymal hematoma	1	0.6
Subarachnoid hemorrhage	6	3.4
Contusion	2	1.2

Table 4 Rates of patients meet the criteria according to groups for patients with GCS 13

Predictor	Group 1	Group 2
Canadian CT* Head Rule		
Positive	3	0
Negative	4	0
New Orleans Criteria		
Positive	3	0
Negative	4	0

analysis was performed with SPSS (version 11.0; SPSS, Inc., Chicago, IL). Results were expressed with number and percentage. Chi-square test was used in comparison of categorical data. ROC analyze was performed to determine the effectiveness of detecting intracranial injury with both decision rules. The sensitivity, specificity, and predictive values with 95% confidence intervals (CIs) for performance of each decision rule for CT scan intracranial traumatic findings were calculated separately for patients having GCS score of 13 and patients having GCS score of 14–15. P < 0.05 was considered statistically significant. When appropriate, CIs were calculated with a 95% confidence level.

Results

During the study period, data were collected for 198 trauma patients who met inclusion criteria. Of these, 21

were excluded because of refusing to be included in the study, 2 were excluded because of missing data, resulting in 175 patients in the data analysis. Table 2 shows the demographic and clinical characteristics of the overall study group. In the enrolled patients, male to female ratio was 1.5. The mean age of the patients was 45 ± 21.3 in group 1 and 49 ± 20.6 in group 2. The most common mechanism of trauma was falling. Headache was the main symptom in both groups (Table 2). CT scan was performed in all of 175 patients; pathologic findings were present in 17 patients (9.71%). The most common intracranial injury was Subarachnoid hemorrhage (Table 3).

Sensitivity, Specificity, PPV, and NPV of both of the criteria of the patients having GCS score 13 were 100%, %0, 42% and 100% respectively (Table 4, Figure 1).

For the patients having GCS score between 14–15; the sensitivity and specificity of CCHR were 78.5% and 42.8% respectively, whereas sensitivity and specificity of NOC were 85.7% and 0.7%. Positive predictive value (PPV) and negative predictive value (NPV) were both higher in CCHR than NOC. PPV and NPV of CCHR were respectively 11.1% and 95.6% whereas PPV and NPV of NOC were 0.7% and 84.6% (Table 5, Figure 2).

Discussion

In the most of the prior studies, motor vehicle accidents were reported to be the most common mechanism of trauma [3,4]. Some other authors also reported the

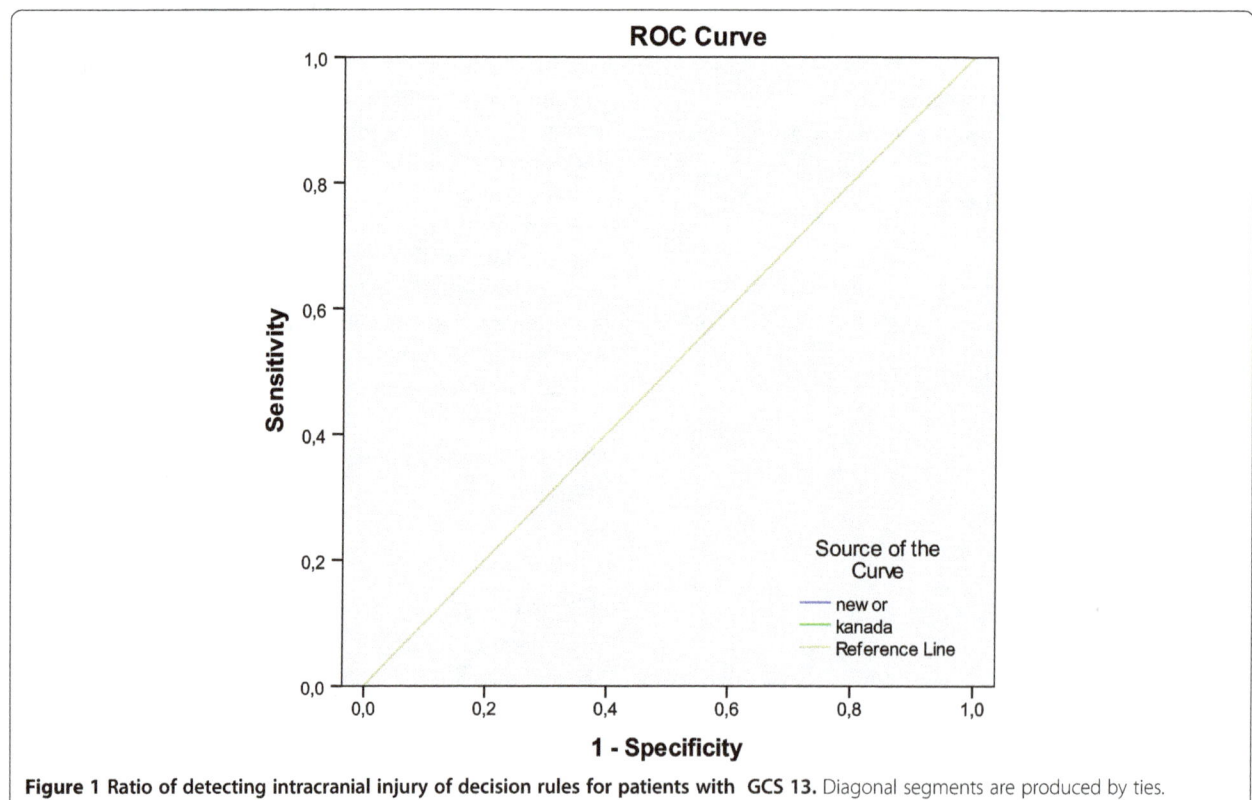

Figure 1 Ratio of detecting intracranial injury of decision rules for patients with GCS 13. Diagonal segments are produced by ties.

Table 5 Rates of patients meet the criteria according to groups for patients with GCS 14-15

Predictor	Group 1	Group 2
Canadian CT* Head Rule		
Positive	11	88
Negative	3	66
New Orleans Criteria		
Positive	12	143
Negative	2	11

*CT= Computed tomography.

falling as the most common trauma mechanism [13]. In the present study, the most common mechanism for trauma was found as falling in accordance with the later study. Assault was the second and motor vehicle accidents were the third most common mechanisms of trauma. Our hospital is in the center of the city, and away from the high ways. This may be the reason for motor vehicle accidents to be the third most common cause. The mechanism of trauma is probably depends on the distance from hospital to high ways, social and economical status and degree or level of hospital as trauma centre. Similar to prior studies, males were the most affected sex group from the trauma in the present study [3,4,13]. This is probably due to men's working in more dangerous jobs, taking more places in active city social

life, being more associated with violence and male drivers being more than females.

In the present study, efficacy of both criteria were found similar in the patients having GCS score 13. In the patients having GCS score 14–15, a comparison of the clinical decision rules for use of CT in patients with MHI showed that both the CCHR and the NOC were sensitive for the outcome measure of any traumatic intracranial lesion on CT which is "clinically important" brain lesion. Although the sensitivity was high in these two decision rules, they both had much lower sensitivities in this study than the original published studies [3,13-15]. Papa et al. and Smits et al. found sensitivities of both rules to reach 100% [13,15]. The cause of lower sensitivities may be explained by our patients' low socioeconomic status and unreliable history. In contrast to previous publications, Ro et al. found lower sensitivities in both decision rules similar to our study results. They also found the sensitivity higher in NOC and specificity higher in CCHR [16]. In the present study, the specificity of CCHR was higher than specificity of NOC (47,1% versus 6.9%). Our results were similar to the results of the study reported by Smits et al. They found the specificity of CCHR higher than the specificity of NOC (39.7% versus 5.6%) [13]. Papa et al. and Stiell et al. also found the specificity of CCHR higher than NOC [3,15]. In the present study, CCHR was found to be superior to NOC

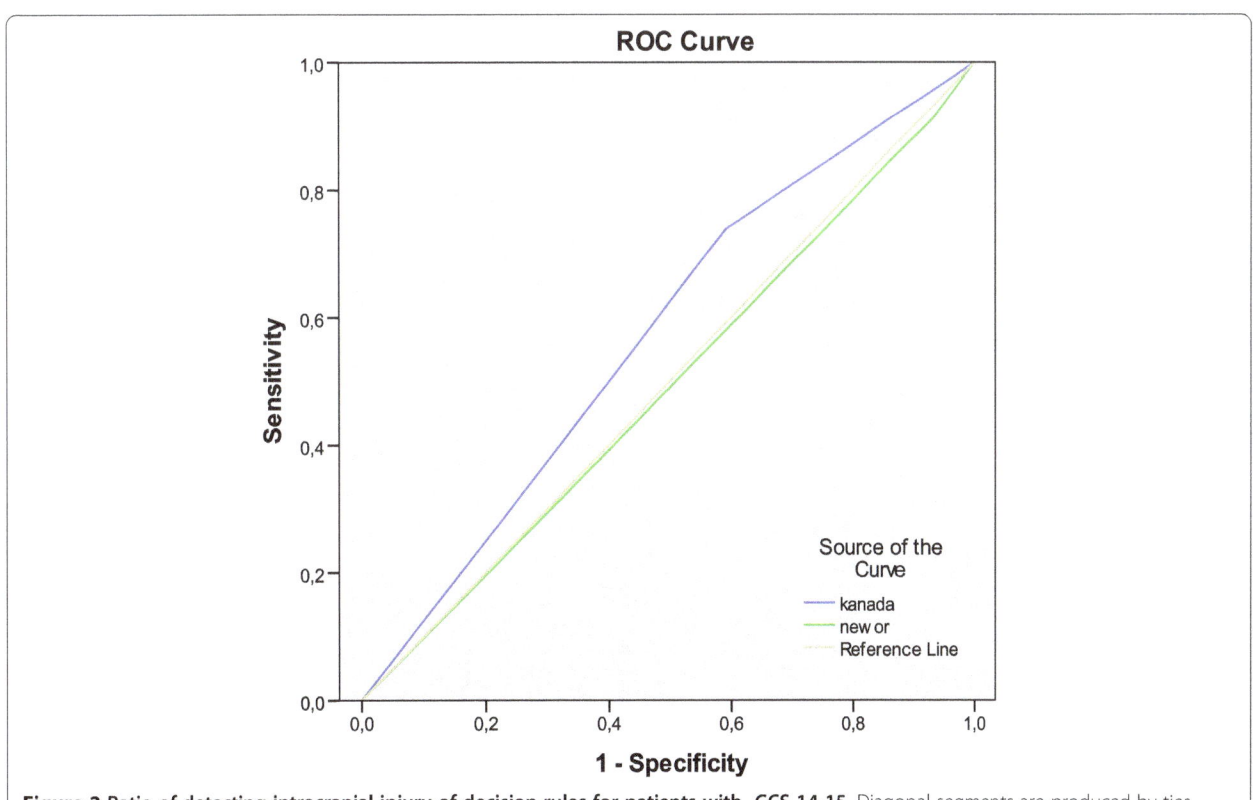

Figure 2 Ratio of detecting intracranial injury of decision rules for patients with GCS 14-15. Diagonal segments are produced by ties.

due to higher specificity, higher PPV and NPV. The only superiority of NOC in our study was the sensitivity with 88.2% while it was 76.4% in CCHR. Many prior studies also found the sensitivity of NOC higher than the sensitivity of CCHR [13,16]. Smits et al. tried to explain this difference in sensitivities for neurocranial traumatic CT findings between the 2 decision rules with more stringent use of the risk factor of external injury in the CCHR. For example in the NOC, this risk factor comprises all external injuries above the clavicles. Despite the NOC having higher sensitivity, specificities for neurocranial traumatic CT findings were low for the NOC decision rule, and higher for the CCHR [13]. In accordance with Smits et al. higher sensitivity of NOC causes the lower specificity and this means an increase in healthcare costs.

Conclusion

In summary, for patients with MHI, the CCHR and the NOC have both high sensitivities for clinically important brain injury although this study reports much lower sensitivities than the prior published studies. Additionally, the CCHR has higher specificity, PPV and NPV for important clinical outcomes than does the NOC. We believe that use of CCHR may result in reduced imaging rates, reduced costs and this would help us to protect our patients from the side effects of radiation.

Limitations

This study is conducted in one center. A multicenter study having larger number of patients and more trauma patients caused by much different mechanism could have been assessed. The study focused only on the two widely accepted clinical decision rules but did not study on other decision rules or aspects.

Our primary outcome measure was any traumatic neurocranial lesions on the CT scan. The third limitation of this study is absence of the second outcome measure which can be defined as findings on the CT scan that led to neurosurgical intervention.

Competing interests
The authors declare that they have no competing interests.

Authors' contributions
The quantitative analysis was planned by CK, MSY, AD. Study data were analyzed by CK,CY,GK and interpreted by BAO, TD, EA, PD. The first version of the manuscript was drafted by AD, GA, BI. All authors contributed to the edition and revision of the manuscript and the final version of the article was reviewed and approved by all authors.

Author details
[1]Emergency Department, Baskent University Faculty of Medicine, Ankara, Turkey. [2]Emergency Department, State hospital, Yozgat, Turkey. [3]Emergency Department, Numune Training and Research Hospital, Ankara, Turkey. [4]Emergency Department, Yenimahalle State hospital, Ankara, Turkey. [5]Anesthesia Department, Yenimahalle State hospital, Ankara, Turkey. [6]Emergency Department, Şişli Hamidiye Etfal Training and Research Hospital, İstanbul, Turkey. [7]Emergency Department, Erciyes University Faculty of Medicine, Kayseri, Turkey. [8]Emergency Department, Keciören Training and Research Hospital, Ankara, Turkey.

References

1. Cassidy JD, Carroll LJ, Peloso PM, Borg J, Von Holst H, Holm L, Kraus J, Coronado VG: Incidence, risk factors and prevention of mild traumatic brain injury: results of the WHO Collaborating Centre Task Force on Mild Traumatic Brain Injury. Collaborating Centre Task Force on Mild Traumatic Brain Injury. *J Rehabil Med* 2004, **43**:28–60.
2. Bazarian JJ, McClung J, Shah MN, Cheng YT, Flesher W, Kraus J: Mild traumatic brain injury in the United States, 1998–2000. *Brain Inj* 2005, **19**(2):85–91.
3. Stiell IG, Clement CM, Rowe BH, Schull MJ, Brison R, Cass D, Eisenhauer MA, McKnight RD, Bandiera G, Holroyd B, Lee JS, Dreyer J, Worthington JR, Reardon M, Greenberg G, Lesiuk H, MacPhail I, Wells GA: Comparison of the Canadian CT Head Rule and the New Orleans Criteria in patients with minor head injury. *JAMA* 2005, **294**(12):1511–1518.
4. Bouida W, Marghli S, Souissi S, Ksibi H, Methammem M, Haguiga H, Khedher S, Boubaker H, Beltaief K, Grissa MH, Trimech MN, Kerkeni W, Chebili N, Halila I, Rejeb I, Boukef R, Rekik N, Bouhaja B, Letaief M, Nouira S: Prediction value of the Canadian CT head rule and the New Orleans criteria for positive head CT scan and acute neurosurgical procedures in minor head trauma: a multicenter external validation study. *Ann Emerg Med* 2013, **61**(5):521–527.
5. Hung RH: Minor Head Injury in Infants and Children. In *Tintinalli's Emergency Medicine*. 7th edition. Edited by Tintinalli JE. New York: Mc Graw- Hill; 2011:888–892.
6. Shackford SR, Wald SL, Ross SE, Cogbill TH, Hoyt DB, Morris JA, Mucha PA, Pachter HL, Sugerman HJ, O'Malley K: The clinical utility of computed tomographic scanning and neurologic examination in the management of patients with minor head injuries. *J Trauma* 1992, **33**(3):385–394.
7. Stein SC, Ross SE: The value of computed tomographic scans in patients with low-risk head injuries. *Neurosurgery* 1990, **26**(4):638–640.
8. Klement W, Wilk S, Michalowski W, Farion KJ, Osmond MH, Verter V: Predicting the need for CT imaging in children with minor head injury using an ensemble of Naive Bayes classifiers. *Artif Intell Med* 2012, **54**(3):163–170.
9. Smits M, Dippel DW, Nederkoorn PJ, Dekker HM, Vos PE, Kool DR: Minor head injury: CT-based strategies for management–a cost-effectiveness analysis. *Radiology* 2010, **254**(2):532–540.
10. Brenner DJ, Hall EJ: Computed tomography – an increasing source of radiation exposure. *N Engl J Med* 2007, **357**(22):2277–2284.
11. Melnick ER, Szlezak CM, Bentley SK, Dziura JD, Kotlyar S, Post LA: CT overuse for mild traumatic brain injury. *Jt Comm J Qual Patient Saf* 2012, **38**(11):483–489.
12. Stiell IG, Wells GA, Vandemheen K, Clement C, Lesiuk H, Laupacis A: The Canadian CT Head Rule for patients with minor head injury. *Lancet* 2001, **357**(9266):1391–1396.
13. Ro YS, Shin SD, Holmes JF, Song KJ, Park JO, Cho JS, Lee SC, Kim SC, Hong KJ, Park CB, Cha WC, Lee EJ, Kim YJ, Ahn KO, Ong ME: Comparison of clinical performance of cranial computed tomography rules in patients with minor head injury: a multicenter prospective study. *Acad Emerg Med* 2011, **18**(6):597–604.
14. Smits M, Dippel DW, De Haan GG, Dekker HM, Vos PE, Kool DR, Nederkoorn PJ, Hofman PA, Twijnstra A, Tanghe HL, Hunink MG: External validation of the Canadian CT Head Rule and the New Orleans Criteria for CT scanning in patients with minor head injury. *JAMA* 2005, **294**(12):1519–1525.
15. Stein SC, Fabbri A, Servadei F, Glick HA: A critical comparison of clinical decision instruments for computed tomographic scanning in mild closed traumatic brain injury in adolescents and adults. *Ann Emerg Med* 2009, **53**(2):180–188.
16. Papa L, Stiell IG, Clement CM, Pawlowicz A, Wolfram A, Braga C, Draviam S, Wells GA: Performance of the Canadian CT Head Rule and the New Orleans Criteria for predicting any traumatic intracranial injury on computed tomography in a United States Level I trauma center. *Acad Emerg Med* 2012, **19**(1):2–10.

20

The risk factors of concomitant intraperitoneal and retroperitoneal hemorrhage in the patients with blunt abdominal trauma

Chun-Yi Wu[†], Shang-Ju Yang[†], Chih-Yuan Fu[*], Chien-Hung Liao, Shih-Ching Kang, Yu-Pao Hsu, Being-Chuan Lin, Kuo-Ching Yuan and Shang-Yu Wang

Abstract

Introduction: Intraperitoneal and retroperitoneal hemorrhages may occur simultaneously in blunt abdominal trauma (BAT) patients. These patients undergo emergency laparotomies because of concomitant unstable hemodynamics and positive sonographic examination results. However, if the associated retroperitoneal hemorrhage is found intraoperatively and cannot be controlled surgically, then the patients require post-laparotomy transcatheter arterial embolization (TAE). In the current study, we attempted to determine the risk factors for post-laparotomy TAE.

Materials and methods: Patients with concomitant BAT and unstable hemodynamic were retrospectively analyzed. The characteristics of the patients who underwent laparotomy or who required post-laparotomy TAE were investigated and compared. The Tile classification system was used to evaluate the pelvic fracture patterns.

Results: Seventy-four patients were enrolled in the study. Fifty-nine (79.7%) patients underwent laparotomy to treat intra-abdominal hemorrhage, and fifteen (20.3%) patients underwent additional post-laparotomy TAE because of concomitant retroperitoneal hemorrhage. Pelvic fracture was present in 80.0% of the post-laparotomy TAE patients. This percentage was significantly greater than that of the laparotomy only patients (80.0% vs. 30.5%, $p < 0.001$). Furthermore, 30 patients (40.5%, 30/74) had concomitant pelvic fracture diagnoses. Of these patients, eighteen (60%, 18/30) underwent laparotomy only, while the other twelve patients (40%, 12/30) required post-laparotomy TAE. Compared with the patients who underwent laparotomy only, more patients with Tile B_1-type pelvic fractures (58.3% vs. 11.1%, $p = 0.013$) required post-laparotomy TAE.

Conclusion: Regarding BAT patient management, the likelihood of post-laparotomy TAE should be considered in patients with concomitant pelvic fractures. Furthermore, more attention should be directed toward patients with Tile B_1-type pelvic fractures because of the specific fracture pattern and impaction force.

Keyword: Pelvic fracture, Laparotomy, Transcatheter arterial embolization, Tile B_1

Introduction

Intraperitoneal and retroperitoneal hemorrhages may occur simultaneously in patients with concomitant blunt abdominal trauma (BAT) and unstable hemodynamics [1-3]. Additionally, BAT management principles have evolved to a non-operative management approach because of advancements in treatment concepts and improvements in

diagnostic modalities [4,5]. however, laparotomies are still necessary in some situations. In contrast, transcatheter arterial embolization (TAE) serves as an effective surgery alternative for retroperitoneal hemorrhage management [6-8]. Therefore, in addition to aggressive resuscitation, either a laparotomy or a TAE is usually needed for the hemostasis management of these patients. Furthermore, some complicated cases require both procedures; however, only limited information is available for hemorrhage origin assessment when only clinical presentation and primary tools are used for the evaluations. Although sonographic examination is utilized in emergency departments (ED)

* Correspondence: drfu5564@yahoo.com.tw

[†]Equal contributors

Department of Trauma and Emergency Surgery, Chang Gung Memorial Hospital, Chang Gung University, 5, Fu-Hsing Street, Kwei Shan Township, Taoyuan, Taiwan

worldwide, it can only detect intraperitoneal hemorrhage and has limitations regarding retroperitoneal hemorrhage surveillence [9-11]. Therefore, it is difficult to identify patients with concomitant intraperitoneal and retroperitoneal hemorrhages during primary evaluations over a short time period.

Patients usually undergo emergency laparotomies because of concomitant unstable hemodynamics and positive sonographic examination results [9,10,12]. However, if associated retroperitoneal hemorrhages are found intraoperatively and cannot be controlled surgically, then post-laparotomy TAE is required. The preparation of an angioembolization suite and the gathering of personnel are usually time-consuming, which may delay definitive hemostasis. Furthermore, transporting these patients between the operation and angiographic rooms is risky under such critical conditions. Therefore, the early identification of these patients is important to ensure that subsequent treatments can be initiated in a timely manner. Additionally, more information may be needed for physicians to predict retroperitoneal hemorrhages and further hemostatic procedure requirements.

In this study, we describe a retrospective observation of the management of patients with concomitant BAT and unstable hemodynamics. The different clinical course characteristics were delineated and compared, and the patients who underwent post-laparotomy TAE were investigated and analyzed. We attempted to determine the risk factors that indicated post-laparotomy TAE and analyzed the critical decision-making processes that occurred when only limited information was available.

Materials and methods

From May 2008 to October 2013, patients with concomitant BAT and unstable hemodynamic were retrospectively analyzed. They were evaluated and treated according to our established algorithm, which is based on the Advanced Trauma Life Support (ATLS) guidelines [13] (Figure 1). The Pelvic X-ray was routinely used as an adjunct to the primary survey in these patients. Unstable hemodynamics were defined as having systolic blood pressure (SBP) < 90 mmHg, without response to 2000 ml of fluid resuscitation. Patients who died in the ED without undergoing other evaluations were not enrolled in the current study. The pelvic circumferential compression device (PCCD) was applied in the ED while the pelvic fracture diagnosed. Then the patients underwent emergency laparotomy and had positive sonographic examination results, which indicated intra-abdominal hemorrhage. Post-laparotomy TAE was indicated for the patients with retroperitoneal hemorrhages that were found intraoperatively. They were moved to an angiographic room after a damage-control laparotomy after intraperitoneal/retroperitoneal packing directly without additional computed

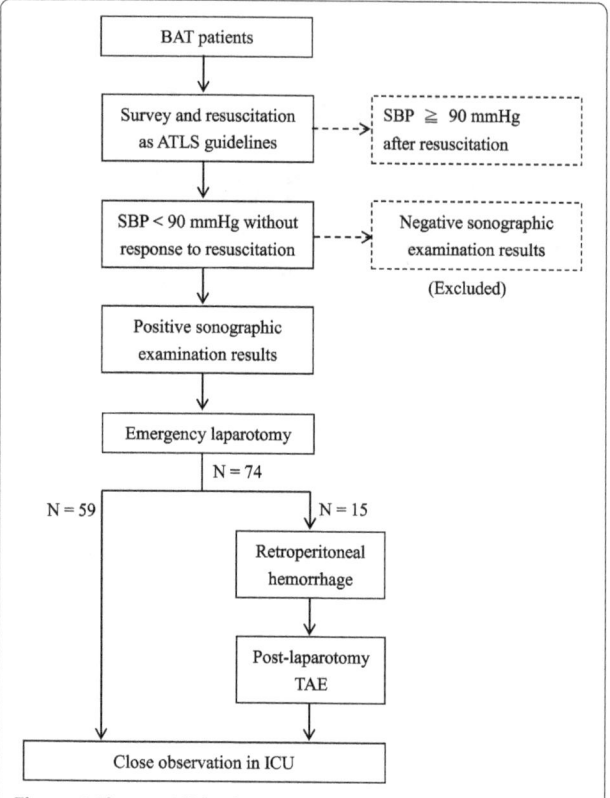

Figure 1 The established BAT patient protocol used at our institution.

tomographic (CT) scan. These patients were taken to the intensive care unit (ICU) for further observation after these hemostasis procedures. In our institution, the operating and angiography rooms were available 24 hours per day, and a TAE could be performed within one hour.

In this study, the characteristics of the patients who required post-laparotomy TAEs were noted and investigated. Patient demographics, Revised Trauma Scores (RTSs), Injury Severity Scores (ISSs) and number of blood transfusions in the ED were routinely recorded. The Tile classification system was used to evaluate the pelvic fracture patterns [14,15]. The pelvic ring has a stable fracture with intact sacroiliac complex in type A injuries. The type B and C injuries were classified as unstable pelvic fracture (B_1: external rotational unstable, B_2: internal rotational unstable, C: both rotational and vertical unstable). The patients who underwent laparotomy only or laparotomy plus post-laparotomy TAE were compared.

All data are presented as patient percentages or means with standard deviations. The numerical data were compared using the Wilcoxon two-sample exact test. Nominal data were compared using Fisher's exact test. Multivariate logistic regression analysis was performed to determine the independent risk factors related to the requirement for post-laparotomy TAE. All statistical analyses were performed using the SPSS computer software package (version 13.0, Chicago, IL, USA). A value of $p < 0.05$ was considered to be significant.

Results

During the 68-month study period, 3,871 patients with BAT diagnoses were sent to our ED. Thirty-nine patients died in the ED without undergoing further evaluations and were excluded. A total of 74 patients with concomitant BAT and unstable hemodynamics without response to 2000 ml of fluid resuscitation were enrolled in this study. The mean patient age was 42.0 years (48 [64.7%] males and 26 [35.3%] females).

The various clinical course distributions for the patients are shown in Figure 1. Fifty-nine (79.7%) patients underwent laparotomy only to treat intra-abdominal hemorrhage, and fifteen (20.3%) patients underwent post-laparotomy TAE because of concomitant retroperitoneal hemorrhage. Table 1 compares the patients who underwent laparotomy only with patients who required post-laparotomy TAE. Pelvic fracture was present in 80.0% of the patients who required post-laparotomy TAE, which was significantly greater than the percentage of the patients who underwent laparotomy only (80.0% vs. 30.5%, $p < 0.001$). These patients had significantly higher ISSs (24.6 ± 24.1 vs. 19.5 ± 20.7, $p = 0.004$), lower RTSs (4.819 ± 1.335 vs. 6.007 ± 0.772, $p = 0.011$) and a greater amount of transfused blood (1356.3 ± 977.6 ml

vs. 887.3 ± 934.9 ml, $p = 0.028$) (Table 1). Multivariate logistic regression analyses revealed that the presence of a pelvic fracture (odds ratio [OR] = 3.4, $p = 0.018$) and an ISS $\geq$ 16 (OR = 2.2, $p = 0.048$) were two significant predictive factors for patients requiring post-laparotomy TAE (Table 2).

In the current study, there were 30 concomitant pelvic fracture diagnoses (40.5%, 30/74). Of these patients, eighteen (60%, 18/30) underwent laparotomy only, while the other twelve patients (40%, 12/30) required post-laparotomy TAE. Compared with the laparotomy-only patients, the post-laparotomy TAE patients required more transfused blood (1542.8 ± 1022.5 ml vs. 914.5 ± 425.9 ml, $p < 0.001$). Additionally, there were more patients with type B_1 pelvic fractures (58.3% vs. 11.1%, $p = 0.013$) or unstable pelvic fractures (75.0% vs. 22.2%, $p = 0.008$) among these patients. Furthermore, the post-laparotomy TAE patients also demonstrated significantly higher ISSs (26.3 ± 14.1 vs. 22.5 ± 20.7, $p = 0.004$) and lower RTSs (4.115 ± 2.431 vs. 5.981 ± 3.212, $p = 0.011$) than the

Table 2 The factors independently associated with post-laparotomy TAE in the overall patient population

Variable	Odds ratio (95% CI)	p-value[j]
Pelvic fracture	3.4 (2.2 ~ 11.4)	0.018
Blood transfusion $\geq$ 1500 ml	8.7 (0.7 ~ 15.2)	0.302
RTS < 5.5	5.2 (0.1 ~ 13.4)	0.272
ISS $\geq$ 16	2.2 (1.6 ~ 9.5)	0.048

[j]Multivariate logistic regression.

Table 1 Comparisons between the patients who underwent laparotomy only and the patients who required post-laparotomy TAE

Variables	Laparotomy only (N = 59)	Laparotomy → TAE (N = 15)	p-value
Age	42.3 ± 24.2	40.6 ± 23.1	0.916[#]
Gender (N)			0.367[$]
Female	19 (32.2%)	7 (46.7%)	
Male	40 (67.8%)	8 (53.3%)	
ISS	19.5 ± 20.7	24.6 ± 24.1	0.004[#]
RTS	6.007 ± 0.772	4.819 ± 1.335	0.011[#]
Blood transfusion (ml)	887.3 ± 934.9	1356.3 ± 977.6	0.028[#]
Pelvic fracture (N)			< 0.001[$]
Yes	18 (30.5%)	12 (80.0%)	
No	41 (69.5%)	3 (20.0%)	
Pelvis stability			< 0.001[$]
Stable (tile A)	55 (93.2%)	6 (40.0%)	
Unstable (tile B/C)	4 (6.8%)	9 (60.0%)	

The variables are expressed as means ± SD.
[#]Wilcoxon two-sample exact test, [$]Fisher's exact test.

Table 3 Comparisons between the pelvic fracture patients who underwent laparotomy only and the patients who required post-laparotomy TAE

Variables	Laparotomy only (N = 18)	Laparotomy → TAE (N = 12)	p-value
Age	41.8 ± 16.7	43.0 ± 22.6	0.854[#]
Gender (N)			1.000[$]
Female	5 (27.8%)	4 (33.3%)	
Male	13 (72.2%)	8 (66.7%)	
ISS	22.5 ± 20.7	26.3 ± 14.1	0.004[#]
RTS	5.981 ± 3.212	4.115 ± 2.431	0.011[#]
Blood transfusion (ml)	914.5 ± 425.9	1542.8 ± 1022.5	< 0.001[#]
Fracture pattern (N)			0.013[$]
Tile B_1	2 (11.1%)	7 (58.3%)	
Non-Tile B_1 ($A + B_2 + C$)	16 (88.9%)	5 (41.7%)	
Pelvis stability			0.008[$]
Stable (tile A)	14 (77.8%)	3 (25.0%)	
Unstable (tile B/C)	4 (22.2%)	9 (75.0%)	

Variables are expressed as means ± SD.
[#]Wilcoxon two-sample exact test, [$]Fisher's exact test.

Table 4 The factors independently associated with post-laparotomy TAE in pelvic fracture patients

Variable	Odds ratio (95% CI)	p-value[j]
Tile B$_1$ pelvic fracture	6.4 (4.0 ~ 15.1)	0.002
Blood transfusion ≧ 1500 ml	2.9 (0.1 ~ 4.6)	0.519
RTS < 5.5	3.3 (0.4 ~ 5.1)	0.238
ISS ≧ 16	5.5 (3.6 ~ 14.2)	0.001

[j]Multivariate logistic regression.

other patients (Table 3). Table 4 shows that a type B$_1$ pelvic fracture (OR = 6.4, p = 0.002) and an ISS > 16 (OR = 5.9, p = 0.002) were two independent risk factors for post-TAE laparotomy.

In current study, there were three patients without pelvic fractures who required post-laparotomy TAE. Their angiographic examinations revealed that all of them had active lumbar arterial hemorrhage.

Discussion

Blunt abdominal trauma may result in intraperitoneal or retroperitoneal hemorrhages, which are both potentially life-threatening and require organized rapid evaluation and treatment [1-3]. An emergency laparotomy is usually indicated for an intraperitoneal hemorrhage that presents as intra-abdominal free fluid during sonography. In the management of the associated retroperitoneal hemorrhage, the PCCD and even the extraperitoneal packing are required to decrease the retroperitoneal hemorrhage before the laparotomy. Then the further TAE could be performed for the definitive hemostasis. However, in these patients, it is difficult to consider the requirement of TAE until persistent expansion of a retroperitoneal hematoma was detected intraoperatively. At that time, the TAE preparation would be initiated. After a damage-control laparotomy, with intraperitoneal/retroperitoneal packing, the patients

would be sent to an angiographic room. Therefore, they would remain in critical condition with an ongoing hemorrhage while waiting for an angioembolization suite to be prepared and for personnel to be gathered.

In the current study, 74 patients underwent emergency laparotomy because of concomitant unstable hemodynamics and positive sonographic examination results. Retroperitoneal hemorrhage was found intraoperatively in 15 of these patients (20.3%); thus, they underwent post-laparotomy TAE. The percentage of these patients with concomitant pelvic fracture was significantly greater than that of the patients who underwent laparotomy only (80.0% vs. 30.5%, p < 0.001). Furthermore, multivariate logistic regression analyses revealed that the presence of a pelvic fracture was a significant factor in predicting the need for post-laparotomy TAE in such patients (OR = 3.4, p = 0.018) (Table 2). Pelvic fractures usually stem from high-kinetic-energy blunt trauma and can result in retroperitoneal hemorrhage. Associated hemodynamic instability was reported in 5–20% of these patients, and the subsequent reported mortality rate was 18–40% [16-20]. Therefore, in addition to intraperitoneal hemorrhage, an associated retroperitoneal hemorrhage should also be considered when managing patients with BAT and unstable hemodynamics with concomitant pelvic fractures.

Previous reports have proposed that unstable pelvic fractures indicate major ligamentous disruptions that are often associated with life threatening arterial bleeding [14,15,21]. Additionally, pelvic fracture patterns were classified into three main groups according to the integrity of the posterior sacroiliac complex by Tile [14,15]. The focused analysis of pelvic fracture patients in the current study revealed that the patients who required post-laparotomy TAE had a significantly greater percentage of unstable pelvises (75.0% vs. 22.2%, p = 0.008) and type B$_1$ (external rotational unstable) pelvic fractures

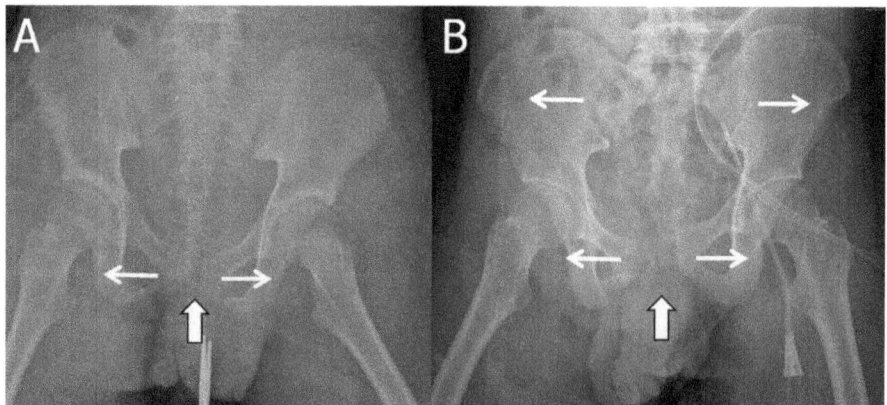

Figure 2 Plain external rotational type pelvic fracture films. The large arrows indicate the disruptive force direction and side of the impact, and the small arrows indicate the splaying of the pubic symphysis **(A)** and further external iliac wing rotation **(B)**.

(58.3% vs. 11.1%, $p = 0.013$) compared with the patients who underwent laparotomy only (Table 3). Furthermore, multiple logistic regression analyses in the current study also revealed that type B_1 pelvic fractures were an independent risk factor for concomitant intraperitoneal and retroperitoneal hemorrhages, with approximately an eight-fold increased risk of requiring post-laparotomy TAE (OR = 6.4, $p = 0.002$) (Table 4).

Unlike other pelvic fractures, type B_1 pelvic fractures create complete anterior pelvis diastases and partial or complete posterior pelvis diastases (Figure 2) [15,18,22]. The tensile and shearing force of such injuries are generally from the middle and front. They tend to open the anterior pelvis, which is thinner than the iliac bone, over the lateral side by pubic ramus fracture or pubic symphysis ligaments rupture mechanisms (Figure 2A). Furthermore, additional external rotational forces may result in splaying of the anterior pelvis and external rotation of the iliac wings, which provide circumferential protection of the intra-abdominal organs (Figure 2B). Therefore, it is reasonable that such impaction, with relative weak protection, may be associated with a greater risk of intraperitoneal injury. Additionally, it was reported that the external rotational pelvic fracture involves greater vessel disruption and more hemorrhaging than other injury mechanisms [22]. Our previous report also indicated its association with bilateral sacroiliac joint injuries and further bilateral arterial injuries [23]. According to the above theories, concomitant intraperitoneal and retroperitoneal hemorrhages may occur in type B_1 pelvic fracture patients. In managing patients with unstable hemodynamics and positive sonographic examinations, associated retroperitoneal hemorrhages should be suspected in patients with concomitant type B_1 pelvic fractures.

Another concern is in evaluating other associated injuries. The ISS has been used to evaluate the severity of other associated injuries [24,25]. This trauma scoring system is a tool that can assist with the triage, prognosis prediction and resource allocation of ED trauma patients. In the current study, the post-laparotomy TAE patients also had significantly higher ISSs than the patients who underwent laparotomy only. Multiple logistic regression analysis also revealed that a higher ISS (≥ 16) was independently associated with an increased risk for post-laparotomy TAE. Although the precise ISS was not available in the ED, the current study results indicate that other associated injuries may increase the risk of subsequent deterioration requiring additional procedures.

The early identification of post-laparotomy TAE patients might shorten the waiting time for TAE. Furthermore, the risk that occurs while patients wait and during transportation could also be reduced. Pelvic fractures can easily be diagnosed on a plain pelvis film; thus, type B_1 pelvic fractures could also be identified accordingly. This fact revealed that concomitant retroperitoneal hemorrhages and the necessity of additional hemostatic procedures for unstable patients could be surmised with primary tool evaluations (e.g., sonographic examinations and plain pelvis films). To save additional time, one suggestion is to simultaneously prepare for TAE while performing laparotomy in type B_1 pelvic fracture patients. This process may diminish the increased risk of injuries associated with concomitant retroperitoneal hemorrhages, which may require post-laparotomy TAE.

The limitations of this study are its retrospective nature and small number of examined cases. Our conclusions may be limited by a possible selection bias. Additionally, the role of CT scan was not discussed in the current study. We agree that CT scan could augment the detection of soft tissue injuries and active arterial bleeding; however, CT scans are not recommended for most patients with unstable hemodynamics [13]. Further studies with larger sample sizes and prospective designs are needed to establish precise treatment plan algorithms in the ED.

Conclusion
In BAT patient management, the likelihood of post-laparotomy TAE should be considered in concomitant pelvic fracture patients. Furthermore, more attention should be directed toward patients with Tile B_1-type pelvic fractures because of its specific fracture pattern and impaction force.

Competing interests
The authors declare that they have no competing interests.

Authors' contributions
CYW: Article writing, data collection. SJY: Article writing, data collection, statistic analysis. CYF: Supervisor of article writing. CHL, SC K, YPH, BCL, KCY, SYW: Data collection. All authors read and approved the final manuscript.

Authors' information
Chun-Yi Wu and Shang-Ju Yang are first author.

References
1. Fang J-F, Shih L-Y, Wong Y-C, Lin B-C, Hsu Y-P. Angioembolization and laparotomy for patients with concomitant pelvic arterial hemorrhage and blunt abdominal trauma. Langenbecks Arch Surg. 2011;396:243–50.
2. Fang J-F, Wong Y-C, B- L, Hsu Y-P, Chen M-F. Usefulness of multidetector computed tomography for the initial assessment of blunt abdominal trauma patients. World J Surg. 2006;30:176–82.
3. Tyburski JG, Wilson RF, Dente C, Steffes C, Carlin AM. Factors affecting mortality rates in patients with abdominal vascular injuries. J Trauma. 2001;50:1020–6. NOM.
4. Raza M, Abbas Y, Devi V, Prasad KV, Rizk KN, Nair PP. Non operative management of abdominal trauma - a 10 years review. World J Emerg Surg. 2013;8:14.
5. Sriussadaporn S, Pak-art R, Tharavej C, Sirichindakul B, Chiamananthapong S. A multidisciplinary approach in the management of hepatic injuries. Injury. 2002;33:309–15.
6. Hauschild O, Aghayev E, von Heyden J, Strohm PC, Culemann U, Pohlemann T, et al. Angioembolization for pelvic hemorrhage control: results from the German pelvic injury register. J Trauma Acute Care Surg. 2012;73:679–84.

7.   Jeske HC, Larndorfer R, Krappinger D, Attal R, Klingensmith M, Lottersberger C, et al. Management of hemorrhage in severe pelvic injuries. J Trauma. 2010;68:415–20.

8.   Miller PR, Moore PS, Mansell E, Meredith JW, Chang MC. External fixation or arteriogram in bleeding pelvic fracture: initial therapy guided by markers of arterial hemorrhage. J Trauma. 2003;54:437–43.

9.   Verbeek DO, Zijlstra IA, van der Leij C, Ponsen KJ, van Delden OM, Goslings JC. The utility of FAST for initial abdominal screening of major pelvic fracture patients. World J Surg. 2014;38:1719–25.

10. Walcher F, Weinlich M, Conrad G, Schweigkofler U, Breitkreutz R, Kirschning T, et al. Prehospital ultrasound imaging improves management of abdominal trauma. Br J Surg. 2006;93:238–42.

11. Tayal VS, Nielsen A, Jones AE, Thomason MH, Kellam J, Norton HJ. Accuracy of trauma ultrasound in major pelvic injury. J Trauma. 2006;61:1453–7.

12. Clarke JR, Trooskin SZ, Doshi PJ, Greenwald L, Mode CJ. Time to laparotomy for intra-abdominal bleeding from trauma does affect survival for delays up to 90 min. J Trauma. 2002;52:420–5.

13. Chapleau W, Al-Khatib J, Haskin D, LeBlanc P, Cardenas G, Borum S, et al. Advanced trauma life support. 9th ed. Chicago, IL: ATLS Subcommittee; American College of Surgeons' Committee on Trauma; International ATLS working group; 2013. J Trauma Acute Care Surg.

14. Pennal GF, Tile M, Waddell JP, Garside H. Pelvic disruption: assessment and classification. Clin Orthop Relat Res. 1980;151:12–21.

15. McMurtry R, Walton D, Dickinson D, Kellam J, Tile M. Pelvic disruption in the polytraumatized patient: a management protocol. Clin Orthop Relat Res. 1980;151:22–30.

16. Starr AJ, Griffin DR, Reinert CM, Frawley WH, Walker J, Whitlock SN, et al. Pelvic ring disruptions: prediction of associated injuries, transfusion requirement, pelvic arteriography, complications, and mortality. J Orthop Trauma. 2002;16:553–61.

17. Smith W, Williams A, Agudelo J, Shannon M, Morgan S, Stahel P, et al. Early predictors of mortality in hemodynamically unstable pelvis fractures. J Orthop Trauma. 2007;21:31–7.

18. Cryer HM, Miller FB, Evers BM, Rouben LR, Seligson DL. Pelvic fracture classification: correlation with hemorrhage. J Trauma. 1988;28:973–80.

19. Brun J, Guillot S, Bouzat P, Broux C, Thony F, Genty C, et al. Detecting active pelvic arterial haemorrhage on admission following serious pelvic fracture in multiple trauma patients. Injury. 2014;45:101–6.

20. Biffl WL, Smith WR, Moore EE, Gonzalez RJ, Morgan SJ, Hennessey T, et al. Evolution of a multidisciplinary clinical pathway for the management of unstable patients with pelvic fracture. Ann Surg. 2001;233:843–50.

21. Fu CY, Wu SC, Chen RJ, Wang YC, Chung PK, Yeh CC, et al. Evaluation of pelvic fracture stability and the need for angioembolization: pelvic instabilities on plain film have an increased probability of requiring angioembolization. Am J Emerg Med. 2009;27:792–6.

22. Dalal SA, Burgess AR, Siegel JH, Young JW, Brumback RJ, Poka A, et al. Pelvic fracture in multiple trauma: classification by mechanism is key to pattern of organ injury, resuscitative requirements, and outcome. J Trauma. 1989;29:981–1000.

23. Fu CY, Hsieh CH, Wu SC, Chen RJ, Wang YC, Shih CH, et al. Anterior-posterior compression pelvic fracture increases the probability of requirement of bilateral embolization. Am J Emerg Med. 2013;31:42–9.

24. Sacco WJ, MacKenzie EJ, Champion HR, Davis EG, Buckman RF. Comparison of alternative methods for assessing injury severity based on anatomic descriptors. J Trauma. 1999;47:441–6.

25. Baker SP, O'Neill B, Haddon Jr W, Long WB. The injury severity score: a method for describing patients with multiple injuries and evaluating emergency care. J Trauma. 1974;14:187–96.

21

Non-heparinized ECMO serves a rescue method in a multitrauma patient combining pulmonary contusion and nonoperative internal bleeding

Pei-Hung Wen[1,2,5*], Wai Hung Chan[1,2*], Ying-Cheng Chen[3], Yao-Li Chen[1,4], Chien-Pin Chan[1,2] and Ping-Yi Lin[4]

Abstract

Pulmonary contusion and acute respiratory distress syndrome (ARDS) is a common manifestation in polytraumatic patients. Although mechanical ventilation is still the first choice of treatment, a group of patients are still unable to maintain their oxygenation. The role of extracorporeal membrane oxygenation (ECMO) has been more clarified when the lung is extensively damaged and when conventional modality failed. ECMO provides the lung an opportunity to rest by permitting reduced ventilator settings and limiting further barotraumas. However, ECMO is still considered contraindicated in polytramatic patients combining pulmonary contusion and other organ hemorrhage because of systemic anticoagulation during the treatment. We herein report a patient who successfully survive a multitrauma combining pulmonary contusion and grade IV liver laceration using non-heparinized venovenous extracorporeal membrane oxygenation (vv-ECMO). The associated literature were reviewed.

Keywords: ECMO, Heparin-free, Polytraumatic, Acute pulmonary contusion, Internal bleeding

Introduction

Acute pulmonary failure is a common manifestation in polytraumatic patients. The mechanism included pulmonary contusion, acute respiratory distress syndrome (ARDS) resulting from any inflammation process such as aspiration pneumonia, or fat embolism because of long bone fracture [1]. The management could be very challenging despite advances in critical care management.

Extracorporeal membrane oxygenation (ECMO) serves as the final method when conventional mechanical ventilation fails to maintain the oxygenation. It helps maintain systemic tissue oxygenation via extracorporeal circuit when the lung function is compromised [2,3]. However, the situation became more complicated when the lung failure combines other vital organ damage and risk of bleeding because of systemic anticoagulation during the treatment.

The introduction of heparin-free ECMO seems to be the possible solution for such dilemma. We report our experience of using heparin-free vv-ECMO to help a patient survive a trauma combining acute pulmonary failure and severe liver subcapsular laceration. The literature regarding the application of ECMO in polytraumatic patients combining acute pulmonary failure and other vital organ damage were reviewed.

Case report

A 19-year-old man suffered from a multi-trauma after a traffic accident when he was riding a motorcycle and collided into a car. Upon arrival at our tertiary trauma center, he initially presented with a Glasgow Coma Score of 8 and severe hypoxia. He was intubated immediately. Large amount of food content was sucked from the endotracheal tube. Primary chest computed tomography (CT) reported right lung consolidation with patchy opacities, which was consistent with a combination of blunt chest contusion and aspiration pneumonia (Figure 1). Abdominal CT showed grade IV laceration over bilateral hemiliver without evident contrast extravasation (Figure 2). The gas

* Correspondence: 144995@cch.org.tw; peihong@mail2000.com.tw
[1]General Surgery Division, Surgery Department, Changhua Christian Hospital, Changhua City, Taiwan
[2]Trauma Division, Surgery Department, Changhua Christian Hospital, 500 No. 135, Nanxiao Street, Changhua City, Taiwan
Full list of author information is available at the end of the article

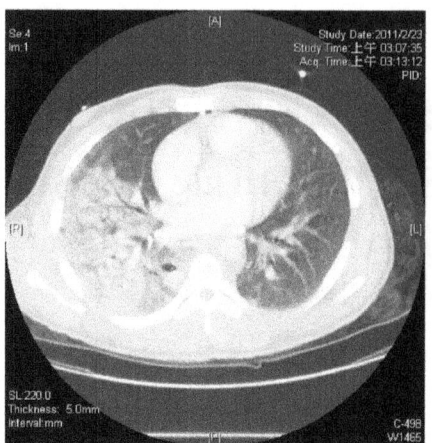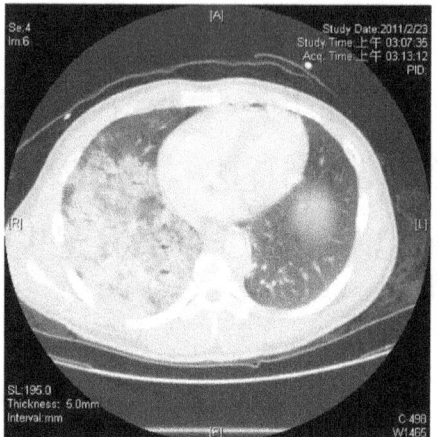

Figure 1 Chest CT showed right lung consolidation with patchy opacities.

exchange did not improve despite of mechanical ventilation, and the patient still presented with severe hypoxemia. The parameter about respiration showed PaO2/FiO2: 70.2 under invasive ventilation (pressure-mode inverse ratio ventilation, I:E 2:1). ECMO was thus recommended for lung contusion, aspiration pneumonia and acute pulmonary failure.

With regards of a polytraumatic patient combining liver laceration, ECMO is contraindicated because the need of systemic anticoagulation may induce further internal bleeding. A heparin-free, vv-ECMO was thus suggested. An extracorporeal circuit was constructed via a venous access through internal jugular vein and femoral vein, using Seldinger technique. The blood flow was set at the rate of 2.42 L/min, and the FiO2 was set at 45%. The oxygenation status improved dramatically after the introduction of ECMO (Table 1). The liver laceration was treated conservatively. The patient weaned from ECMO five days later, and was extubated nine days later.

The total intensive care unit stay was 10 days, and he discharged after a sixteen-day hospitalization. There was no ECMO related complications during the course.

Literature review

We searched the PubMed (2000–2013) database for case reports about the launch of ECMO regardless of heparin-containing or heparin-free in multi-trauma patients. The abstracts of all articles published in English were screened. The full texts of articles published in other languages but with an abstract in English were analyzed. Articles were selected for review if they included the following patient data: age, sex, clinical presentation, combined injury besides acute pulmonary failure, the details of ECMO treatment, and the outcome.

There were six case reports containing 11 patients described in detail, and one clinical paper containing 10 cases found in the literature, which are listed in Table 2.

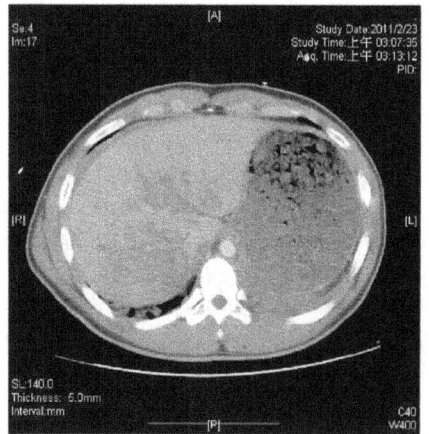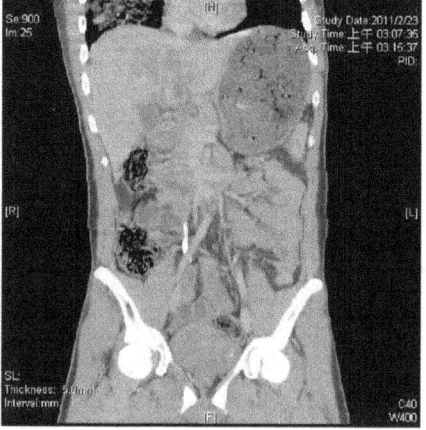

Figure 2 The coronal view and saggital view of abdominal CT showed grade IV laceration over bilateral hemiliver without evident contrast extravasation.

Table 1 Oxygenation status before and after ECMO introduction

	Pre-ECMO	Post-ECMO	Pre-weaning
pH	7.231	7.352	7.440
pCO2 (mmHg)	58.4	39.2	30.4
pO2 (mmHg)	70.2	147.2	91.5
O2 Saturation (%)	89.5	98.5	97.9

Discussion

Despite of the various mechanical ventilation technique and the improved knowledge of the adjustment of ventilation parameters, a group of patients with traumatic pulmonary contusion or ARDS are still unable to benefit from these technique. ECMO has been proved to be an rescue therapy when conventional methods are ineffective. ECMO was also reported to be effective in polytraumatic patients combining pulmonary contusion and other organ damage including bronchial rupture [2,4], endobronchial hemorrhage [5], blunt abdominal trauma (BAT) with internal bleeding necessitating exploratory laparotomy [6], or traumatic brain injury [7-10]. However, the use of ECMO on patients with a preexisting bleeding risk without need of immediate operation is still rarely reported.

The application of heparin-free ECMO has been proposed recently to overcome the dilemma. Muellenbach et al. reported three successful cases of heparin-free vv-ECMO on a patient with traumatic lung failure and severe traumatic brain injury [9]. Matthias et al. reported that six of ten polytraumatic patients with coexisting pulmonary failure or cardiopulmonary failure and bleeding shock survived using a heparin-free ECMO, which is by far the only largest series in the literature [6]. However, ECMO is still a controversy on a multitrauma combining pulmonary failure and blunt abdominal trauma needing only nonoperative management. Of the total 11 cases reported in detail in the literature (Table 2), six patients had concurrent BAT with liver or spleen laceration [2,4,8,9]. Only one received successful nonoperative treatment for grade III liver laceration [4].

The improvement of ECMO technique including centrifugal pumps and heparin-coated circuits reduced the amount of heparin needed. However, with regards to a patient who had spontaneous hemostasis on liver laceration, we still chose the heparin-free method to reduce the risk of rebleeding. Based on the hemodynamic stability and the daily improvement of lung condition, we did not used additional method to prevent clotting of the circuit except the close monitor of ACT. The duration

Table 2 ECMO in polytraumatic patients combining acute pulmonary failure and other vital organ damage: literature review

References	Case no.	Combined injury besides pulmonary failure	Intervention	ECMO	Heparin	ECMO duration	Outcome
Madershahian et al. [2]	1, 19/F	Spleen, Liver	Laparotomy	v-a[5]	(+)	138 hours	Survived
		Right main bronchus	Thoracotomy				
	2, 48/M	Vertebra and long bone Fracture	Osteosynthesis	v-a	(+)	120 hours	Survived
	3, 26/M	Spleen	Splenectomy	v-va[6]	(+)	84 hours	Survived
		Brain					
Yuan et al. [5]	4, 18/M	Liver, Gr. III	Conservative	v-v	(+)	10 days	Survived
		Endobronchial hemorrhage					
	5, 38/M	Brain SDH[1]	Conservative	v-v	(+)	5 days	Survived
Campione et al. [4]	6, 14/M	Bronchial Disruption	Right bilobectomy of lung	v-v	(+)	3 days	Survived
Yen et al. [7]	7, 21/M	Brain EDH[2]	Decompressive craniotomy	v-a	(+)	49 hours	Survived
Friesenecker, et al. [8]	8, 34/M	Liver, Spleen	Laparotomy	v-v	(+)	17 days	Survived
		Brain ICH[3] with edema	Decompressive craniotomy				
Muellenbach et al. [9]	9, 53/M	Liver	Laparotomy	v-v	(−)	8 days	Survived
		Traumatic brain injury	ICP[4] Monitoring				
	10, 16/M	Traumatic brain injury		v-v	(−)	3 days	Survived
	11, 28/M	Spleen	Splenectomy	v-v	(−)	2 days	Survived
		Traumatic brain injury					
Arlt et al. [6]	10 Cases	Bleeding shock	-	7 v-v	All (−)	Mean 5 days	6/10 Survived
				3 v-a			

[1]SDH: Subdural hemorrhage; [2]EDH: Epidural hemorrhage; [3]ICH: Intracerebral hemorrhage; [4]ICP: Intracerebral pressure; [5]V-a: Venoarterial ; [6]V-va: veno-venoarterial.

of ECMO was five days, which is comparable to other report.

Conclusion

ECMO can serve as a rescue method to provide the traumatic lung to rest. Although it was previously regarded to be contraindicated in polytraumatic patient with coexisting organ hemorrhage, there are growing successful experiences reported recently. We report a heparin-free, vv-ECMO method for patients combining acute pulmonary failure and nonoperative liver laceration, which may extend the feasibility of ECMO in polytraumatic patients.

Consent

Written informed consent was obtained from the patient for the publication of this report and any accompanying images.

Abbreviations

ECMO: Extracorporeal membrane oxygenation; ARDS: Acute respiratory distress syndrome; v-v ECMO: Venovenous ECMO; CT: Computed tomography; FiO_2: Fraction of inspired oxygen; BAT: Blunt abdominal trauma; SDH: Subdural hemorrhage; EDH: Epidural hemorrhage; ICH: Intracerebral hemorrhage; ICP: Intracerebral pressure; V-a ECMO: Venoarterial ECMO; V-va ECMO: Veno-venoarterial ECMO.

Competing interests

The authors declare that they have no competing interests.

Authors' contributions

PHW is the first author who reviewed the medical records and wrote the main article. WHC is the visiting staff who was in charge of the patient during the hospitalization, and serves as the corresponding author. YCC is the vascular surgeon responsible for the ECMO use. YLC is the chief of the surgery department and the vice superintendent of Changhua Christian Hospital who coordinated between the department. CPC is the chief of the trauma department who coordinated the trauma team. PYL is the doctor in research department responsible for article review. All authors read and approved the final manuscript.

Author details

[1]General Surgery Division, Surgery Department, Changhua Christian Hospital, Changhua City, Taiwan. [2]Trauma Division, Surgery Department, Changhua Christian Hospital, 500 No. 135, Nanxiao Street, Changhua City, Taiwan. [3]Cardiovascular Division, Surgery Department, Changhua Christian Hospital, Changhua City, Taiwan. [4]Transplant Medicine and Surgery Research Centre, Changhua Christian Hospital, Changhua City, Taiwan. [5]Surgery Department, Cishan Hospital, 84247 No. 60, Zhongxue Rd., Cishan District, Kaohsiung City, Taiwan.

References

1. Cordell-Smith JA, Roberts N, Peek GJ, Firmin RK. Traumatic lung injury treated by extracorporeal membrane oxygenation (ECMO). Int J Care Injured. 2006;37:29–32.
2. Madershahian N, Wittwer T, Strauch J, Franke UF, Wippermann J, Kaluza M, et al. Application of ECMO in multitrauma patients with ARDS as rescue therapy. J Card Surg. 2007;22:180–4.
3. Michaels AJ, Schriener RJ, Kolla S, Awad SS, Rich PB, Reickert C, et al. Extracorporeal life support in pulmonary failure after trauma. J Trauma Inj Infect Crit Care. 1999;46:638–45.
4. Campione A, Agostini M, Portolan M, Alloisio A, Fino C, Vassallo G. Extracorporeal membrane oxygenation in respiratory failure for pulmonary contusion and bronchial disruption after trauma. J Thorac Cardiovasc Surg. 2007;133:1673–4.
5. Yuan K-C, Fang J-F, Chen M-F. Treatment of endobronchial hemorrhage after blunt chest trauma with extracorporeal membrane oxygenation (ECMO). J Trauma. 2008;65:1151–4.
6. Arlt M, Philipp A, Voelkel S, Rupprecht L, Mueller T, Hilker M, et al. Extracorporeal membrane oxygenation in severe trauma patients with bleeding shock. Resuscitation. 2010;81:804–9.
7. Yen T-S, Liau C-C, Chenc Y-S, Chaoa A. Extracorporeal membrane oxygenation resuscitation for traumatic brain injury after decompressive craniotomy. Clin Neurol Neurosurg. 2008;110:295–7.
8. Friesenecker BE, Peer R, Rieder J, Lirk P, Knotzer H, Hasibeder WR, et al. Craniotomy during ECMO in a severely traumatized patient. Acta Neurochir. 2005;147:993–6.
9. Muellenbach RM, Kredel M, Kunze E, Kranke P, Kuestermann J, Brack A, et al. Prolonged heparin-free extracorporeal membrane oxygenation in multiple injured acute respiratory distress syndrome patients with traumatic brain injury. J Trauma Acute Care Surg. 2012;72:1444–7.
10. Muellenbach RM, Redel A, Kuestermann J, Brack A, Gorski A, Rosner T, et al. Extracorporeal membrane oxygenation and severe traumatic brain injury. Is the ECMO-therapy in traumatic lung failure and severe traumatic brain injury really contraindicated? Anaesthesist. 2011;60:647–52.

22

Assessment of maxillofacial trauma in emergency department

Engin D Arslan[1*], Alper G Solakoglu[1], Erdal Komut[3], Cemil Kavalci[2], Fevzi Yilmaz[1], Evvah Karakilic[1], Tamer Durdu[1] and Muge Sonmez[1]

Abstract

Introduction: The incidence and epidemiological causes of maxillofacial (MF) trauma varies widely. The objective of this study is to point out maxillofacial trauma patients' epidemiological properties and trauma patterns with simultaneous injuries in different areas of the body that may help emergency physicians to deliver more accurate diagnosis and decisions.

Methods: In this study we analyze etiology and pattern of MF trauma and coexisting injuries if any, in patients whose maxillofacial CT scans was obtained in a three year period, retrospectively.

Results: 754 patients included in the study consisting of 73.7% male and 26.3% female, and the male-to-female ratio was 2.8:1. Mean age was 40.3 ± 17.2 years with a range of 18 to 97. 57.4% of the patients were between the ages of 18–39 years and predominantly male. Above 60 years of age, referrals were mostly woman. The most common cause of injuries were violence, accounting for 39.7% of the sample, followed by falls 27.9% and road traffic accidents 27.2%. The primary cause of injuries were violence between ages 20 and 49 and falls after 50. Bone fractures found in 56,0% of individuals. Of the total of 701 fractured bones in 422 patients the most frequent was maxillary bone 28,0% followed by nasal bone 25,3%, zygoma 20,2%, mandible 8,4%, frontal bone 8,1% and nasoethmoidoorbital bone 3,1%. Fractures to maxillary bone were uppermost in each age group.

8, 9% of the patients had brain injury and only frontal fractures is significantly associated to TBI ($p < 0.05$) if coexisting facial bone fracture occurred. Male gender has statistically stronger association for suffering TBI than female ($p < 0, 05$). Most common cause of TBI in MF trauma patients was violence (47, 8%).

158 of the 754 patients had consumed alcohol before trauma. No statistically significant data were revealed between alcohol consumption gender and presence of fracture. Violence is statistically significant ($p < 0.05$) in these patients.

Conclusion: Studies subjected maxillofacial traumas yield various etiologic factors, demographic properties and fracture patterns probably due to social, cultural and governmental differences. Young males subjected to maxillofacial trauma more commonly as a result of interpersonal violence.

Keywords: Maxillofacial trauma, Mid face fracture, Emergency department

Introduction

The incidence and epidemiological causes of maxillofacial (MF) trauma and facial fractures varies widely in different regions of the world due to social, economical, cultural consequences, awareness of traffic regulations and alcohol consumption. Reports from distinct regions in Turkey also have different etiological findings [1,2].

According to the studies in developed countries assault is the leading cause of facial fractures followed mostly by motor vehicle accidents, pedestrian collisions, stumbling, sports and industrial accidents but the leading cause shifts to road traffic accidents in underdeveloped or developing areas of the world followed by assaults and other reasons including warfare [3-9].

Diagnosis and management facial injuries are a challenge particularly in the setting of coexisting polytrauma in emergency department. Our goal is to broaden clinical data of MF trauma patients for public health measures. It

* Correspondence: engindeniz.arslan@gmail.com
[1]Emergency Department, Ankara Numune Training and Research Hospital, Altındağ, 06100 Ankara, Turkey

is our credence that broader knowledge of MF trauma patients' epidemiological properties and trauma patterns with simultaneous injuries in different areas of the body may help emergency physicians to deliver more accurate diagnosis and decisions. In this study we analyze etiology and pattern of MF trauma and coexisting injuries if any.

Patients and methods

In the study MF injuries were diagnosed after evaluation of the patients' history, physical examination, forensic record and radiological studies. Patients with isolated nasal and dentoalveolar fracture were excluded and in patients with suspected more severe facial injuries, maxillofacial CT scans were performed as proposed by our hospitals clinical policy. We retrospectively evaluated patients referred to our emergency department (ED) between 2010 March and 2013 March whose maxillofacial CT scans were obtained. Our study's variables are presented as; age, gender, cause of injury, site of injury, alcohol consumption, coexisting intracranial, cervical, orthopedic, abdominal injuries and mortality if any. During the analyses Mid-face region injuries were classified as Le Fort I, Le Fort II, Le Fort III, blow out, zygomaticomaxillary complex, nasorbitoethmoid complex and zygomatic arc fractures. Pan-facial fracture is defined as fractures affecting all three parts of face (Frontal, mid-face and mandible at the same time). If the patient suffered from multiple fractures, each fracture was analyzed separately and if the patient had traumatic brain injury Glasgow Coma Scale (GCS) was evaluated and GCS was grouped as mild (14–15), moderate (8–13) and severe (3–8). All data was documented on SPSS v.17 and analyzed. Comparisons were made with chi-square test with%95 confidence interval and p values <0, 05 were considered as statistically significant. All authors obey the rules

of Helsinki Declaration and no ethic problem exist in the manuscript.

Results

Demographic pattern of the patients and trauma mechanisms

556 (73.7%) male and 198(26.3%) female patients were included in the study and the male-to-female ratio was 2.8:1. Mean age was 40.3 ± 17.2 years with a range of 18 to 97 years also mean age of patients with MF fractures were almost the same (40, 06 ± 17, 2). Majority of the patients (n = 432, 57.4%) were between the ages of 18–39 years and predominantly male. Above 60 years of age, referrals were mostly woman.

The most common cause of injuries were violence, accounting for 39.7% (n = 299) of the sample, followed by falls 27.9% (n = 210) and road traffic accidents 27.2% (n = 205). In patients between 20 to 49 years violence was the main cause of injuries, whereas after 50 years old falls were the primary cause of injuries. These associations were found to be statistically significant (p < 0, 0001).

When road traffic accidents were subdivided, motor vehicle accidents have the ratio of 17.7% (n = 134) of all patients, followed by vehicle-pedestrian collisions 8.1% (n = 61) and motorcycle accidents (n = 9) 1.2%. No statistically relevant data were identified between gender, age group and trauma causes. Table 1 illustrates age, gender and trauma mechanism relationships.

MF injury and fracture analyses
Fracture, injury patterns, age and cause of injury classification

Soft-tissue injuries accounted for 44,0% (n = 332), while bone fractures 56,0% (n = 422). Of the total of 701 fractured bones in 422 patients the most frequent was

Table 1 Trauma mechanisms according to age and gender

Ages	Gender	Violence	Stumble and fall	Road traffic accidents	Strike by object	Occupational	Explosion	Total (%)
19–30	Male	99	32	59	13	0	1	204 (27.1)
	Female	16	9	17	1	0	0	43 (5.7)
31–40	Male	85	22	30	6	8	2	153 (20.3)
	Female	9	9	13	0	0	1	32 (4.2)
41–50	Male	52	23	19	1	1	0	96 (12.7)
	Female	5	8	13	2	0	0	28 (3.7)
51–60	Male	16	27	14	2	0	0	59 (7.8)
	Female	6	10	17	1	0	0	34 (4.9)
61–70	Male	8	8	5	1	0	0	22 (2.9)
	Female	0	11	4	0	0	0	15 (2.0)
70+	Male	2	13	7	0	0	0	22 (2.9)
	Female	1	38	7	0	0	0	46 (6.1)
Total (%)		299 (39.7)	210 (27.9)	205 (27.2)	27 (3.6)	9 (1.2)	4 (0.5)	754

maxillary bone n = 211(28,0%) followed by nasal bone n = 191 (25,3%), zygoma n = 152 (20,2%), the mandible n = 63 (%8,4) frontal bone n = 61 (8,1%) and nasoethmoidoorbital bone n = 23(%3,1). Fractures to maxillary bone were uppermost in each age group. Figure 1 illustrates facial fractures according to anatomical sites and Figure 2 explains the relationship of fractures with trauma mechanisms.

Violence was mostly the cause of nasal, maxillary, zygoma and frontal bone fractures whereas for mandibular fractures main cause was falls. Statistically important trauma mechanism causing any facial bone fractures was not displayed.

Fracture analyses according to anatomical sites

Mid-facial fractures In this study there were 385 patients with fractures of the mid-face. Most frequent mid-face fractures were maxillary fractures (27,4%) followed by nasal bone (25,8%) and zygoma (20,2%) fractures. Simultaneous fractures of mid-face including multiple zygoma, maxillary, nasal fractures are classified as combined fractures and constitute 11,7% of patients. For combined fractures most common cause is falls. Isolated zygomatic arch fractures were often as a result of violence and falls and related in 19-30 age group with (p <0, 0001). Table 2 details the relationship with trauma mechanism and fracture sites with special considerations. Multiple facial bone fractures in same patients must be considered.

Mandibular fractures A total of 63 patients with mandibular fractures were documented. The main fracture site was mandibular corpus (28,5%) followed by ramus (23,8%). Ratio of patients suffering from fractures affecting more than one anatomical mandibular sites is 26,9%. Most common combined fracture of mandible was

ramus and angle fracture, effecting 17, 4% of patients. The fractures were generally caused by falls (34.5%), followed by violence (31.1%).

Fractures and coexisting traumas
MF traumas coexisting with traumatic brain injury and skull fractures

Of all the patients 8, 9% had brain injury whereas RTA patients had ratio of 13, 7%. Only frontal fractures are significantly associated to Traumatic Brain Injury (TBI) (p < 0.05) if coexisting facial bone fracture occurred and Cramer's V and Phi value is above 0.3. Male gender has statistically stronger association for suffering TBI than female (p < 0, 05). Most common cause of TBI in MF trauma patients was violence (47, 8%) followed by falls (28, 4%) and road traffic accidents (RTA) (20, 9%). Most common TBI was subarachnoid hemorrhage (44,8%), followed by contusions (22,4%), epidural hematoma (20,9%), pnemocephalus (19,4%), subdural hematoma (16,4%) and diffuse axonal injury (6%). Of the 68 patients with TBI 17 patients had suffered from severe brain traumatic brain injury and 6 of them died of TBI. 33 patients had mild and 18 had moderate brain trauma and admitted to brain surgery ward for observation and surgery if necessary. Multiple TBI patterns in same patients must be considered.

Traumas to non-facial areas and hospital mortality

172 (22,8%) patients suffered from 232 total injuries both to cranium and body. Additional body trauma rather than cranium occurred in 15, 4% (n = 116) of patients. Of these; injuries to upper extremity, lower extremity, chest, pelvis and abdomen were seen in 5,8% (n = 44), 4,6% (n = 35), 4% (n = 30), 1, 9% (n = 17) and 1, 6% (n = 12) of patients respectively.

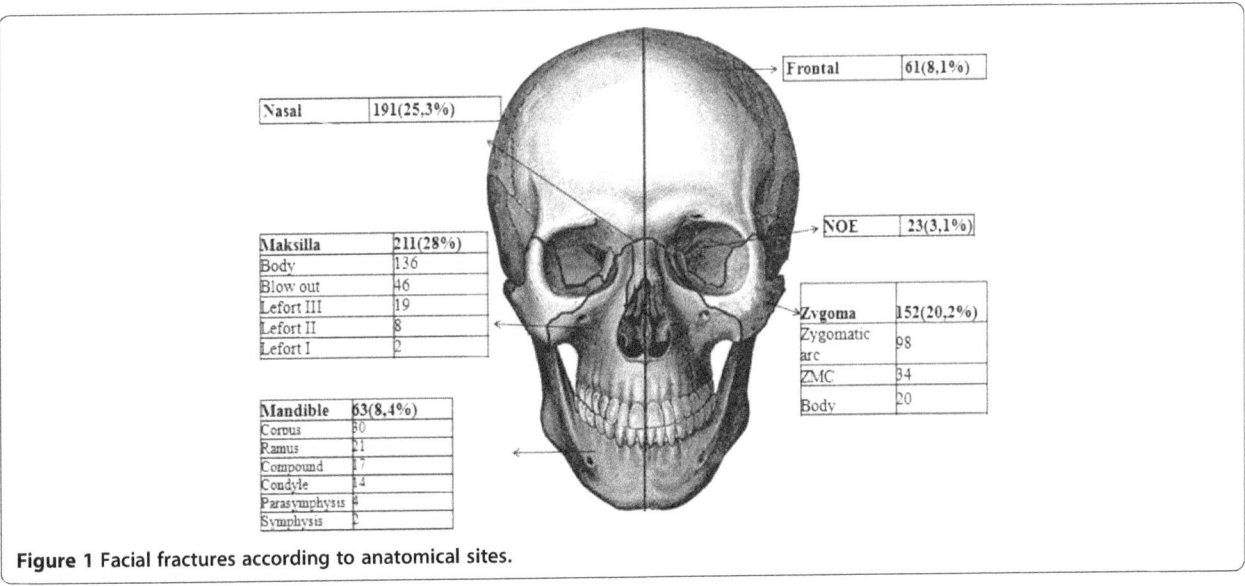

Figure 1 Facial fractures according to anatomical sites.

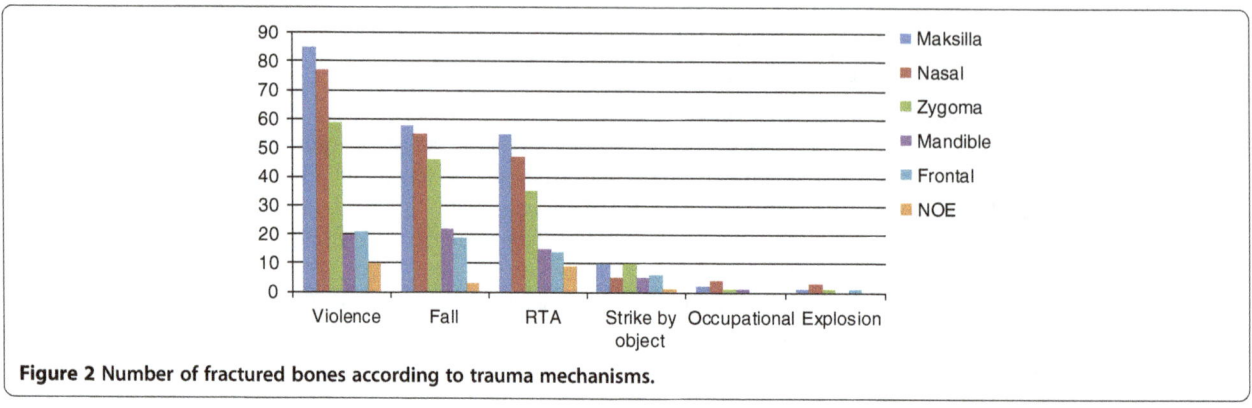

Figure 2 Number of fractured bones according to trauma mechanisms.

In RTA victims the ratios vary, total of 30,7% (n = 63) patients suffered from coexisting trauma and injury of the upper extremity was noticed in 12, 2% (n = 25), followed by injury to lower extremity in 11, 7% (n = 24) chest in 10, 7% (n = 22) pelvis in 4, 9% (n = 10), abdomen in 3, 9% (n = 8). Table 3 illustrates details of injury patterns with co-existing trauma.

A total of 24 patients were intubated during the study period. 17 patients were intubated because of severe traumatic brain injury and 7 from trauma complications such as pnemothoraces, hemorrhagic shock etc. Of the 17 severe TBI patients only 2 of them had isolated sagittal maxillary fracture and 1 had soft tissue injury. 3 of the patients had panfacial trauma with Lefort III type maxillary fracture where as 11 patients had compound midfacial and/or mandibular fracture.

6 of the admitted patients died from TBI, 1 from ICU complication and 2 from internal bleeding.

Injury and association with alcohol consumption

158 of the 754 patients had consumed alcohol before trauma. No statistically significant data were revealed between alcohol consumption gender and presence of fracture. Trauma mechanism of facial injury in intoxicated patients was distributed almost evenly, most common cause is violence and compared to other causes, suffering from violence is statistically higher (p < 0.05) furthermore young male group (age between 19-30) is

consuming more alcohol compared to other age groups in same gender (p < 0.001).

Discussion

Trauma is the leading cause of deaths occurred in first 40 years of life and it is well known that MF injuries are frequently seen in polytrauma victims. MF region includes organs executing essential functions of the body like respiration, speech, mastication, vision, smelling so special attention must be paid in case of facial trauma. Advanced trauma life support (ATLS) principles must be applied for the initial assessment of all MF injury victims as in any trauma patient. The most important sequence of ATLS is maintenance of airway patency in these patients. Airway compromise should occur due to tongue falling back, hemorrhage to oropharyngeal region, foreign bodies, mid facial fractures themselves. If possible endotracheal intubation is the preferred method to establish airway patency as no chance to intubate, crichothyroidotomy can be performed particularly in comatose patients [10].

In this study we assessed the epidemiology of MF injuries in emergency department as first contact of injured patients and analyzed 754 patients with facial injuries caused by various mechanisms. According to the Turkish Statistical Institute's data in 2013, Ankara has a population of 4.965.552 and is the second largest city in Turkey. Our Research and Training hospital is one of the historical

Table 2 Special midfacial fractures according to trauma mechanism

	RTA	Violence	Occupational	Falls	Explosion	Struck by object	Total
Lefort I	0	1	0	0	0	0	1
Lefort II	6	1	0	1	0	0	8
Lefort III	9	5	0	5	0	0	19
Blowout	14	15	3	10	1	3	46
ZMC	10	7	0	16	0	1	34
Zygomatic arc	25	34	1	35	0	3	98
NOE	8	8	1	6	0	0	23

Table 3 Fractures and injury patterns in patients with coexisting maxillofacial trauma

		n of patients	% of patients
Orthopaedic injuries	Hand/wrist	17	9,8
	Forearm	16	9,3
	Femur	16	9,3
	Tibia/Fibula	16	9,3
	Humerus	11	6,3
	Clavicle/Scapula	10	5,8
	Foot/Ankle	9	5,2
	Lumber vertebra	3	1,7
Abdominal/Pelvic	Pelvis fracture	13	7,5
	Spleen hematoma	5	2,9
	Liver hematoma	4	2,3
	Pelvis hematoma	2	1,1
	Gastric perforation	2	1,1
	Retroperitoneal hematoma	1	0,5
Torso injuries	Clavicle/Scapula fracture	10	5,8
	Pnemothorax/Hemothorax	11	6,3
	Costa fracture	7	4,0
	Pulmonary contusion	2	1,1
		n	% of patients with TBI
TBI's	Subarachnoid haemorrhage	30	44.1
	Brain contusion	15	22
	Epidural haemorrhage	14	20.5
	Pnemocephalus	13	19.1
	Subdural haemorrhage	11	16.1
	Diffuse axonal injury	4	5.8

hospitals in Ankara with a level-1 trauma center and gets referrals from Ankara and other neighboring cities. Our population and trauma mechanisms are distinct from other studies executed in Middle East countries. There were 556 (%73.7) male and 198 (%26.3) female and the male-to-female ratio was 2.8:1 and assaults are seen as primary cause of trauma mechanism. In our neighboring Middle East countries male to female ratios varies from 4.5:1 to 11:1 [9,11-13]. Segregation of women from social life in these countries may be the cause of disproportionate gender distribution. Our gender distribution is more likely to urbanized European countries particularly since woman rights are relatively well established in Turkey [5,6].

Most common age group encountering MF trauma is 19–30 age group and that seems to be correlated with the other studies and as exposed by the other studies higher age is more correlated to falls and younger age is more inclined to assaults and road traffic accidents [5,8]. In our investigation falls are the primary cause of injury in females accounting for 42,9% of the samples whereas assaults lead in males (%47, 1).

Our trauma mechanism analyses are also characteristic for Turkey's unique sociocultural background. Studies mentioned above from eastern countries reveal that most common trauma mechanism is road traffic accidents. We believe lack of traffic regulations in these countries may be the cause of high ratio of RTA's. In our study most common trauma mechanisms are assaults followed by falls. But our populations' assault rate is not as high as our western neighbor Bulgaria [6]. Another study in Ankara, conducted in our hospitals plastic surgery department by Aksoy et all at late 1990's revealed notable differences with our study that trauma pattern shifted from road traffic accidents to assaults in our hospital [1]. For the past 20 years Turkey is adopting traffic regulation laws including seat belt usage and driver side airbag implantation on cars which is shown by Mouzakes et al to protect patients from MF trauma [14]. Although it seems hard to postulate we estimate that people's compliance to new laws may be relatively lower than European countries.

Plenty of studies were executed for fracture patterns in MF trauma in oral and facial departments throughout the world [6,7,9,13,15]. These studies including the Aksoy et al reported that mainly mandibular and zygomatic bones were fractured bones [1]. In our study we found that most frequent fractured bone was maxillary bone (28, 0%) followed by the nasal bone (25, 3%). To minimalize the missing mid-facial fractures that cannot be diagnosed by physical examination or conventional direct graphs, we confirmed the fractures by coronal and axial maxillofacial CT scans but we did not perform CT scan in patients whom we consider mild facial trauma. We believe that's the basis of relatively low ratio of nasal fracture for ER patient sample.

Zygoma fractures are mostly seen in young male patients whose life style are at high risk for trauma and in our study we observed that isolated zygomatic arch fractures were usually because of violence and falls. Also zygomatic arc fractures are associated in young male age group. Another study from Brazil focusing on zygoma fractures demonstrated that falls and assaults were the leading cause of injuries, compatible with our study. Age group and gender distribution is alike with Brazil study [16].

EDs serve as the first point of entry into the hospital system for a significant percentage of patients seeking treatment for MF injuries [17]. Furthermore we suppose that majority of emergency physicians deal with simple maxillary and nasal bone fractures without consultations that may explain the differences in fracture distribution between ED and oral and facial surgery departments. One of the few studies from ED was performed in Tehran explains about facial trauma epidemiology [18]. Contrary to our results they have found that mandibular and nasal bones fractures were most common. We believe this difference is due to their patient universe which includes more severe trauma patients who requires 24 hour observation period.

A few study tried to correlate TBI with facial lesions to open a pathway to emergency physicians' clinical decisions. In our study there was no association between, trauma mechanism and gender to TBI. Frontal fractures with coexisting fractures in mid face and mandible caries higher risk for TBI so should be managed cautiously.

There is also a lack of studies involving MF trauma to non-facial areas of body and mortality, in our study we have found total of 15.3% of patients suffered coexisting trauma. Study from India [19] points out that mostly head and orthopedic injuries are seen in MF trauma patients. Indian study reports high coexisting trauma rate of 25.6%. We believe that this ratio is due to high ratio of road traffic accident victims in that study. In our study road traffic accident patients have ratio of 30, 7%

additional trauma with high ratio of orthopedic and head injuries in line with Indian study.

Alcohol use is another reason for MF traumas leading to hostile behavior causing violence and careless driving causing RTA in addition to that intoxicated patients are usually difficult to examine and small fractures in intoxicated patients can easily be misdiagnosed. Reduction of drunk drivers reduces MF trauma severity and the association of alcohol and interpersonal violence is well recognized [20,21]. We have found that 158 of the 754 patients were intoxicated before trauma. This relatively high ratio for a highly Muslim populated country can be explained by our hospitals place which is famous for its night-life like Jeju [3]. Alcohol consumption declines rapidly in our eastern neighbors [22].

Conclusion

MF trauma management is sometimes challenging in emergency room. Knowing the MF trauma presentations, concomitant non facial injuries and TBI patterns are important for emergent management. To our knowledge common literature lacks studies from ED. We believe for MF trauma epidemiology, ED study results are more reliable in the light of information above. Further studies are needed to improve our hypothesis.

Abbreviations
ED: Emergency department; MF: Maxillofacial; RTA: Road traffic accidents; TBI: Traumatic brain injury.

Competing interests
The authors declare that they have no competing interests.

Authors' contributions
EDA and AS conceived of the study, participated in the design of the study and drafted the manuscript. CK and EK participated in the sequence alignment and performed the statistical analysis EK carried out the imagining studies, and helped to draft the manuscript. FY, TD, MS participated in its design and coordination. All authors read and approved the final manuscript.

Author details
[1]Emergency Department, Ankara Numune Training and Research Hospital, Altındağ, 06100 Ankara, Turkey. [2]Emergency Department, Başkent Univercity Hospital, Çankaya, 06350 Ankara, Turkey. [3]Radiology Department, Ankara Numune Training and Research Hospital, Altındağ, 06100 Ankara, Turkey.

References
1. Aksoy E, Unlu E, Sensoz O: A retrospective study on epidemiology and treatment of maxillofacial fractures. J Craniofac Surg 2002, 13(6):772–775.
2. Erol B, Tanrikulu R, Gorgun B: Maxillofacial fractures. Analysis of demographic distribution and treatment in 2901 patients (25-year experience). J Craniomaxillofac Surg 2004, 32(5):308–313.
3. Lee JH, Cho BK, Park WJ: A 4-year retrospective study of facial fractures on Jeju, Korea. J Craniomaxillofac Surg 2010, 38(3):192–196.
4. Gassner R, et al: Cranio-maxillofacial trauma: a 10 year review of 9,543 cases with 21,067 injuries. J Craniomaxillofac Surg 2003, 31(1):51–61.
5. van den Bergh B, et al: Aetiology and incidence of maxillofacial trauma in Amsterdam: a retrospective analysis of 579 patients. J Craniomaxillofac Surg 2012, 40(6):e165–e169.

6. Bakardjiev A, Pechalova P: **Maxillofacial fractures in Southern Bulgaria - a retrospective study of 1706 cases.** *J Craniomaxillofac Surg* 2007, **35**(3):147–150.

7. Iida S, *et al*: **Retrospective analysis of 1502 patients with facial fractures.** *Int J Oral Maxillofac Surg* 2001, **30**(4):286–290.

8. Ramli R, *et al*: **A retrospective study of oral and maxillofacial injuries in Seremban Hospital, Malaysia.** *Dent Traumatol* 2011, **27**(2):122–126.

9. Motamedi MH: **An assessment of maxillofacial fractures: a 5-year study of 237 patients.** *J Oral Maxillofac Surg* 2003, **61**(1):61–64.

10. Ceallaigh PO, *et al*: **Diagnosis and management of common maxillofacial injuries in the emergency department. Part 1: advanced trauma life support.** *Emerg Med J* 2006, **23**(10):796–797.

11. Mohajerani SH, Asghari S: **Pattern of mid-facial fractures in Tehran, Iran.** *Dent Traumatol* 2011, **27**(2):131–134.

12. Al Ahmed HE, *et al*: **The pattern of maxillofacial fractures in Sharjah, United Arab Emirates: a review of 230 cases.** *Oral Surg Oral Med Oral Pathol Oral Radiol Endod* 2004, **98**(2):166–170.

13. Klenk G, Kovacs A: **Etiology and patterns of facial fractures in the United Arab Emirates.** *J Craniofac Surg* 2003, **14**(1):78–84.

14. Mouzakes J, *et al*: **The impact of airbags and seat belts on the incidence and severity of maxillofacial injuries in automobile accidents in New York State.** *Arch Otolaryngol Head Neck Surg* 2001, **127**(10):1189–1193.

15. Naveen Shankar A, *et al*: **The pattern of the maxillofacial fractures - a multicentre retrospective study.** *J Craniomaxillofac Surg* 2012, **40**(8):675–679.

16. Gomes PP, Passeri LA, Barbosa JR: **A 5-year retrospective study of zygomatico-orbital complex and zygomatic arch fractures in Sao Paulo State, Brazil.** *J Oral Maxillofac Surg* 2006, **64**(1):63–67.

17. Allareddy V, Nalliah RP: **Epidemiology of facial fracture injuries.** *J Oral Maxillofac Surg* 2011, **69**(10):2613–2618.

18. Zargar M, *et al*: **Epidemiology study of facial injuries during a 13 month of trauma registry in Tehran.** *Indian J Med Sci* 2004, **58**(3):109–114.

19. Gandhi S, *et al*: **Pattern of maxillofacial fractures at a tertiary hospital in northern India: a 4-year retrospective study of 718 patients.** *Dent Traumatol* 2011, **27**(4):257–262.

20. Telfer MR, Jones GM, Shepherd JP: **Trends in the aetiology of maxillofacial fractures in the United Kingdom (1977-1987).** *Br J Oral Maxillofac Surg* 1991, **29**(4):250–255.

21. Laverick S, Patel N, Jones DC: **Maxillofacial trauma and the role of alcohol.** *Br J Oral Maxillofac Surg* 2008, **46**(7):542–546.

22. Hashemi HM, Beshkar M: **The prevalence of maxillofacial fractures due to domestic violence–a retrospective study in a hospital in Tehran, Iran.** *Dent Traumatol* 2011, **27**(5):385–388.

23

Study of the occurrence of intra-abdominal hypertension and abdominal compartment syndrome in patients of blunt abdominal trauma and its correlation with the clinical outcome in the above patients

Ajeet Ramamani Tiwari and Jayashri Sanjay Pandya[*]

Abstract

Background: Intra-abdominal pressure (IAP) measurements have been identified as essential for diagnosis and management of both intra-abdominal hypertension (IAH) and Abdominal compartment syndrome (ACS). It has gained prominent status in ICUs worldwide. We aimed to evaluate the utility of measurement of rise in bladder pressure to assess IAP levels in blunt abdominal trauma (BAT) patients.

Patients and methods: Thirty patients of BAT with solid organ injuries were included in this study. Intra-abdominal pressure was measured through a Foleys bladder catheter throughout their stay. Bladder pressure was compared with clinical parameters like mean arterial pressures(MAP), respiratory rate(RR), serum creatinine(SC) and abdominal girth(AG) and also with outcome in terms of intervention whether operative(OI) or non-operative(NOI).

Results: Bladder pressure showed significant correlation with MAP (R = −0.418; P = 0.022), AG (R = 0.755; P = 0.000), SC (R = 0.689; P = 0.000) and RR (R = 0.537; P = 0.002). Bladder pressure (R = 0.851; P = 0.000), SC (R = 0.625; P = 0.000), MAP (R = −0.350; P = 0.058) and maximum AG difference (R = 0.634; P = 0.000) showed significant correlation with intervention. In total, 17 patients (56 %) required intervention, 9 patients (30 %) underwent NOI (pigtailing or aspiration) while 8 (27 %) needed OI. More than 3 derailed parameters were associated with 100 % intervention (Mean 3.47, SD-1.23). High APACHE III score on admission (>40) was associated with increased intervention (p = 0.001). Intervention correlates well with Grade of injury (p = 0.000) and not with number of organs injured (p = 0.061). Blood transfusion of 2 or more units of blood was associated with increased intervention (p = 0.000).

(Continued on next page)

* Correspondence: smruti63@hotmail.com
Department of General Surgery, Topiwala National Medical College and Bai
Yamunabai Laxman Nair Charitable Hospital, Mumbai Central 400008, India

(Continued from previous page)

Conclusion: Increased bladder pressure and other clinical parameters (MAP, SC, RR and change in AG) correlates well with intervention. Elevated bladder pressure correlates well with other clinical parameters in patients with BAT. Bladder pressure, SC, MAP, RR and AG difference can be used to determine the group of patients that can be managed conservatively and those that would benefit with minimal intervention or exploration. During Non-operative management (NOM) of patients with BAT and multiple solid organ injuries, IAP monitoring may be a simple and objective guideline to suggest further intervention whether NOI or OI. Although routine bladder pressure measurements will result in unnecessary monitoring of large number of patients it is hoped that patients with IAH can be detected early and subsequent ACS with morbid abdominal exploration can be prevented. However the criterion for non-operative failure and the point of decompression needs further refinement to prevent an increase of nontherapeutic operations.

Keywords: Blunt abdominal trauma, Intra-abdominal pressure, Abdominal compartment syndrome, Intra-abdominal hypertension, Bladder pressure, Non-operative management

Background

Since 19th century, intra-abdominal hypertension (IAH) and abdominal compartment syndrome (ACS) have been recognized. ACS has been indicated as a complication in serious blunt abdominal trauma (BAT) for more than 50 years. It develops as a consequence of increased intra-abdominal pressure (IAP) not only in abdominal trauma, but also in intestinal obstructions with serous edema of the bowels or a chronically growing ascites [1, 2]. IAH and ACS are major factors responsible for significant morbidity and mortality among the critically ill patients and their role has been appreciated in last 15 years [3–5].

The incidence of IAH in critical care patients is reported to be 50 %, of these 50 %, 32.1 % develop IAH and 4.2 % develop ACS within their first day of ICU [6, 7]. Historically physical observation and measurement of abdominal girth were used to determine the presence of IAH. This method of measurement is inaccurate due to a high risk of variability and low reliability. A range of approaches to measure IAP include intra gastric, intra rectal, inferior vena cava and via a urinary indwelling catheter pressure monitoring systems [5, 8–11].

Continuous bladder IAP measurements are more reliable to intermittent measurements. This technique was first described by *Kron* et al. which involves placing a Foley catheter in the urinary bladder. It is considered as the 'gold standard' for indirect clinical measurement of IAP [12–15].

Non Operative Management (NOM) is the treatment of choice for BAT since last few decades because of increased evidence of surgery related complications [16, 17]. NOM consists of five therapeutic strategies to overcome IAH/ACS, includes evacuation of intra luminal content, evacuation of intra-abdominal space occupying lesions, improvement in abdominal wall compliance, optimization of fluid administration and tissue perfusion by serially monitoring of patients with the help of different imaging techniques [18].

Monitoring these patients during NOM requires precise clinical skills taking into account various clinical and laboratory parameters. Most of these standard clinical parameters monitored during NOM collectively help the surgeon to take decisions that are very subjective in nature. Many of these patients develop distension of abdomen following few days of trauma which might be due to trivial causes such as continued slow hemorrhage and bile leak causing peritoneal irritation and excessive fluid secretion with bowel edema. However the distension might also be due to serious complications like massive re-bleeding, delayed bowel perforation or frank biliary peritonitis. While monitoring these patients in critical care unit with parameters like pulse, blood pressure, hemogram, ABG, abdominal girth at small time intervals the surgeon always has a dilemma as to whether the deteriorating clinical condition is either due to these trivial causes or serious ones that would mandate an open exploration. Repeat imaging with CT scan might help sometimes for serious complications like delayed perforation or massive re-bleeds however they are not specific in the event of development of ACS for trivial causes. None of the above clinical parameters objectively help the surgeon to define occurrence of ACS in these patients which many times can be tackled with plain decompression via less invasive means like aspiration and pigtailing rather than ending up with morbid negative abdominal explorations.

In the quest to objectively define development of ACS in the patients of BAT managed with NOM, we serially measured their bladder pressures while they were being treated in their respective surgical units. At the end of the treatment we tried to correlate different clinical parameters and bladder pressures to propose that serial bladder pressure monitoring should be a part of clinical assessment of these patients for early diagnosis and timely intervention in the event of development of ACS.

Methods

This was a prospective descriptive observational study carried out at our tertiary center after obtaining permission from the Institutional Ethics Committee. 30 patients of BAT with solid organ injuries were included in the study. However patients with head and spinal injury, urinary bladder injury, history of neurogenic bladder or previous bladder surgery were excluded from the study as above conditions would cause variations in bladder pressure measurements. At presentation patient's/Patient's legally accepted relative's consent was obtained for inclusion into the study.

Patients were admitted in one of the 6 surgical units of the hospital depending upon the day they presented to the hospital. All patient's APACHE III score was calculated at admission as per departmental policy and patients were managed as per surgical unit's trauma management protocols. The common management protocol for all the 6 surgical units were initial resuscitation as per ATLS protocols, CT abdomen when vitally stable, blood, FFP and crystalloid transfusion when required, hourly monitoring of pulse, BP, CVP, respiratory rate, abdominal girth, urinary output, serum creatinine, 6 hourly monitoring of ABG, hemoglobin, hematocrit and strict immobilization for a minimum of 3 days with continued limb mobilization, compression stockings and chest physiotherapy. However the decision of operative management of these patients, who deteriorated upon a trial of NOM, was solely made by surgical unit head, after taking into account the above mentioned clinical and laboratory parameters. The bladder pressures of all the patients who fit into the inclusion criteria was monitored 6 hourly from the time of admission when the patients were catheterized. The end point was removal of Foley's catheter either before discharge or upon death. Intra-abdominal pressure was measured through a Foleys bladder catheter using water column measurement at pubic symphysis.

At the end of the study, sequential bladder pressure was compared to the outcome in terms of intervention whether operative (OI) or non-operative (NOI) and raised bladder pressures correlated with clinical parameters like mean arterial pressures (MAP), respiratory rate (RR), serum creatinine (SC) and abdominal girth (AG). Statistical analysis was performed by software SPSS20.0. Chi square test and spearman correlation was calculated to correlate various clinical parameters with intervention and increased bladder pressure. Descriptive analysis performed to assess demographic data.

Results

Out of the 30 patients included in the study, 28 (93 %) were males and 2 (7 %) were female patients between 18 to 60 years (mean-32, SD-12.17) of age. The minimal APACHE III score was 8 while maximum was 94 (mean-45.4, SD-22.80) at entry level. 13 (43 %) patients required no intervention and settled with conservative management while 17 (57 %) patients required intervention. Out of 17, 9 (53 %) patients underwent NOI while 8 (47 %) needed OI. The mean hospital stay was 11 days (minimum 6 and maximum 16). During hospital stay, 24 patients required blood transfusion at some point. One patient succumbed to her injuries while rest of the patients were discharged after treatment.

The cut off values were, AG change of more than or equal to 3 cm from the time of admission, SC more than or equal to 2 mg/dl, MAP less than or equal to 70 mmHg, RR more than or equal to 24 per minute and bladder pressure more than or equal to 25 cm H2O as abnormal. Correlation was obtained when these parameters were compared at time of intervention. Parameters with respect to their cut off values were statistically analyzed with intervention. Bladder pressure ($R = 0.851$; $P = 0.000$), SC ($R = 0.625$; $P = 0.000$), MAP ($R = -0.350$; $P = 0.058$) and maximum AG difference ($R = 0.634$; $P = 0.000$) showed significant correlation with intervention. (Table 1, Fig. 1).

Statistical correlation analysis of change in SC, MAP, RR and AG was performed with increase in bladder pressure. MAP ($R = -0.418$; $P = 0.022$), AG ($R = 0.755$; $P = 0.00$), SC ($R = 0.689$; $P = 0.000$) and RR ($R = 0.537$; $P = 0.002$) showed significant Spearman correlation with respect to rise in bladder pressure. More than 3 derailed parameters were associated with 100 % intervention (Mean 3.47, SD-1.23). (Table 1, Fig. 1).

Increased APACHE III score (>40) was associated with increased intervention ($p = 0.001$). Intervention correlates well with grade of injury ($p = 0.000$) and not with number of organs injured. Blood transfusion of 2 or more units of blood correlates with intervention ($p = 0.000$) (Table 2).

Discussion

Abdominal trauma can result in the increase of IAP for a variety of reasons, including the accumulation of blood or free fluid in the peritoneal cavity, edema of the intestinal wall, retroperitoneal hematoma or abdominal packing for hemorrhage control. Therefore the continuing hepatic hemorrhage and increasing amounts of bloody ascites found in failed NOM can lead to an elevation in IAP [19]. ACS with multiple organ dysfunction is a consequence of the effects of IAH on multiple organ systems. Elevated IAP results in impaired physiology and organ functions due to the limited abdominal wall compliance [20]. In patients with severe trauma the incidence of ACS has been reported at 14 % – 15 % after damage control laparotomies. To date there are very few reports describing the changes in IAP or the development of IAH or ACS while the patients are receiving NOM after BAT [19]. NOM has been established as the

Table 1 Correlation between bladder pressure, abdominal Girth (AG) difference, mean arterial pressure, serum creatinine, respiratory rate and intervention during the course of treatment for blunt abdominal trauma

			Maximum bladder pressure	Intervention vs no intervention
Spearman's rho	Maximum bladder pressure	Correlation coefficient	1.000	0.851
		Sig. (2-tailed)		.000
	Maximum AG difference (cm)	Correlation coefficient	.755	0.634
		Sig. (2-tailed)	.000	.000
	Lowest mean arterial pressure	Correlation coefficient	-.418	−0.350
		Sig. (2-tailed)	.022	.058
	Maximum serum creatinine	Correlation coefficient	.689	0.625
		Sig. (2-tailed)	.000	.000
	Maximum respiratory rate	Correlation coefficient	.537	0.445
		Sig. (2-tailed)	.002	.014
	Intervention vs no intervention	Correlation coefficient	-.851	1.000
		Sig. (2-tailed)	.000	

treatment of choice for most of the patients with BAT with solid organ injury.

Similar to Croce et al. who reported mean transfusion requirement in first 48 h to be 1.9 units our overall mean transfusion requirement was 1.93 units however no limitation of transfusion requirement was mentioned [21]. Most authors favor the ultimate decisive factor of NOM should be hemodynamic stability of the patient. However no definitive limitation of transfusion requirement to maintain the hemodynamic stability in such patients has been documented. In our study 2 or more units of blood transfusion was associated with increased intervention. A falling hematocrit presents the surgeon with a dilemma as to whether the liver laceration is the cause of the ongoing bleeding especially in patients with multiple solid organ injuries. Although the CT scan study can objectively demonstrate the change in solid organ lesions and the amount of hemoperitoneum, this diagnostic modality is not readily available. Moreover, the hepatic and splenic lesion may be confused with the initial ingress of interstitial fluid between the lacerations [19].

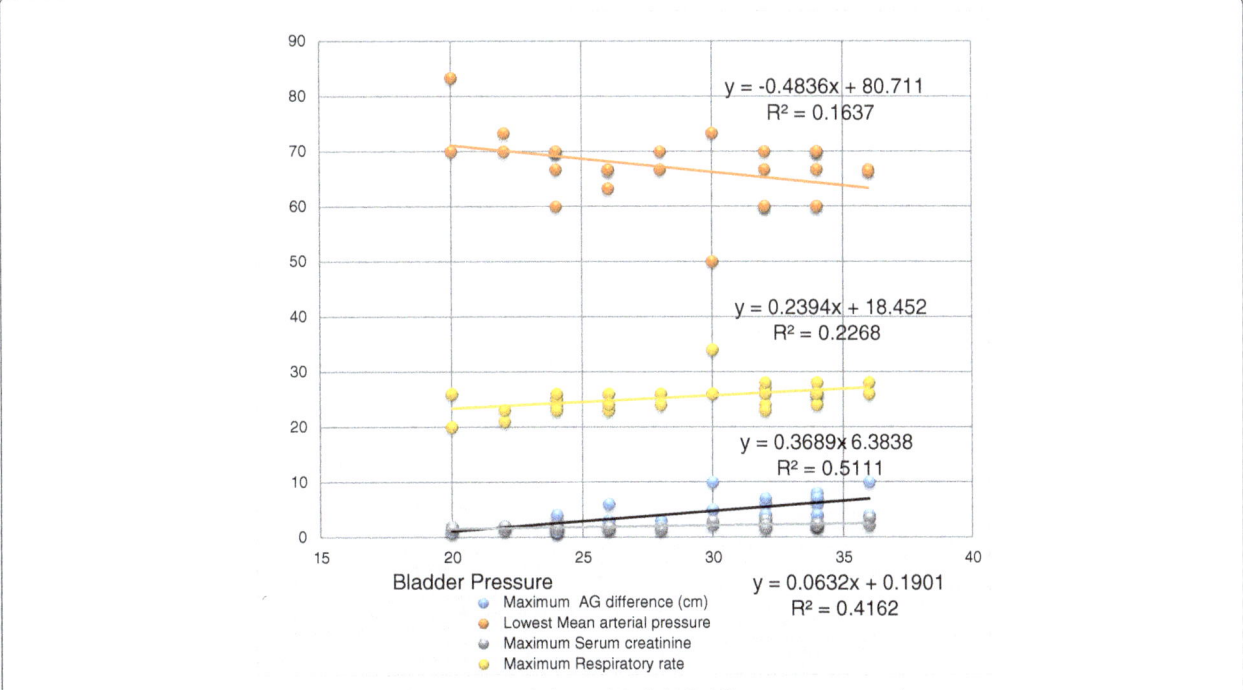

Fig. 1 Chart showing correlation between Bladder pressure, abdominal Girth (AG) difference, mean arterial pressure, serum creatinine, respiratory rate and Intervention during the course of treatment for blunt abdominal trauma

Table 2 Cross table showing relation between Apache III score, grades of injury, number of organs injured, blood transfusion and intervention

Apache III score	No intervention	Intervention	Chi square value	P value
<=40	11	5	11.808	0.001
>40	1	13		
Grades of injury				
1,2	8	0	16.364	0.000
3,4	4	18		
Number of organs injured				
> = 2	4	13	4.434	0.061
1	8	5		
Blood transfusion (units)				
<2	11	1	22.245	0.000
> = 2	1	17		

Since no adverse effects of IAP below 25 cm H2O were reported this value was therefore used as a cutoff point for our study. Ray-Jade Chen et al. studied ACS in patients with hepatic injuries in BAT and using IAP of 25 cm H2O as cutoff point compared the two groups with respect to estimated liver related transfusions, PaO2/FiO2 and peritoneal signs. All patients with IAP of 25 cm of H2O or greater had exacerbation of peritoneal signs before operation and a strong correlation between the IAP value and presence of peritoneal signs was found [19]. In our study we did not use peritoneal signs as they are highly subjective and examiner dependent. It can be confused by concomitant thoraco-abdominal or pelvic injuries and variable pain responses from different points. In our study we included patients of not only hepatic injuries but other solid organ injuries due to BAT to have a more broad generalization of ACS in this group of patients as not just hepatic injuries but other solid organ injuries too are managed conservatively and have equal probability of developing ACS. This notion is supported from our finding that it is not the number of organs that are injured (*p* = 0.061) but the grade of injury of the solid organ injured (*p* = 0.000) that causes increased intervention (Table 2). Despite the popularity of NOM no known parameters can precisely reflect the ongoing hemorrhage and predict whether the hemodynamic instability is due to continued bleeding or development of ACS. Hence in our study we included simple bedside clinical parameters i.e. Bladder pressure, RR, MAP, SC and change in AG, that are routinely used to monitor these patients with BAT undergoing NOM and found that more than 3 deranged parameters was associated with 100 % intervention.

In NOM of patients with solid organ injuries the continuing hemorrhage and increasing amount of ascites (bloody

or secretory) can lead to an increase in IAP. Resuscitation and edema formation after shock or relative ischemia may result in a cyclic process that perpetuates IAP elevation. Hence for aggressive resuscitation in the patients sustaining solid organ injuries the probability of hemodynamic derangement from IAP elevation is high. A further increase of the IAP will subsequently compromise the hemodynamics and result in non-operative failure. A negative abdominal exploration in these patients can be avoided if ACS due to excessive fluid can be recognized at an early stage by continuous monitoring of bladder pressures. Burch et al. developed a working grade system for ACS on the basis of urinary bladder pressure measurements. They recommended that in patients after celiotomy with bladder pressure of 26 to 35 cm H2O decompression is necessary and with bladder pressure exceeding 35 cm H2O reexploration is mandatory [22]. These findings match with our study in which Bladder pressure more than 25 cm of H2O was statistically significant when compared to time of intervention. In our study we found that more than 3 deranged clinical parameters (out of Bladder pressure, SC, RR, MAP and AG) was associated with 100 % intervention.

Ray-Jade Chen et al. described the failure of NOM in their study as those that- 1. Manifested hemodynamic derangement (systolic pressure < 90 mm Hg) despite resuscitation, or 2. Had stable hemodynamics but with an IAP of 25 cm H2O or greater. Of the 25 patients of BAT with liver injuries that Ray-Jade Chen et al. studied, 5 developed IAP greater than 25 cm H2O and underwent laparoscopy for decompression [19]. In our study we did not use laparoscopy instead decompression was achieved through pigtailing and multiple aspirations of the intra-abdominal collections in 9 patients who underwent NOI (Table 3). 19 patients(76 %) were successfully treated non operatively in Ray-Jade Chen et al. study that matched with our finding of 22 patients out of 30 (73 %).

Table 3 Data showing types of intervention in patients with different organ injuries

		Intervention			Total
		Operative	Non operative	None	
Solid organ injury	Liver	0	1	6	7
	Liver/Kidney	0	0	1	1
	Liver/Pancreas	0	1	0	1
	Liver/Spleen	4	5	3	12
	Liver/Spleen/Kidney	0	1	0	1
	Liver/Spleen/Pancreas	1	0	0	1
	Liver/Spleen/Pancreas/Kidney	0	1	0	1
	Spleen	3	0	3	6
Total		8	9	13	30

Of the 17 patients that required intervention 9 of them underwent NOI and the morbidity of negative abdominal exploration was avoided by simple procedures like pigtailing and aspiration (Table 3). In a study by Cheatham et.al, percutaneous catheter decompression (PCD) was compared with open abdominal decompression in treatment of IAH and ACS. PCD potentially avoided the need for subsequent open abdominal decompression in 25 of 31 patients (81 %) treated [23]. The lower mortality found in our study suggests that IAH and ACS can be managed using non-operative methods, which will prevent morbidity associated with exploratory laparotomy. However L. Pleva et al. suggested that in the event of any suspicion for acute elevation of IAP and development of ACS the performance of decompression laparotomy is indicated even with the assumption of negative preoperative finding [24]. Nevertheless identification of this group of patients by continuous bladder pressure monitoring who develop ACS due to increased fluid inside the abdominal cavity and not due to ongoing hemorrhage is essential as the morbidity of a negative exploration can be avoided by simple decompressive NOI and can buy some more time for successful completion of NOM.

Limitations of our study was non utilization of complex physiologic monitoring of hemodynamic and pulmonary dysfunction in ACS like the oxygen delivery index and peak airway pressures as Swan Ganz catheter was not routinely used in our trauma units. Also while they were receiving NOM the cardiac output index and oxygen transport variables were not measured. Our preliminary study was small and the criterion of decompression needs further evaluation.

Conclusion

Increased bladder pressure and other clinical parameters (MAP, SC, RR and change in AG) correlates well with intervention. Elevated bladder pressure correlates well with other clinical parameters in patients with BAT. Bladder pressure, SC, MAP, RR and AG difference can be used to determine the group of patients that can be managed conservatively and those that would benefit with minimal intervention or exploration. It is the grade of injury to solid organs that determine intervention and not the number of solid organs injured. During NOM of patients with BAT and multiple solid organ injuries, IAP monitoring may be a simple and objective guideline that might be in future included in Trauma Severity Scales to suggest further intervention whether NOI or OI. Although routine bladder pressure measurements will result in unnecessary monitoring of large number of patients it is hoped that patients with IAH can be detected early and subsequent ACS with morbid abdominal exploration can be prevented. However the criterion for non-operative failure and the point of decompression

needs further refinement to prevent an increase of non-therapeutic operations.

Competing interests
The authors declare that they have no competing interests.

Authors' contributions
Dr. ART conceived and designed the study, acquired and analysed data and drafted the manuscript. Dr. JSP revised the manuscript and gave final approval for publication.

Acknowledgement
We would like to thank Dr. Aparna Deshpande for her valuable inputs during the course of the study, Dr. Amar Udare for technical assistance and Dr. Durgesh Sahoo for statistical analysis.

References
1. Coombs HC. The mechanism of the regulation of intra-abdominal pressure. Am J Phsyiol. 1920;61:159–63.
2. Ivatury RR, Poter JM, Simon RJ, et al. Intra-abdominal hypertension after life-threatening penetrating abdominal trauma: prophylaxis, incidence, and clinical relevance to gastric mucosal pH and abdominal compartment syndrome. J Trauma. 1998;44:1016–21.
3. Leanne H, Frost SA, Ken H, Newton PJ, Davidson PM. Management of intra-abdominal hypertension and abdominal compartment syndrome: a review. J Trauma Manage Outcomes. 2014;8:2.
4. Cheatham ML, Safcsak K. Is the evolving management of intra-abdominal hypertension and abdominal compartment syndrome improving survival? Crit Care Med. 2010;38(2):402–7.
5. Cheatham ML. Abdominal compartment syndrome. Curr Opin Crit Care. 2009;15(2):154–62.
6. Malbrain ML, Cheatham ML, Kirkpatrick A, Sugrue M, De Waele J, Ivatury R. Abdominal compartment syndrome: it's time to pay attention! Intensive Care Med. 2006;32(11):1912–4.
7. Kim I, Prowle J, Baldwin I, Bellomo R. Incidence, risk factors and outcome associations of intra-abdominal hypertension in critically ill patients. Anaesth Intensive Care. 2012;40(1):79–89.
8. Malbrain MLNG, Cheatham ML, Kirkpatrick A, Sugrue M, Parr M, De Waele J, et al. Results from the international conference of experts on intra-abdominal hypertension and abdominal compartment syndrome. I. definitions. Intensive Care Med. 2006;32(11):1722–32.
9. Cheatham ML. Intra-abdominal pressure monitoring during fluid resuscitation. Curr Opin Crit Care. 2008;14(3):327–33.
10. Malbrain M, Jones F. Intra-abdominal pressure measurement techniques. In: Ivatury R, Cheatham M, Malbrain M, Sugrue M, editors. Abdominal compartment syndrome. Texas: Landes Bioscience; 2006.
11. Sugrue M, Bauman A, Jones F, Bishop G, Flabouris A, Parr M. Clinical examination is an inaccurate predictor of intra-abdominal pressure. World J Surg. 2002;26(12):1428–31.
12. Malbrain M, De Laet I, Viaene D, Schoonheydt K, Dits H. In vitro validation of a novel method for continuous intra-abdominal pressure monitoring. Intensive Care Med. 2008;34(4):740–5.
13. Kron IL, Harman PK, Nolan SP. The measurement of intra-abdominal pressure as a criterion for abdominal re-exploration. Ann Surg. 1984;199(1):28–30.
14. Malbrain M. Abdominal compartment syndrome. F1000 Med Reports. 2009;1:86.
15. Wendon J, Biancofiore G, Auzinger G. Intra-abdominal hypertension and the liver. In: Ivatury RR, Cheatham ML, Malbrain M, Sugrue M, editors. Abdominal Compartment Syndrome. Georgetown, TX: Landis Bioscience; 2006. p. 138–43.
16. Velmahos GC, Toutouzas KG, Radin R, Chan L, Demetriades D. Non-operative treatment of blunt injury to solid abdominal organs:a prospective study. Arch Surg. 2003;138(8):844–51.
17. Giannopoulos GA, Katsoulis EI, Tzanakis NE, Panayotis AP, Digalakis M. Non-operative management of blunt abdominal trauma. Is it safe and feasible in a district general hospital? J Trauma Resuscitation Emerg Med. 2009;17:22–8.

18. Cheatham ML. Non-operative Management of Intra-abdominal Hypertension and Abdominal Compartment Syndrome. World J Surg. 2009;33(6):1116–22.

19. Chen RJ, Fang JF, Chen MF. Intra-abdominal pressure monitoring as a guideline in the non-operative management of blunt hepatic trauma. J Trauma. 2001;51(1):44–50. PubMed.

20. Barnes GE, Laine GA, Giam PY, Smith EE, Granger HJ. Cardiovascular responses to elevation of intra-abdominal hydrostatic pressure. Am J Physiol. 1985;248:R209–13.

21. Croce MA, Fabian TC, Menke PG, Waddle-Smith L, Minard G, Kudsk KA, et al. Non-operative management of blunt hepatic trauma is the treatment of choice for hemodynamically stable patients. Results of a prospective trial. Ann Surg. 1995;221(6):744–53. PubMed PMID: 7794078, PubMed Central PMCID: PMC1234706, discussion 753–5. Review.

22. Burch JM, Moore EE, Moore FA, Franciose R. The abdominal compartment syndrome. Surg Clin North Am. 1996;76(4):833–42. Review. PubMed.

23. Cheatham ML, Safcsak K. Percutaneous catheter decompression in the treatment of elevated intra-abdominal pressure. Chest. 2011;140(6):1428–35.

24. Pleva L, Sír M, Mayzlík J. Abdominal compartment syndrome in polytrauma. Biomed Pap Med Fac Univ Palacky Olomouc Czech Repub. 2004;148(1):81–4. PubMed.

24

Non-invasive hemodynamic monitoring in trauma patients

Matthias Kuster[1], Aristomenis Exadaktylos[2] and Beat Schnüriger[1,3*]

Abstract

Background: The assessment of hemodynamic status is a crucial task in the initial evaluation of trauma patients. However, blood pressure and heart rate are often misleading, as multiple variables may impact these conventional parameters. More reliable methods such as pulmonary artery thermodilution for cardiac output measuring would be necessary, but its applicability in the Emergency Department is questionable due to their invasive nature. Non-invasive cardiac output monitoring devices may be a feasible alternative.

Methods: A systematic literature review was conducted. Only studies that explicitly investigated non-invasive hemodynamic monitoring devices in trauma patients were considered.

Results: A total of 7 studies were identified as suitable and were included into this review. These studies evaluated in a total of 1,197 trauma patients the accuracy of non-invasive hemodynamic monitoring devices by comparing measurements to pulmonary artery thermodilution, which is the gold standard for cardiac output measuring. The correlation coefficients r between the two methods ranged from 0.79 to 0.92. Bias and precision analysis ranged from -0.02 +/- 0.78 l/min/m^2 to -0.14 +/- 0.73 l/min/m^2. Additionally, data on practicality, limitations and clinical impact of the devices were collected.

Conclusion: The accuracy of non-invasive cardiac output monitoring devices in trauma patients is broadly satisfactory. As the devices can be applied very early in the shock room or even preclinically, hemodynamic shock may be recognized much earlier and therapeutic interventions could be applied more rapidly and more adequately. The devices can be used in the daily routine of a busy ED, as they are non-invasive and easy to master.

Keywords: Initial care, Hypovolemic shock, Non-invasive hemodynamic monitoring, Trauma

Introduction

When managing trauma patients, it is crucial to evaluate the hemodynamic status to exclude hemorrhage. During the initial assessment, blood pressure and heart rate are commonly used to estimate blood loss. However, these parameters may be altered due to pain, hypothermia, neurogenic or cardiogenic shock or other factors related to the patient or to the injury. Moreover, analgesic, sedative or relaxing drugs may interfere with these conventional vital signs, thus making their interpretation difficult.

* Correspondence: beat.schnuriger@gmail.com
[1]Department of Visceral and Transplant Surgery, Bern University Hospital, Bern, Switzerland
[3]Department of Visceral Surgery and Medicine, Bern University Hospital, Bern, Switzerland

Therefore, other diagnostic tools are required for hemorrhage detection. It has been shown that cardiac output is substantially different in hypotensive patients with or without blood loss. Low cardiac output then indicates blood loss, whereas normal or elevated cardiac output implies that blood loss is unlikely and that there may be other reasons for hypotension [1]. This is in accordance with many studies that have demonstrated that surviving patients exhibit significantly different hemodynamic patterns from non-survivors, and that these differences are already apparent in the Emergency Department (ED). For example, it has been repeatedly shown that cardiac index is higher in survivors than in non-survivors [2-8].

Pulmonary artery catheter thermodilution is considered to be the gold standard for cardiac output measurement [9]. Unfortunately, the invasive nature of this method means that it is not applicable during the initial phase in the ED [9,10]. Thus, thermodilution often cannot be used early in the evaluation of trauma patients.

A non-invasive device that permits advanced hemodynamic monitoring as soon as the patient arrives in the ED or even preclinically would be of great benefit in the assessment of the hemodynamic state. However, before such a new device is introduced into clinical routine, it needs to be assessed in controlled clinical trials.

The purpose of this review is to evaluate the accuracy and clinical applicability of non-invasive hemodynamic monitoring devices in the early assessment of trauma patients.

Methods
Search strategy
A systematic literature search was conducted using PubMed as its primary source. Studies from January 1966 to July 2014 were considered. Multiple searches were performed using the following keywords: non-invasive hemodynamic monitoring AND/OR non-invasive cardiac output monitoring AND/OR thoracic electrical bioimpedance AND/OR impedance cardiography AND/OR bioreactance AND/OR NICOM AND trauma. In PubMed, the 'related articles' algorithm was employed to identify additional articles. Moreover, bibliographies of original reports and reviews were screened for additional citations. Preliminary screening was performed utilizing titles and abstracts. The full-length articles of potentially appropriate studies were retrieved for further screening.

Inclusion and exclusion criteria
Only those studies were considered for inclusion that explicitly investigated the accuracy of non-invasive hemodynamic monitoring devices in trauma patients by comparing it to the pulmonary artery catheter thermodilution method (Figure 1). Devices were examined that measure at least cardiac output through thoracic electrical bioimpedance, or through variations of this technology, such as bioreactance. Both prospective and retrospective studies were considered for inclusion. Studies in languages other than English, reviews, case reports or case series of <10 patients, were not considered for inclusion.

Data extraction
Data was extracted on the accuracy of non-invasive hemodynamic monitoring devices. The devices measurements had to be compared to pulmonary artery catheter thermodilution, the gold standard for cardiac output measuring [9]. Correlation coefficients were taken from the articles, together with bias and precision analysis between the non-invasive hemodynamic monitoring device

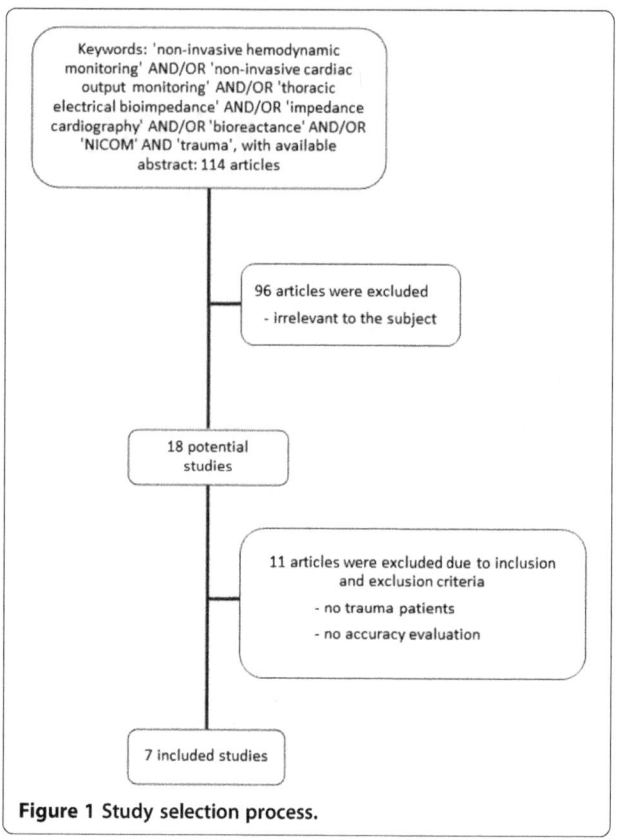

Figure 1 Study selection process.

and pulmonary artery catheter thermodilution. If obtainable, the limits of agreement were also extracted.

Besides data on accuracy, attention was paid to the device's usability in the ED, including advantages and limitations due to the device's mode of operations and its mode of displaying data. Finally, the new devices' possible clinical impact in the ED was considered.

Characteristics of devices
For non-invasive hemodynamic monitoring, the most commonly used method is the thoracic electrical bioimpedance technology. Eleven non-invasive disposable prewired hydrogen electrodes need to be placed on predefined locations on the skin. Three electrodes function as electrocardiography leads and are placed across the precordium and left shoulder [2,4-8,11-13]. The other eight are positioned in pairs so that they lie over the top and bottom of the lung [5,11]. Each pair consists of an injecting and a sensing electrode. Two injecting electrodes are placed on the lateral side of the neck, opposing each other, and the other two on each side of the chest at the level of the xiphisternal joint. The injecting electrodes send a 100-kHz, 4-mA alternating current through the patient's thorax, and the sensing electrodes measure voltage differences which change during the cardiac cycle. Each contraction of the hearth ejects the stroke volume into the aorta, which reduces the impedance (resistance) across the chest, as the

electrical signals preferentially travel down the aorta, rather than passing through the aerated alveoli of the lung. Thus, an electrical pulsatile impedance curve is captured by the sensing electrodes. This curve is used to calculate the baseline impedance (Zo) and the first derivative of the impedance waveform (dZ/dt). The bioimpedance signals and the electrocardiogram are filtered with an all-integer-coefficient filtering technology to decrease processing time. The digital signal processing also uses time-frequency distributions to increase signal-to-noise ratios. Thus, the device is able to calculate stroke volume, which is multiplied by heart rate to get cardiac output [11].

The bioreactance method is a modification of the thoracic electrical bioimpedance technology [10]. It is based on an analysis of relative phase shifts of an oscillating current that occur when this current traverses the thoracic cavity. Four dual-electrode stickers need to be placed on the skin. Each sticker consists of an outer injecting electrode that emits a high-frequency sine wave into the body, and an inner receiver electrode that is used by the voltage input amplifier. Two stickers are placed left and right on the upper thorax, while the other two are placed on the lower thorax. The stickers on a given side of the body are paired, so that the currents are passed between the outer electrodes of the pair and voltages are recorded from the inner electrodes. The system detects the phase shift of the input signal relative to the injected signal. The change in the phase shift over time is correlated with the blood volume in the aorta, which fluctuates with the cardiac cycle. This allows the calculation of stroke volume [14].

Results

Study selection

Figure 1 shows the study selection process. A total of 114 studies were identified using the aforementioned search strategy. The abstracts were screened, which revealed 18 studies with the potential for inclusion. After obtaining the full-length articles, a total of 7 studies were included [2,3,5,6,11,13,15]. Their publication dates ranged from 1996 to 2006. All these studies compared the performance of a non-invasive hemodynamic monitoring device to the invasive pulmonary artery thermodilution method. They are summarized in Table 1.

The seven studies used devices that are based on thoracic electrical bioimpedance methodology [2,3,5,6,11,13,15]. These devices included a system from Renaissance Technologies, Newtown, Pennsylvania, the IQ System from Wantagh Inc., Bristol, Pennsylvania, the IQ Model 101 from Noninvasive Medical Technologies LLC, Las Vegas, Nevada, and the PhysioFlow from VasoCOM, Bristol, Pennsylvania.

Accuracy of devices

Seven studies evaluated the accuracy of the cardiac output measurements by a thoracic electrical bioimpedance device and correlated this with the measurements of the invasive pulmonary artery catheter thermodilution method [2,3,5,6,11,13,15]. Table 1 gives an overview of the studies designs, the devices used and the data that was extracted.

All authors calculated the correlation coefficient, by comparing the cardiac output measured by the thoracic electrical bioimpedance device to the invasive thermodilution method. Moreover, all but one study conducted a bias and precision analysis [3,5,6,11,13,15]. The newest study also calculated the limits of agreement between the two methods [5].

Four studies published between 1996 and 1999 used a "new thoracic electrical bioimpedance device", developed by Renaissance Technology, Newtown, Pennsylvania

Table 1 Evaluation studies on the accuracy of thoracic electrical bioimpedance devices

Author, year	Study design	Device	Patients	Correlation coefficient r	r^2	Bias and precision (l/min/m^2)
Bishop et al. 1996 [15]	Prospective	Renaissance Technologies	54 patients with gunshot wounds	0.79	0.62	−0.011
Shoemaker et al. 1998 [11]	Retrospective	Renaissance Technologies	268 (139 trauma patients)	0.83	0.68	−0.058 +/- 0.78
Velmahos et al. 1999 [2]	Prospective	Renaissance Technologies	38 severely traumatized patients	0.91	0.83	-
Velmahos et al. 1999 [3]	Prospective	Renaissance Technologies	134 blunt trauma patients	0.83	0.69	−0.02 +/- 0.78
Shoemaker et al. 2001 [6]	Prospective	IQ System; Wantagh Inc.	151 trauma patients	0.91	0.83	−0.3 +/- 1.1
Brown et al. 2005 [13]	Retrospective	IQ System; Wantagh Inc.	285 critically injured patients	0.84	0.71	−0.14 +/-0.73
Shoemaker et al. 2006 [5]	Prospective	IQ Model 101; Noninvasive Medical Technologies LLC or PhysioFlow; VasoCOM	267 trauma patients	0.92	0.84	−0.07 +/- 0.47

[2,3,11,15]. The first study was conducted by Bishop et al. in 1996 [15]. Here, patients with gunshot wounds were assessed. The correlation was $r = 0.79$, $r^2 = 0.62$. Bias was -0.011 $l/min/m^2$. Only a fraction of the cardiac output measurements were performed in the ED, and most came from the intensive care unit (ICU) [15].

In a study by Shoemaker et al. published in 1998, correlations between the pulmonary artery thermodilution method and the thoracic electrical bioimpedance device by Renaissance Technologies were calculated separately in the ED, the ICU, and the Operating Room (OR) [11]. However, this series did not consist of trauma patients only. 52% (139 of 268) of the subjects had trauma-related injuries, while the rest consisted of medical, non-trauma emergencies. The correlation coefficient for the entire population in the ED was $r = 0.83$, $r^2 = 0.68$. Bias and precision were -0.058 +/- 0.78 $l/min/m^2$. In the OR, these values improved to $r = 0.88$, $r^2 = 0.77$, bias and precision = -0.027 +/-0.46 $l/min/m^2$, but these differences were not statistically significant. The authors considered that the overall performance was satisfactory [11].

In 1999, Velmahos et al. evaluated 38 severely traumatized patients on arrival in the ICU with the thoracic electrical bioimpedance device from Renaissance Technologies, Newtown, Pennsylvania [2]. The investigators calculated a correlation coefficient of $r = 0.91$, $r^2 = 0.83$, which they regarded as reasonably satisfactory. However, as the pulmonary artery thermodilution method was initiated after ICU arrival, these findings do not reflect the device's performance in the ED [2]. A second study by the same author included 134 patients with blunt trauma who were assessed with the same devices on arrival in the ED. A correlation coefficient of $r = 0.83$, $r^2 = 0.69$ was found. Bias and precision were -0.02 +/- 0.78 $l/min/m^2$ [3].

The IQ System from Wantagh Inc., Bristol, Pennsylvania is also based on the electrical bioimpedance technology and was evaluated in two studies.[6,13] One was published in 2001 by Shoemaker et al. [6]. These investigators calculated a correlation coefficient of $r = 0.91$, $r^2 = 0.83$. Bias and precision were -0.3 +/- 1.1 $l/min/m^2$. The population in this study consisted of 151 trauma patients and the measurements were performed in the ED [6]. The second study using the IQ System was executed by Brown et al. in 2005 and included 285 critically injured patients, with either blunt (85%) or penetrating traumas (15%) [13]. In this study, the influence of the patient's age on the performance of non-invasive cardiac output measurement was specifically evaluated. The investigators were concerned that atherosclerosis and a rigid thoracic aorta could falsify the results. The study population was stratified into three age groups: <55, 55-70, and >70 years old. The correlation coefficients were 0.82, 0.87, and 0.80, respectively, while bias and precision were -0.17 +/- 0.76 $l/min/m^2$, -0.04 +/- 0.61 $l/min/m^2$,

and -0.04 +/-0.60 $l/min/m^2$, respectively. Thus, good correlations between the cardiac output values of the IQ System and the pulmonary artery thermodilution method were found, and no statistically significant differences were detected between younger and older patients [13].

Shoemaker et al. published a study in 2006 which evaluated the IQ model 101 from Noninvasive Medical Technologies LLC, Las Vegas, Nevada, and the Physio-Flow from VasoCOM, Bristol, Pennsylvania [5]. Both devices are based on thoracic electrical bioimpedance. The correlation coefficient was $r = 0.915$, $r^2 = 0.84$. Bias and precision was -0.07 +/- 0.47 $l/min/m^2$. This was the only study to calculate the limits of agreement (accuracy) between the bioimpedance and thermodilution methods, which was 19.7% and considered to be acceptable [5]. It has been suggested that limits of agreement up to +/- 30% should be accepted when evaluating cardiac output monitoring devices, because pulmonary artery thermodilution itself has an inherent measurement error of 10 to 20% [16,17].

Discussion

A total of five prospective observational and 2 retrospective studies investigating the accuracy of non-invasive hemodynamic monitoring devices in trauma patients are currently available. The thoracic electrical bioimpedance methodology was used in all of these studies. The accuracy of non-invasive cardiac output monitoring was broadly satisfactory.

Practicability and limitations of devices

Accuracy remains the most important aspect when evaluating a new method or technology in patients' hemodynamic monitoring. However, its limitations, usability and convenience in daily clinical routine are also important.

There are important limitations to non-invasive cardiac output measurement that have been identified in the past by several authors. Motion artifacts, restlessness, shivering, anxiety, hyperventilation and agitation can interfere with the measurements [5,6,11]. However, all these circumstances may also limit the accuracy of pulmonary artery thermodilution and most other hemodynamic monitoring techniques [8,11]. Faulty electrode placement can obviously prevent good monitoring [5,6].

Moreover, extensive pulmonary edema, pleural effusion, valvular heart disease, dysrhythmias, extensive chest wall edema, and chest tubes parallel to the aorta can reduce the impedance measured by the device, and lead to false data [5,6,8,11]. In this case, the device's measurements do not provide a reliable basis for clinical decisions [11].

Besides the limitations, some authors have described specific advantages of the non-invasive hemodynamic monitoring devices. One is the continuous, on-line display of measurements [2,3,5,6,8,11,15,18]. This and the real-time data presentation are very convenient [3,5,8,18]. It allows instant recognition of circulatory deterioration and supports clinical decisions [2-4,11-13,15].

Another point that has been emphasized is that non-invasive devices can be applied very early in the ED [2-4,7,8,11,13,18]. The safety of the technology for both patients and staff has been emphasized by many authors [3,5,7,8,11,13,18]. The devices are very mobile and convenient, which allows their use at the bedside [7,8,11,18]. Their use is easy, quick and user-friendly [1,3,6,11,15]. Finally, feasibility is good, as the learning curve is short [3,5].

Clinical impact

Most investigators have used the bioimpedance device with other non-invasive techniques, such as pulse oximetry, or measurements of transcutaneous oxygen and carbon dioxide tension and non-invasive blood pressure [2-8,11,12,18]. Thus, the clinician has indicators of cardiac function (cardiac output, stroke volume), pulmonary function (oxygen saturation) and tissue perfusion (oxygen and carbon dioxide tension) [2,4].

The aforementioned early applicability of non-invasive monitoring devices may solve a key problem of invasive hemodynamic monitoring. It is known that invasive hemodynamic techniques have important limitations, especially in the treatment of trauma patients. For example, inserting pulmonary artery catheters is time-consuming, susceptible to complications, and personnel-intensive, and may be difficult in severely injured patients [1-3]. Moreover, these catheters require a sterile critical care environment and the cessation of other — possibly more urgent — interventions [2-5,7]. In contrast, non-invasive methods may be applied very early in the initial evaluation of the trauma patient, even preclinically [2,11]. Moreover, they do not interfere with clinical management [3]. The continuous real-time display of measurements permits early recognition of circulatory abnormalities or deterioration, which makes it possible to perform early therapeutic interventions and to recognize their hemodynamic effects [2,11]. Shoemaker et al. concluded that non-invasive monitoring is of great value as a "front end" device and may bridge the time to invasive monitoring [11]. Moreover, the physiological parameters measured by the device may permit early recognition of shock and hypotension [3,5,6]. Earlier therapeutic intervention could then be facilitated when time is crucial [2,6]. Furthermore, non-invasive monitoring can be used to titrate therapy to appropriate therapeutic goals [5].

Dunham et al. conducted a study on 270 consecutive trauma activation patients in which they evaluated a non-invasive cardiac output monitoring device [1]. These investigators concluded that the multiple associations of cardiac output with patient conditions imply that non-invasive hemodynamic monitoring provides an objective and clinically valid, relevant, and discriminate measure of cardiac function in acutely injured trauma activation patients. Moreover, they stated, that the use of non-invasive hemodynamic monitoring may be associated with a shorter length of stay in surviving patients with complex injuries [1].

Shoemaker et al. considered that non-invasive monitoring could provide a means to develop an organized coherent therapeutic plan based on physiological criteria measured in the ED. This plan would accompany the patient as he/she proceeds to the OR, the radiology department or the ICU [6].

Future outlook

New devices with potentially better accuracy are emerging. These devices should be evaluated for their impact in routine work when taking care of traumatized patients.

Early differential diagnosis of hypotension in the initial evaluation of trauma patient might be an important advantage of non-invasive hemodynamic monitoring. Knowing the patient's cardiac index early may help the physician to differentiate between blood loss and other causes of hypotension [1]. Thus, these devices may help in determining the etiology of the illness.

If more were known about the hemodynamic changes in bleeding trauma patients, this would help the clinician in using the information gained by non-invasive devices. Therefore, more data is required to interpret the measurements performed early in the ED, e.g. for estimating blood loss.

Conclusion

The accuracy of non-invasive cardiac output monitoring devices in trauma patients is broadly satisfactory. As the devices can be applied very early in the shock room or even preclinically, hemodynamic shock may be recognized much earlier and therapeutic interventions could be applied more rapidly and more adequately. The devices can be used in the daily routine of a busy ED, as they are non-invasive and easy to master. However, the impact of non-invasive cardiac output monitoring on patients' outcome is uncertain and more clinical experience is warranted.

Competing interests
The authors declare that they have no competing interests.

Authors' contributions

MK planed and conducted the literature search, evaluated the literature, drafted and composed the manuscript. AE revised the manuscript critically. BS conceived the review, participated in the planning of the literature search, and revised the manuscript critically. All authors read and approved the final manuscript.

Author details

[1]Department of Visceral and Transplant Surgery, Bern University Hospital, Bern, Switzerland. [2]Department of Emergency Medicine, Bern University Hospital, Bern, Switzerland. [3]Department of Visceral Surgery and Medicine, Bern University Hospital, Bern, Switzerland.

References

1. Dunham CM, Chirichella TJ, Gruber BS, Ferrari JP, Martin JA, Luchs BA, et al. Emergency department noninvasive (NICOM) cardiac outputs are associated with trauma activation, patient injury severity and host conditions and mortality. J Trauma Acute Care Surg. 2012;73:479–85.
2. Velmahos GC, Wo CC, Demetriades D, Shoemaker WC. Early continuous noninvasive haemodynamic monitoring after severe blunt trauma. Injury. 1999;30:209–14.
3. Velmahos GC, Wo CC, Demetriades D, Murray JA, Cornwell 3rd EE, Asensio JA, et al. Invasive and non-invasive physiological monitoring of blunt trauma patients in the early period after emergency admission. Int Surg. 1999;84:354–60.
4. Tatevossian RG, Shoemaker WC, Wo CC, Dang AB, Velmahos GC, Demetriades D. Noninvasive hemodynamic monitoring for early warning of adult respiratory distress syndrome in trauma patients. J Crit Care. 2000;15:151–9.
5. Shoemaker WC, Wo CC, Chien LC, Lu K, Ahmadpour N, Belzberg H, et al. Evaluation of invasive and noninvasive hemodynamic monitoring in trauma patients. J Trauma. 2006;61:844–53. discussion 853-844.
6. Shoemaker WC, Wo CC, Chan L, Ramicone E, Kamel ES, Velmahos GC, et al. Outcome prediction of emergency patients by noninvasive hemodynamic monitoring. Chest. 2001;120:528–37.
7. Lu KJ, Chien LC, Wo CC, Demetriades D, Shoemaker WC. Hemodynamic patterns of blunt and penetrating injuries. J Am Coll Surg. 2006;203:899–907.
8. Colombo J, Shoemaker WC, Belzberg H, Hatzakis G, Fathizadeh P, Demetriades D. Noninvasive monitoring of the autonomic nervous system and hemodynamics of patients with blunt and penetrating trauma. J Trauma. 2008;65:1364–73.
9. Compton F, Schafer JH. Noninvasive cardiac output determination: broadening the applicability of hemodynamic monitoring. Semin Cardiothorac Vasc Anesth. 2009;13:44–55.
10. Chamos C, Vele L, Hamilton M, Cecconi M. Less invasive methods of advanced hemodynamic monitoring: principles, devices, and their role in the perioperative hemodynamic optimization. Perioper Med (Lond). 2013;2:19.
11. Shoemaker WC, Belzberg H, Wo CC, Milzman DP, Pasquale MD, Baga L, et al. Multicenter study of noninvasive monitoring systems as alternatives to invasive monitoring of acutely ill emergency patients. Chest. 1998;114:1643–52.
12. Nicholls TP, Shoemaker WC, Wo CC, Gruen JP, Amar A, Dang AB. Survival, hemodynamics, and tissue oxygenation after head trauma. J Am Coll Surg. 2006;202:120–30.
13. Brown CV, Shoemaker WC, Wo CC, Chan L, Demetriades D. Is noninvasive hemodynamic monitoring appropriate for the elderly critically injured patient? J Trauma. 2005;58:102–7.
14. Keren H, Burkhoff D, Squara P. Evaluation of a noninvasive continuous cardiac output monitoring system based on thoracic bioreactance. Am J Physiol Heart Circ Physiol. 2007;293:H583–9.
15. Bishop MH, Shoemaker WC, Shuleshko J, Wo CC. Noninvasive cardiac index monitoring in gunshot wound victims. Acad Emerg Med. 1996;3:682–8.
16. Pugsley J, Lerner AB. Cardiac output monitoring: is there a gold standard and how do the newer technologies compare? Semin Cardiothorac Vasc Anesth. 2010;14:274–82.
17. Critchley LA, Critchley JA. A meta-analysis of studies using bias and precision statistics to compare cardiac output measurement techniques. J Clin Monit Comput. 1999;15:85 91.
18. Martin M, Brown C, Bayard D, Demetriades D, Salim A, Gertz R, et al. Continuous noninvasive monitoring of cardiac performance and tissue perfusion in pediatric trauma patients. J Pediatr Surg. 2005;40:1957–63.

25

Non-iatrogenic esophageal injury: a retrospective analysis from the National Trauma Data Bank

Alberto Aiolfi[1]* (iD), Kenji Inaba[2], Gustavo Recinos[2], Desmond Khor[2], Elizabeth R. Benjamin[2], Lydia Lam[2], Aaron Strumwasser[2], Emanuele Asti[1], Luigi Bonavina[1] and Demetrios Demetriades[2]

Abstract

Background: Traumatic, non-iatrogenic esophageal injuries, despite their rarity, are associated with significant morbidity and mortality. The optimal management of these esophageal perforations remains largely debated. To date, only a few small case series are available with contrasting results. The purpose of this study was to examine a large contemporary experience with traumatic esophageal injury management and to analyze risk factors associated with mortality.

Methods: This National Trauma Data Bank (NTDB) database study included patients with non-iatrogenic esophageal injuries. Variables abstracted were demographics, comorbidities, mechanism of injury, Abbreviated Injury Scale (AIS), esophageal Organ Injury Scale (OIS), Injury Severity Score (ISS), level of injury, vital signs, and treatment. Multivariate analysis was used to identify independent predictors for mortality and overall complications.

Results: A total of 944 patients with non-iatrogenic esophageal injury were included in the final analysis. The cervical segment of the esophagus was injured in 331 (35%) patients. The unadjusted 24-h mortality (8.2 vs. 14%, $p = 0.008$), 30-day mortality (4.2 vs. 9.3%, $p = 0.005$), and overall mortality (7.9 vs. 13.5%, $p = 0.009$) were significantly lower in the group of patients with a cervical injury. The overall complication rate was also lower in the cervical group (19.8 vs. 27.1%, $p = 0.024$). Multilogistic regression analysis identified age >50, thoracic injury, high-grade esophageal injury (OIS IV–V), hypotension on admission, and GCS <9 as independent risk factors associated with increased mortality. Treatment within the first 24 h was found to be protective (OR 0.284; 95% CI, 0.148–0.546; $p < 0.001$). Injury to the thoracic esophagus was also an independent risk factor for overall complications (OR 1.637; 95% CI, 1.06–2.53; $p = 0.026$).

Conclusions: Despite improvements in surgical technique and critical care support, the overall mortality for traumatic esophageal injury remains high. The presence of a thoracic esophageal injury and extensive esophageal damage are the major independent risk factors for mortality. Early surgical treatment, within the first 24 h of admission, is associated with improved survival.

Keywords: Esophageal trauma, Non-iatrogenic esophageal injury, Primary suture, Outcomes

* Correspondence: alberto.aiolfi86@gmail.com
[1]Department of Biomedical Sciences for Health, University of Milan, IRCCS Policlinico San Donato, Piazza Edmondo Malan, 1, 20097 Milan, Italy
Full list of author information is available at the end of the article

Background

The management of iatrogenic and spontaneous perforations of the esophagus has well-established risk factors and treatment guidelines. In this setting, thoracic perforations are associated with poor outcomes because of the association with systemic sepsis and multi-organ failure [1–5]. In contrast, small and well-contained cervical perforations are associated with better outcomes [6]. Prompt diagnosis and early treatment have been shown to improve outcomes [7–9].

Despite its rarity, traumatic esophageal injury is associated with a significant morbidity and mortality burden. To date, only a few small series are available in the literature addressing management and outcomes with contrasting results. As a result, our current understanding of the optimal treatment for these injuries is unclear.

The purpose of this study was to examine a large contemporary experience with traumatic esophageal injury management, to compare cervical and thoracic injury, and to analyze risk factors associated with mortality.

Methods

After Institutional Review Board approval, the National Trauma Data Bank (NTDB) was queried to identify all patients 16 years and older who sustained a traumatic esophageal injury (ICD-9 codes 862.22 and 862.32) over a 7-year period (2007–2014). Patients transferred from an outside hospital and those who died upon arrival were excluded from the study. Spontaneous (Boerhaave syndrome) and iatrogenic esophageal perforations that occurred during upper gastrointestinal endoscopy were also excluded from the final analysis.

Variables extracted from the NTDB included demographics, comorbidities, mechanism of injury, Abbreviated Injury Scale (AIS), Injury Severity Score (ISS), Organ Injury Scale (OIS), and vital signs in the emergency department. The location of the esophageal injury (cervical vs. thoracic), treatment modalities (primary repair vs. esophagectomy vs. esophagostomy), and timing of surgical treatment were abstracted. Outcomes of interest included in-hospital mortality, complications, ventilation days, ICU length of stay, and hospital length of stay.

The study population was further subdivided and analyzed by the level of esophageal injury: cervical or thoracic. Severe injury was defined as AIS 3 or higher in any body region. Early surgical treatment was defined as operative intervention performed in the first 24 h. Isolated esophageal injury was defined as an esophageal injury with no other associated injuries with an AIS ≥3.

Statistical analysis

Categorical variables were reported as percentages, while continuous variables were reported as medians with interquartile range (IQR). Continuous variables were also dichotomized using clinically relevant cut-off points. Univariate analysis was performed to identify differences between outcomes in groups of interest. The Mann-Whitney U test was used to compare continuous variables while Fisher's exact or Pearson's chi-squared test was used to compare proportions for categorical variables. Variables with $p < 0.2$ in univariate analysis were included into a forward stepwise logistic regression to identify independent predictors for mortality and the development of complications. Multicollinearity testing was performed to identify the correlation between variables. The accuracy of the test is calculated using the area under the curve with a 95% confidence interval. Variables with a p value <0.05 were considered significant. All statistical analysis was performed using SPSS for Windows version 23.0 (SPSS Inc. Chicago, IL).

Results

During the study period, a total of 1603 patients were identified from the NTDB as having a traumatic esophageal injury, with an overall prevalence of 0.02% (1603/ 5,774,836). Due to an unspecified description of the esophageal injury, 659 patients (41.1%) were excluded from the final analysis leaving a final study population of 944 patients (Fig. 1).

Demographics

Patients with an esophageal injury were more likely to be males (77.6%), with a median age of 35 years (IQR 24–52) and 27.4% were over 50 years of age. On admission, 9.4% of the cases were identified as being hypotensive (systolic blood pressure <90 mmHg), with a median heart rate of 97 (IQR 80–112), and a Glasgow Coma Scale (GCS) <9 was seen in 23.1% of cases.

Mechanism of injury

Approximately half of the esophageal injuries were due to a penetrating injury mechanism (50.6%). Gunshot wounds, seen in 337 (35.7%) of patients, were the most common mechanism of injury for patients with a penetrating injury, followed by stab wounds in 14.9%. For patients sustaining blunt injuries, motor vehicle crash (MVC) was the most common mechanism of injury seen in 179 (19%) patients, followed by falls in 7.7%, and assault in 4.1% (Table 1).

Injury description

Patients presenting to the emergency department with an esophageal injury had a median ISS of 24 (IQR 16–33), with 80.6% having an ISS >15. Associated severe head, chest, and abdominal injuries were documented in 28.6, 91.1, and 17.1% of patients, respectively.

Injury to the thoracic esophagus occurred in 64.9% of patients, and the remaining 35.1% had a cervical

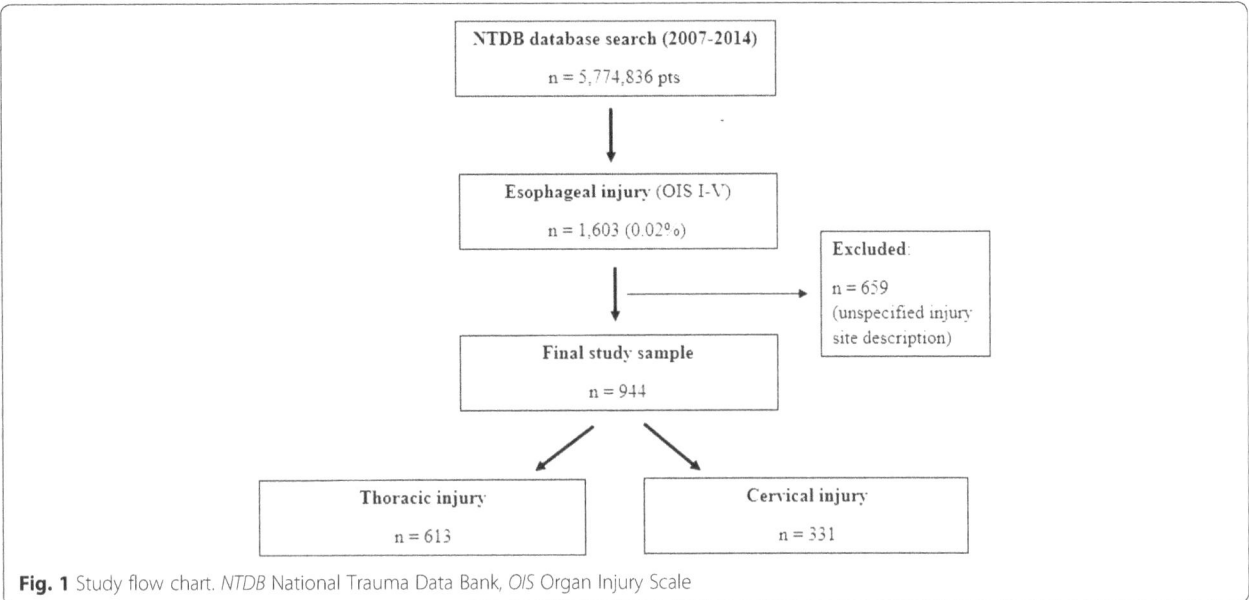

Fig. 1 Study flow chart. *NTDB* National Trauma Data Bank, *OIS* Organ Injury Scale

esophageal injury. Patients with a cervical injury were also more likely to have an associated tracheal injury requiring surgical repair and needing tracheostomy (17.5 vs. 7.3%, *p* < 0.001 and 26 vs. 18.4%, *p* = 0.007, respectively). High-grade injury with full-thickness perforation occurred in 56.5% of patients (OIS III: *n* = 466, 49.4%; OIS IV/V: *n* = 68, 7.2%); low-grade esophageal injury occurred in 43.4% of patients (OIS I/II: *n* = 410). Overall, 218 patients (23.1%) had an isolated esophageal injury, and half of these had a low-grade injury (OIS I/II: *n* = 120, 55%).

Cervical esophageal injuries were more likely to occur following a penetrating mechanism (60.4 vs. 45.4%, *p* < 0.001) (Table 1). Compared to thoracic injuries, cervical injuries were less frequent after MVC (13.9 vs. 21.7%, *p* = 0.004) and less likely to have associated severe abdominal trauma (8.8 vs. 21.5%, *p* < 0.001). No difference in the median ISS, systolic blood pressure, GCS, and ISS >15 were noted in the two study groups (Table 1).

Outcomes

Overall, 345 (36.5%) patients went to the operating room for exploration and 275 (79.7%) had a surgical intervention within the first 24 h of admission. Primary suture repair was performed in 317 (91.9%) patients. Patients with a cervical injury were more likely to undergo a primary repair (37.8 vs. 31.3%, *p* = 0.045). A drainage procedure was performed in 160 (16.9%) patients, and an esophageal stent was placed in 11 (1.2%) patients (Table 2). In the remaining 425 (45%) patients, the treatment was either non-operative or unspecified. Esophageal resection and diversion were more likely to be performed in patients with a grade III, IV, and V esophageal injury (Table 3).

The overall mortality was significantly higher in patients who sustained a blunt esophageal injury compared to patients with a penetrating injury (18.8 vs. 9.8%, *p* < 0.001). Thoracic esophageal injury was associated with significantly higher overall (14 vs. 8.2%, *p* = 0.008), 24-h (9.3 vs. 4.2%, *p* = 0.005), and 30-day mortality (13.5 vs. 7.9%, *p* = 0.009). No significant differences were noted in terms of hospital length of stay, ICU length of stay, and ventilation days. Pneumonia was the most commonly reported complication with a trend toward a higher incidence in the thoracic group (9.5 vs. 5.8%, *p* = 0.072). Sepsis and pulmonary embolism were higher in patients who sustained a thoracic injury (4.8 vs. 1.1%, *p* = 0.006 and 2.5 vs. 0%, *p* = 0.008, respectively), and the overall complication rate was higher in the thoracic esophageal group (27.1 vs. 19.8%, *p* = 0.024) (Table 4).

Forward stepwise logistic regression analysis identified thoracic injury, age >50 years old, high-grade esophageal rupture (OIS IV–V), hypotension on admission, GCS <9, and severe head injury (AIS ≥3) as independent factors associated with increased mortality (Table 5). Treatment within the first 24 h was found to be a protective factor for mortality (OR 0.284; 95% CI, 0.148–0.546; *p* < 0.001) (Table 5). Injury to the thoracic esophagus with open perforation into the mediastinum was found to be an independent risk factor associated with an increased overall complication rate (OR 1.637; 95% CI, 1.06–2.53; *p* = 0.026).

Discussion

The purpose of this study was to examine a large contemporary experience with traumatic esophageal injury, specifically with regard to the management, outcomes, and risk factors for mortality. Injury to the thoracic

Table 1 Demographics and clinical data according to the location of the esophageal injury

	Total (n = 944)	Thoracic (n = 613)	Cervical (n = 331)	p
Demographics				
Age (years), median (IQR)	35 (24–52)	35 (24–53)	36 (25–49)	0.885
Age >50 year	259 (27.4)	180 (29.4)	79 (23.9)	0.071
Gender, male	731 (77.6)	469 (76.8)	262 (79.2)	0.4
Race/ethnicity				
White	534 (56.6)	342 (55.8)	192 (58)	0.512
Black	240 (25.4)	148 (24.1)	92 (27.8)	0.219
Mechanism				<0.001
Blunt	335 (35.5)	241 (39.3)	94 (28.4)	
Penetrating	478 (50.6)	278 (45.4)	200 (60.4)	
GSW	337 (35.7)	210 (34.3)	127 (38.4)	0.208
SW	141 (14.9)	68 (11.1)	73 (22.1)	<0.001
MVC	179 (19)	133 (21.7)	46 (13.9)	0.004
AVP	12 (1.3)	10 (1.6)	2 (0.6)	0.179
Fall	73 (7.7)	51 (8.3)	22 (6.6)	0.358
MCC	26 (2.8)	18 (2.9)	8 (2.4)	0.642
Assault	39 (4.1)	26 (4.2)	13 (3.9)	0.817
Comorbidities				
Current smoker	141 (14.9)	72 (11.7)	69 (20.8)	<0.001
Chronic renal failure	4 (0.4)	2 (0.3)	2 (0.6)	0.53
Diabetes mellitus	51 (5.4)	34 (5.5)	17 (5.1)	0.79
Myocardial infarction	6 (0.6)	6 (1)	0 (0)	0.096
Hypertension	149 (15.8)	96 (15.7)	53 (16)	0.888
Obesity	48 (5.1)	25 (4.1)	23 (6.9)	0.055
Respiratory disease	62 (6.6)	32 (5.2)	30 (9.1)	0.023
Cirrhosis	2 (0.2)	2 (0.3)	0 (0)	0.544
ED vitals				
SBP <90 mmHg	89 (9.4)	63 (10.3)	26 (7.9)	0.224
HR (bpm), median (IQR)	97 (80–112)	97 (80–114)	96 (80–109)	0.258
GCS score <9	218 (23.1)	139 (22.7)	79 (23.9)	0.678
Injury description				
ISS, median (IQR)	24 (16–33)	24 (16–34)	21 (16–29)	0.181
ISS >15	761 (80.6)	495 (80.8)	266 (80.4)	0.886
Associated injuries (AIS ≥3)				
Head	270 (28.6)	167 (27.2)	103 (31.1)	0.209
Chest	860 (91.1)	559 (91.2)	301 (90.9)	0.896
Abdomen	161 (17.1)	132 (21.5)	29 (8.8)	<0.001
Extremities	119 (12.6)	86 (14)	33 (10)	0.073
Isolated esophageal injury	218 (23.1)	133 (21.7)	85 (25.7)	0.166
Esophageal OIS				0.103
OIS I–II	410 (43.4)	280 (45.7)	130 (39.3)	
OIS III	466 (49.4)	287 (46.8)	179 (54.1)	
OIS IV–V	68 (7.2)	46 (7.5)	22 (6.6)	

Table 1 Demographics and clinical data according to the location of the esophageal injury *(Continued)*

Procedures			
Tracheostomy	199 (21.1)	113 (18.4)	86 (26)	0.007
Trachea repair	103 (10.9)	45 (7.3)	58 (17.5)	<0.001
Surgical treatment	345 (36.5)	208 (33.9)	137 (41.4)	0.023
Early treatment (≤24 h)	275 (29.1)	163 (26.6)	112 (33.8)	0.019

Values are presented as median (IQR) and *n* (%)
GSW gunshot wound, *SW* stab wound, *MVC* motor vehicle collision, *AVP* auto versus pedestrian, *MCC* motorcycle collision, *SBP* systolic blood pressure, *HR* heart rate, *GCS* Glasgow Coma Scale, *ISS* Injury Severity Score, *AIS* Abbreviated Injury Scale, *OIS* Organ Injury Scale, *IQR* interquartile range

segment of the esophagus was found to be a major risk factor for mortality. Early treatment, within 24 h from admission, was independently associated with improved survival.

Traumatic esophageal injury is rare and associated with high morbidity and mortality. While previous studies have tried to describe outcomes, management, and risk factors for mortality, the limited sample size remained a major weakness.

In our study of more than 900 cases, the overall mortality rate was 12%. This is slightly lower compared to a 2001 retrospective multicenter study that analyzed patients with a penetrating esophageal injury (19%) [9]. This finding likely reflects recent improvements in the treatment and critical care management of such patients. In accordance with a retrospective 2013 database study of 227 patients who sustained a penetrating esophageal injury, the majority of deaths (62.8%) occurred in the first 24 h of admission due to the severity of associated injuries [10]. In our study, the mortality rate for cervical injuries was significantly lower than thoracic injuries. This result is in keeping with the current data showing that cervical injuries are associated with lower mortality [11]. This may be due to the protected anatomical location of the cervical esophagus which limits lateral bacterial spillage avoiding downward mediastinal contamination [12]. In contrast, injury to the thoracic segment of the esophagus is often associated with extensive, non-contained bacterial spillage with mediastinitis, pleural effusion, empyema, systemic sepsis, and multi-organ failure [13]. Moreover, the negative intrathoracic pressure can exacerbate the bacterial spillage from the esophageal lumen into the thoracic cavity [14].

Primary repair was the most commonly adopted surgical approach. Debridement of necrotic tissue, complete exposure of the mucosal layer, and a tension-free repair is recommended whenever feasible. Massive destructive injuries may require a more aggressive approach using esophageal resection or diversion [11]. In our study, the more invasive surgical procedures were performed for extensive esophageal injury. An early surgical procedure was performed in 79.7% of patients who underwent an operation. It has been previously advocated that early treatment is associated with improved outcomes because of limited bacterial spillage and less systemic inflammatory response. Brinster et al. in a 2004 literature review on 559 patients with esophageal perforation found that a treatment delay greater than 24 h can result in a doubled risk of mortality [7]. Similarly, Asensio et al., in a retrospective multicenter study, found that a treatment delay of greater than 13 h was associated with a significant increase in the overall complication rate and worse outcomes [9]. Discordant results were reported in a small retrospective single center study of 119 patients who sustained an iatrogenic or spontaneous perforation, with no difference in terms of mortality when comparing early and late treatment [15].

Non-operative management has been advocated for selected patients in the setting of iatrogenic and spontaneous esophageal perforation [16]. Markar et al. in a large 12-year retrospective multicenter study of 2564 patients demonstrated a significant reduction in the

Table 2 Different operative strategies according to the location of the esophageal injury

	Thoracic (*n* = 613)	Cervical (*n* = 331)	*p*
Primary suture (*n* = 317)	192 (31.3)	125 (37.8)	0.045
Esophagectomy (*n* = 15)	8 (1.3)	7 (2.1)	0.342
Esophageal diversion/esophagostomy (*n* = 13)	6 (1)	7 (2.1)	0.24
Esophageal stent (*n* = 11)	7 (1.1)	4 (1.2)	1
Perivisceral drainage (*n* = 160)	115 (18.8)	45 (13.6)	0.044

Values are presented as *n* (%)

Table 3 Different operative strategies according to the esophageal Organ Injury Scale (OIS)

	OIS I–II (*n* = 410)	OIS III (*n* = 466)	OIS IV–V (*n* = 68)	*p*
Primary suture (*n* = 317)	71 (17.3)	220 (47.2)	26 (38.2)	<0.001
Esophagectomy (*n* = 15)	0 (0)	13 (2.8)	2 (2.9)	0.003
Esophageal diversion/ esophagostomy (*n* = 13)	0 (0)	9 (1.9)	4 (5.9)	<0.001
Esophageal stent (*n* = 11)	2 (0.5%)	9 (1.9%)	0 (0)	0.116
Perivisceral drainage (*n* = 160)	77 (18.8)	70 (15)	13 (19.1)	0.296

Values are presented as *n* (%)

Table 4 Outcome comparison between patients with a thoracic and cervical esophageal injury

	Total		Thoracic		Cervical		p
	(n = 944)		(n = 613)		(n = 331)		
Mortality	113	(12.0)	86	(14.0)	27	(8.2)	0.008
1-day mortality	71	(7.5)	57	(9.3)	14	(4.2)	0.005
30-day mortality	109	(11.5)	83	(13.5)	26	(7.9)	0.009
Mechanical ventilation (days)[a], median (IQR)	5	(2–14)	6	(2–15)	4	(2–11)	0.124
ICU stay (days)[a], median (IQR)	7	(3–15)	7	(3–16)	6	(3–13)	0.157
Hospital length of stay (days)[a], median (IQR)	12	(5–23)	13	(5–25)	11	(5–22)	0.131
Complications[b]							
Acute kidney injury	19	(2.5)	12	(2.5)	7	(2.5)	0.998
ARDS	43	(5.7)	31	(6.5)	12	(4.3)	0.21
Deep SSI	19	(2.5)	14	(2.9)	5	(1.8)	0.334
Pneumonia	61	(8.1)	45	(9.5)	16	(5.8)	0.072
DVT	27	(3.6)	20	(4.2)	7	(2.5)	0.23
Sepsis	26	(3.4)	23	(4.8)	3	(1.1)	0.006
PE	12	(1.6)	12	(2.5)	0	(0.0)	0.008
Cardiac arrest	16	(2.1)	10	(2.1)	6	(2.2)	0.958
Organ/space SSI	17	(2.3)	12	(2.5)	5	(1.8)	0.519
Stroke/CVA	8	(1.1)	6	(1.3)	2	(0.7)	0.717
Superficial SSI	20	(2.7)	15	(3.2)	5	(1.8)	0.265
UTI	25	(3.3)	16	(3.4)	9	(3.2)	0.927
Catheter related Blood infection	3	(0.4)	2	(0.4)	1	(0.4)	1
Overall complication	184	(24.4)	129	(27.1)	55	(19.8)	0.024
Overall infectious complication	127	(16.8)	88	(18.5)	39	(14.0)	0.115

Values are presented as median (IQR) and n (%)

ICU intensive care unit, *ARDS* acute respiratory distress syndrome, *SSI* surgical site infection, *DVT* deep vein thrombosis, *PE* pulmonary embolism, *CVA* cerebrovascular accident, *UTI* urinary tract infection, *IQR* interquartile range

[a]Include only patients without mortality (n = 831)

[b]Include only patients with hospital length of stay >2 days (n = 754)

Table 5 Independent risk factors for mortality

	Mortality			
	Adjusted p	OR	95% CI for OR	
Age >50 year	0.032	1.686	(1.045 –	2.723)
OIS I-II	Reference	Reference		
OIS III	0.578	1.151	(0.701 –	1.888)
OIS IV-V	0.03	2.256	(1.081 –	4.709)
Severe head injury (AIS ≥3)	<0.001	2.839	(1.794 –	4.493)
Thoracic injury	0.028	1.757	(1.062 –	2.907)
GCS score <9	<0.001	3.553	(2.247 –	5.618)
Hypotension	<0.001	6.087	(3.475 –	10.659)
Early treatment (≤24h)	<0.001	0.284	(0.148 –	0.546)

Logistic regression was performed with potentially causative variables (in gray) in which p value was <0.2 in univariate analysis. Multicollinearity test was checked before doing multivariate analysis

Hosmer-Lemeshow Goodness-of-Fit Test p=0.326, Cox & Snell R2=0.153, Nagelkerke R2=0.294

AUC=0.829 (95% CI=0.786-0.871, p<0.001)

OR Odds Ratio, *CI* Confidence Interval

overall number of surgical procedures with a concomitant increase in non-operative management [17]. Minimally invasive endoscopic stenting or clipping for iatrogenic perforation has also been proposed for small discontinuities with viable, non-necrotic edges [18, 19]. These strategies may be useful in selected, hemodynamically stable trauma patients with a contained leak [20].

Because of the rarity of traumatic esophageal injury, limited data is available. For this reason, we chose to use the NTDB databank to collect a large study population, reducing the risk of a type II error. Exclusion of iatrogenic and spontaneous perforation makes our study population homogeneous, focusing only on traumatic esophageal injury. The major weaknesses of our study are related to its retrospective nature and to the fact that treatment delay of the esophageal injury may have been due to prioritizing treatment of other life-threatening injuries. We were not able to analyze the patient status in detail, and the elapsed time from the onset of symptoms to treatment was also unavailable in this administrative database. Moreover, the lack of specific details regarding the surgical procedure was a limitation.

Conclusions

Despite improvements in surgical technique and critical care support, the overall mortality for traumatic esophageal injury remains high. The presence of a thoracic injury and extensive esophageal damage are the major independent risk factors for mortality. Early surgical treatment is associated with improved survival.

Acknowledgements
None.

Funding
None.

Authors' contributions
AA and EA did the literature search. AA, KI, and LB formed the study design. The data collection was done by AA. AA, GR, and DK analyzed the data. AA, KI, GR, and DD interpreted the data. AA, KI, and LB wrote the manuscript. KI, EB, LL, AS, LB, and DD critically reviewed the manuscript. All authors read and approved the final manuscript.

Competing interests
The authors declare that they have no competing interests.

Author details
[1]Department of Biomedical Sciences for Health, University of Milan, IRCCS Policlinico San Donato, Piazza Edmondo Malan, 1, 20097 Milan, Italy. [2]Division of Trauma and Surgical Critical Care, LAC+USC Medical Center, University of Southern California, 2051 Marengo Street, Los Angeles, CA 90033, USA.

References
1. Makhani M, Midani D, Goldberg A, Friedenberg FK. Pathogenesis and outcomes of traumatic injuries of the esophagus. Dis Esophagus. 2014;27:630–6.
2. Griffiths EA, Yap N, Poulter J, Hendrickse MT, Khurshid M. Thirty-four cases of esophageal perforation: the experience of a district general hospital in the UK. Dis Esophagus. 2009;22:616–25.
3. Vogel SB, Rout WR, Martin TD, Abbitt PL. Esophageal perforation in adults: aggressive, conservative treatment lowers morbidity and mortality. Ann Surg. 2005;241:1016–21.
4. Onat S, Ulku R, Cigdem KM, Avci A, Ozcelik C. Factors affecting the outcome of surgically treated non-iatrogenic traumatic cervical esophageal perforation: 28-years' experience at a single center. J Cardiothorac Surg. 2010;5:46.
5. Attar S, Hankins JR, Suter CM, Coughlin TR, Sequeira A, McLaughlin JS. Esophageal perforation: a therapeutic challenge. Ann Thorac Surg. 1990;50:45–9.
6. Jones II WG, Ginsberg RJ. Esophageal perforation: a continuing challenge. Ann Thorac Surg. 1992;53:534–43.
7. Brinster CJ, Singhal S, Lee L, Marshall MB, Kaiser LR, Kucharczuk JC. Evolving options in the management of esophageal perforation. Ann Thorac Surg. 2004;77:1475–83.
8. Rubesin SE, Levine MS. Radiological diagnosis of gastrointestinal perforation. Radiol Clin North Am. 2003;41:1095–115.
9. Asensio JA, Chahwan S, Forno W, MacKersie R, Wall M, Lake J, et al. Penetrating esophageal injuries: multicenter study of the American Association for the Surgery of Trauma. J Trauma. 2001;50:289–96.
10. Patel MS, Malinoski DJ, Zhou L, Neal ML, Hoyt DB. Penetrating oesophageal injury: a contemporary analysis of the National Trauma Data Bank. Injury. 2013;44:48–55.
11. Biffl WL, Moore EE, Feliciano DV, Albrecht RA, Croce M, Karmy-Jones R, et al. Western Trauma Association critical decisions in trauma: diagnosis and management of esophageal injuries. J Trauma Acute Care Surg. 2015;79:1089–95.
12. Barrett N, Allison PR, Johnstone AS, Bonham-Carter RE. Discussion on unusual aspects of esophageal disease. Proc R Soc Med. 1956;49:529.
13. Muir AD, White J, McGuigan JA, McManus KG, Graham AN. Treatment and outcomes of oesophageal perforation in a tertiary referral centre. Eur J Cardiothorac Surg. 2003;23:799–804.
14. Parsons S, Black E. Traumatic injury to the oesophagus. Surgery: Oesophagus and Stomach. 2006;24:101–4.
15. Bhatia P, Fortin D, Inculet RI, Malthaner RA. Current concepts in the management of esophageal perforations: a twenty-seven year Canadian experience. Ann Thorac Surg. 2011;92:209–15.
16. Ivatury RR, Moore FA, Biffl W, Leppeniemi A, Ansaloni L, Catena F, et al. Oesophageal injuries: position paper, WSES, 2013. World J Emerg Surg. 2014;9(1):9.
17. Markar SR, Mackenzie H, Wiggins T, Askari A, Faiz O, Zaninotto G, et al. Management and outcomes of esophageal perforation: a national study of 2,564 patients in England. Am J Gastroenterol. 2015;110:1559–66.
18. Dasari BV, Neely D, Kennedy A, Spence G, Rice P, Mackle E, et al. The role of esophageal stents in the management of esophageal anastomotic leaks and benign esophageal perforations. Ann Surg. 2014;259:852–60.
19. Biancari F, Saarnio J, Mennander A, Hypén L, Salminen P, Kuttila K, et al. Outcome of patients with esophageal perforations: a multicenter study. World J Surg. 2014;38:902–9.
20. Sudarshan M, Elharram M, Spicer J, Mulder D, Ferri LE. Management of esophageal perforation in the endoscopic era: is operative repair still relevant? Surgery. 2016;160:1104–10.

26

Retrospective study of the effectiveness of Intra-Aortic Balloon Occlusion (IABO) for traumatic haemorrhagic shock

Takayuki Irahara[1], Norio Sato[2*], Yuuta Moroe[3], Reo Fukuda[3], Yusuke Iwai[3] and Kyoko Unemoto[3]

Abstract

Introduction: Intra-aortic balloon occlusion (IABO) is useful for proximal vascular control, by clamping the descending aorta, in traumatic haemorrhagic shock. However, there are limited clinical studies regarding its effectiveness. This study aimed at investigating the effectiveness of IABO for traumatic haemorrhagic shock.

Methods: This retrospective, observational study included trauma patients who underwent IABO at the Emergency and Critical Care Center of Nippon Medical School Tama-Nagayama Hospital between January 2009 and March 2013. 14 patients were included to this study who were in shock on arrival (systolic blood pressure [SBP] <90 mmHg or shock index ≥1), underwent IABO for resuscitation and temporary haemostasis, and subsequently underwent haemostatic intervention (operation or transcatheter arterial embolization). Patient characteristics, physiological status, SBP, heart rate (HR), initial fluid and blood transfusion, time course, and total occlusion time were compared before and after IABO as well as between the survived (n = 5) and non-survived (n = 9) groups.

Results: The majority of patients experienced blunt injuries, with an average injury severity score of 29.5. The liver, pelvis, spleen, and mesenterium represented the majority of injured organs. SBP, but not HR, was significantly higher after IABO than before IABO (123.1 vs. 65.5 mmHg, P = 0.0001). The revised trauma score and probability of survival were significantly different between the survived and non-survived groups (both, P = 0.04). The survived group required significantly less blood transfusion volume than the non-survived group (20 vs. 33.7 red blood cell units, P = 0.04). In addition, the survived group required a significantly shorter total occlusion time than the non-survived group (46.2 vs. 224.1 min, P = 0.002).

Conclusions: IABO was used for relatively severe trauma patients. SBP was significantly higher after IABO, but was not related to survival. However, blood transfusion volume and total occlusion time were related to survival; therefore, it is important to reduce or shorten these parameters, i.e., immediate definitive haemostasis. IABO is effective for traumatic haemorrhagic shock; however, it is also important to consider these points and potential complications.

Keywords: Trauma, Haemorrhagic shock, Proximal vascular control, Intra-aortic balloon occlusion (IABO)

Introduction

It has been reported that an emergent laparotomy in injured hypotensive patients with massive hemoperitoneum frequently results in cardiac arrest as the abdominal wall tamponade is released. Occlusion of the descending aorta before laparotomy is reportedly necessary for proximal vascular control [1,2] and can temporarily decrease intra-abdominal bleeding and maintain blood flow to the brain and heart.

Although left thoracotomy with direct clamping of the descending aorta is considered the primary method, it is very invasive, with reported complications such as anterior spinal artery injury or persistent bleeding from intercostal arteries after recovery from shock. In comparison, occlusion of the descending aorta by intra-aortic balloon occlusion (IABO) is less invasive, and the inflation volume and duration can be controlled in response to vital signs. As a result, the latter method is increasingly being used.

* Correspondence: drnori@kuhp.kyoto-u.ac.jp
[2]Department of Primary Care and Emergency Medicine, Kyoto University, Kyoto, Japan

IABO, which was developed by Edwards et al. in 1953 [3], was initially intended for surgical treatment of abdominal aortic aneurysms and was later applied to traumatic haemorrhagic shock. It is reportedly effective not only for blunt abdominal injuries but also for retro-peritoneal haemorrhage from a pelvic fracture [4], penetrating abdominal trauma [5], and non-traumatic cases such as post-partum haemorrhage [6]. Stannard et al. described the following IABO steps: (1) arterial access, (2) balloon selection and positioning, (3) balloon inflation, (4) balloon deflation, and (5) sheath removal [7].

The opportunities for IABO use are increasing; however, there have been only a few case reports [6,8] or experimental studies of animal models (e.g., porcine and dog) [9-14]. Furthermore, there are limited clinical studies regarding its effectiveness. Therefore, this study aimed to retrospectively investigate the effectiveness of IABO for traumatic haemorrhagic shock based on our clinical experiences.

Materials and methods

Patients

This retrospective, observational study included trauma patients who underwent IABO at the Emergency and Critical Care Center of Nippon Medical School Tama-Nagayama Hospital between January 2009 and March 2013. Of all trauma patients in this period (n = 540), 21 patients underwent IABO without cardiopulmonary arrest on arrival. Furthermore, 7 patients were excluded if the IABO was inserted as a standby without inflation, inserted preventively for non-shock patients and inflated during haemostatic intervention. The remaining 14 patients were included to this study who were in shock on arrival (systolic blood pressure <90 mmHg or shock index ≥1), underwent IABO for resuscitation and temporary haemostasis, and subsequently achieved haemostatic intervention (operation or transcatheter arterial embolization).

Indication and procedure

General indication of IABO in our hospital is haemorrhagic shock due to any of the following: (1) intra-abdominal haemorrhage (e.g., liver or splenic injury); (2) retroperitoneal haemorrhage (e.g., renal injury or pelvic fracture); or (3) non-traumatic haemorrhage (e.g., obstetric or gastrointestinal bleeding). In this study, we analysed only trauma patients in case of (1) and/or (2).

During the procedure, generally, the emergency physician inserted the aortic occlusion balloon (Block Balloon™; Senko Medical Instrument Mfg. Co., Ltd., Tokyo, Japan) without radiographic assistance. A 10-Fr sheath was retained in the femoral artery (generally left), the balloon catheter was inserted above the bleeding point and >2 cm below the bifurcation of subclavian artery, and normal saline was injected to inflate the balloon. The procedure was performed with minimum inflation, with monitoring via blood

Table 1 Characteristics of trauma patients who underwent intra-aortic balloon occlusion

	Values for the entire sample (n = 14)
Age (years)	46.9 ± 5.2
Sex (Men:Women)	10:4
Mechanism of injury (Blunt:Stabbing)	13:1
Primary injured organ (n)	
Liver	6
Pelvis	3
Spleen	2
Mesenterium	2
Kidney	1
Femoral artery	1
ISS	29.5 ± 3.6
RTS	5.414 ± 0.308
Ps	0.62 ± 0.09
Location of insertion (n)	
Emergency room	14
Vascular approach	
Right femoral artery	7
Left femoral artery	7

The primary injured organ was defined as the main bleeding organ.
ISS, injury severity score; RTS, revised trauma score; Ps, probability of survival.
Values are mean ± SE.

pressure in the upper arm, and minimal occlusion time, achieved by incomplete or intermittent occlusion.

Data collection

Data were extracted from medical records. The 14 patients were divided into the survived group (n = 5) and non-survived group (n = 9) based on the final recorded outcome. Data regarding the patient characteristics and physiological status in each group were collected. In addition, systolic blood pressure (SBP), heart rate (HR), initial fluid and blood transfusion, time course, and total occlusion time before and after IABO were collected.

Base excess, body temperature, and prothrombin time were collected from the initial data on arrival. Initial fluid and blood transfusion represent the crystalloid volume and red blood cell (RBC) units within 24 hours of arrival, respectively. The injury severity score, revised trauma score (RTS), and probability of survival (Ps) were calculated with commonly used formulas.

Statistical analysis

Patient characteristics, physiological status, SBP, HR, initial fluid and blood transfusion, time course, and total occlusion time were compared between pre- and post-IABO as well as between the survived group (n = 5) and

Table 2 Physiological status of trauma patients who underwent IABO, based on survival

	Survived (n = 5)	Non-survived (n = 9)	P value
Age (years)	33.6 ± 4.8	54.3 ± 6.5	0.079
ISS	26.0 ± 6.3	31.4 ± 4.6	0.498
RTS	6.280 ± 0.306	4.933 ± 0.364	0.04
Ps	0.86 ± 0.06	0.48 ± 0.11	0.04
Base excess (mmol/L)	-4.9 ± 2.0	-13 ± 2.9	0.064
Body temperature (°C)	34.9 ± 0.34	35.7 ± 0.31	0.191
Prothrombin time (%)	75.1 ± 11.1	60.5 ± 10.5	0.521

ISS, injury severity score; RTS, revised trauma score; Ps, probability of survival.
Values are mean ± SE.

non-survived group (n = 9) using Wilcoxon signed rank tests and Mann-Whitney U tests, respectively. Statistical analyses were conducted using GraphPad Prism 6 (GraphPad Software, Inc., San Diego, CA), and P < 0.05 was considered significant.

Results

Patient characteristics
The mean age was 46.9 years old, 71% of the patients were men, and the majority experienced blunt injuries (Table 1).

Physiological status
Of the measures for physiological status, significant differences were only present between the survived and non-survived groups in the RTS and Ps (both, P = 0.04; Table 2).

Systolic blood pressure and heart rate
SBP was significantly higher after IABO than before IABO, in the entire sample (123.1 ± 10.5 vs. 65.5 ± 4.7 mmHg, P = 0.0001) (Figure 1A). Between the survived and non-survived groups, the change in SBP (ΔSBP) was not significantly different (65.8 ± 17.1 vs. 53.1 ± 15.6 mmHg, P = 0.517) (Figure 1B).

The HR after IABO was not significantly different from that before IABO (98.4 ± 5.7 vs. 109.9 ± 4.5 beats per minute [BPM], P = 0.051) (Figure 2A). The change in HR (ΔHR) was also not significantly different between the survived and non-survived groups (-5.8 ± 10.9 vs. -14.8 ± 6.7 BPM, P = 0.79) (Figure 2B).

Initial fluid and blood transfusion
The initial fluid transition was not significantly different between the survived and non-survived groups (2250 ± 512 vs. 2083 ± 417 mL, P = 0.595) (Figure 3A). However, the survived group required a significantly lower blood volume than the non-survived group (20.0 ± 3.4 vs. 33.7 ± 3.9 RBC units, P = 0.04) (Figure 3B).

Time course and total occlusion time
The comparisons of time course and total occlusion time are shown in Figures 4 and 5.

Between the survived and non-survived groups, there were no significant differences in time from injury to IABO insertion (107.2 ± 17.9 vs. 98.7 ± 7.2 min, P = 0.923) (Figure 4A), time from arrival to IABO insertion (68.4 ± 18.1 vs. 57.9 ± 6.9, P = 0.771) (Figure 4B), or time from IABO insertion to the start of the intervention (52.6 ± 8.2 vs. 42.8 ± 6.3, P = 0.495) (Figure 4C). However, there was a significantly shorter total occlusion time in the survived

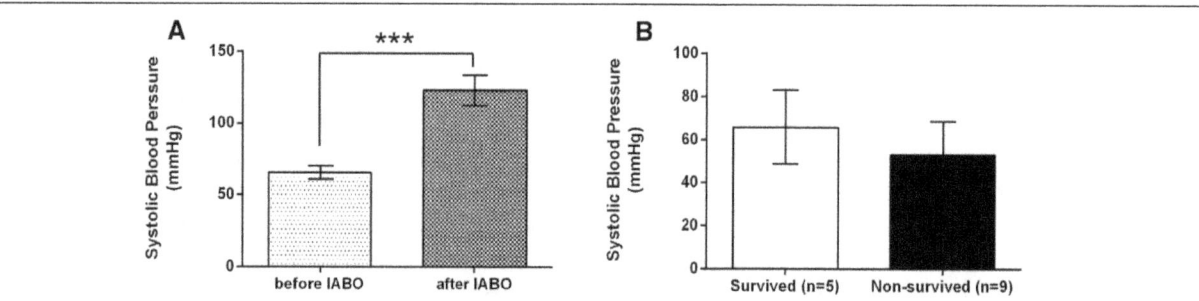

Figure 1 Comparison of systolic blood pressure (SBP) of trauma patients who underwent intra-aortic balloon occlusion (IABO). A: Comparison of SBP before and after IABO in all cases (n = 14). **B**: Comparison of the change in SBP (ΔSBP) between the survived group (n = 5) and non-survived group (n = 9). Values are reported as mean ± SE, analysed using a Wilcoxon signed rank test **(A)** or Mann-Whitney U test **(B)**. *P < 0.05, **P < 0.01, ***P < 0.001.

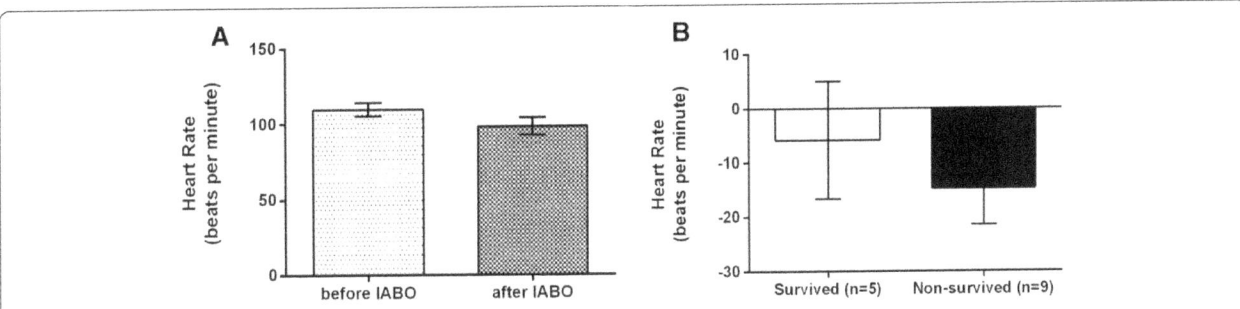

Figure 2 Comparison of heart rate (HR) of trauma patients who underwent intra-aortic balloon occlusion (IABO). A: Comparison of HR before and after IABO in all cases (n = 14). **B**: Comparison of the change in HR (ΔHR) between the survived group (n = 5) and non-survived group (n = 9). Values are reported as mean ± SE, analysed using a Wilcoxon signed rank test **(A)** or Mann-Whitney U test **(B)**.

group than in the non-survived group (46.2 ± 15.0 vs. 224.1 ± 52.1 min, P = 0.002) (Figure 5).

Discussion

This study demonstrated that IABO was used for relatively severe trauma patients, with an significant increase in SBP after IABO. Similar effects have been shown in other the majority of reports, indicating that IABO is effective for achieving hemodynamic stability. However, based on the significant differences in the blood transfusion volume within 24 hours after arrival between survived and non-survived groups, IABO might only have a temporary haemostatic effect. If definitive haemostasis is not achieved, additional blood transfusion is required, with poorer outcomes.

Therefore, survival depends on lower blood transfusion volumes, by immediate definitive haemostasis, and shorter total occlusion times, by deflating the IABO. It should be noted that poorer outcomes may result from delayed definitive haemostasis, which could occur because of a sense of comfort from the temporary improvement of haemodynamics by IABO. For example, enhanced computed tomography (CT) is often used to search for injury sites, but this could unnecessarily delay definitive haemostasis. Actually we performed enhanced

CT after IABO 1 of 5 in survived group and 4 of 9 in non-survived group. Each occlusion time was over 200 minutes in non-survived patients who performed CT. However, the situation may differ by hospital; time is required for the procedure, and IABO has to be deflated temporarily for the injection of contrast medium. As a result, there is a risk that haemodynamics could worsen. Although enhanced CT is necessary when the point of bleeding is unclear and the search for retroperitoneal haemorrhage is unavoidable, the time should be as short as possible.

Physiological status of survived or non-survived patients indicates that IABO was used for relatively more severe trauma patients. Although blood pressure was significantly higher after IABO, it does not appear to be related to survival or have an effect on shock.

Regarding the time course of IABO insertion, it does not appear to be related to survival. Therefore, IABO does not have to be inserted immediately after arrival nor does the intervention need to immediately follow IABO insertion. Instead, the total occlusion time is more important for survival outcomes, as already discussed.

Although patients who were not experiencing shock and underwent IABO for preventive reasons were excluded from this study, we experienced a case of a 46-

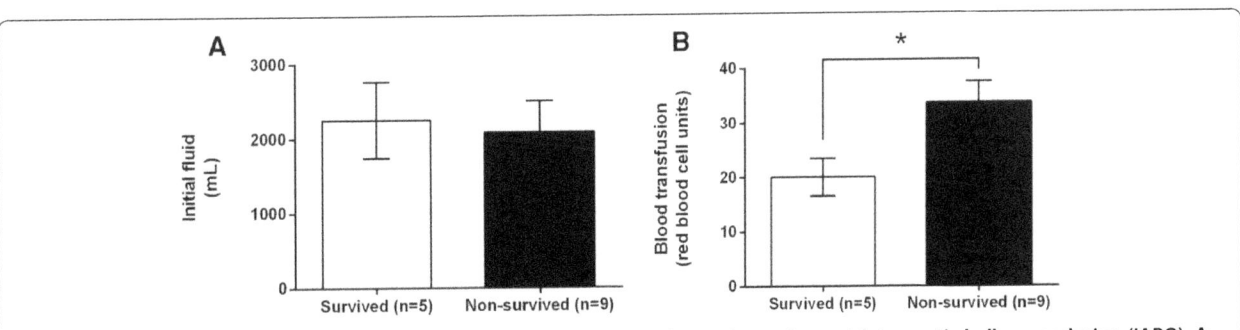

Figure 3 Comparison of initial fluid and blood transfusion in trauma patients who underwent intra-aortic balloon occlusion (IABO). A: Comparison of initial fluid (crystalloid volume within 24 hours of arrival) between the survived group (n = 5) and non-survived group (n = 9). **B**: Comparison of blood transfusion (red blood cell [RBC] units within 24 hours of arrival) requirements between the survived group (n = 5) and non-survived group (n = 9). Values are reported as mean ± SE, analysed using a Mann-Whitney U test. *P < 0.05.

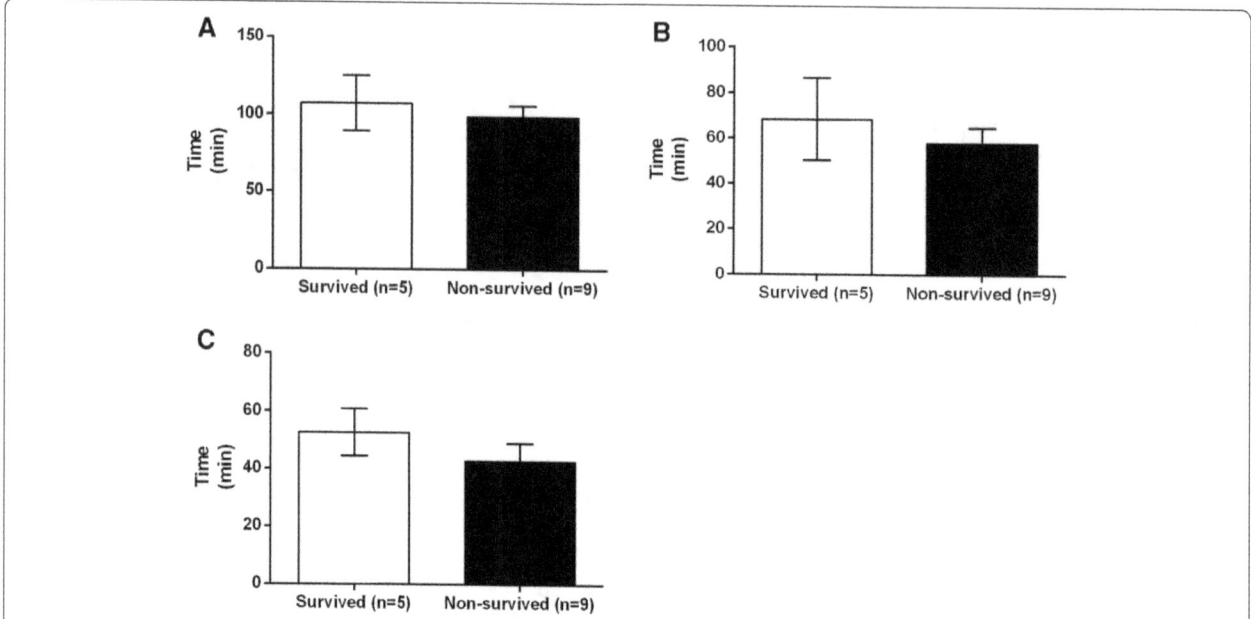

Figure 4 Comparison of the time course in trauma patients who underwent intra-aortic balloon occlusion (IABO). **A**: Comparison of time from injury to IABO insertion between the survived group (n = 5) and non-survived group (n = 9); **B**: Comparison of time from arrival to IABO insertion between the survived group (n = 5) and non-survived group (n = 9); **C**: Comparison of time from IABO insertion to intervention start between the survived group (n = 5) and non-survived group (n = 9). Values are reported as mean ± SE, analysed using a Mann-Whitney U test.

year-old man with an abdominal stab wound in which IABO was extremely effective for maintaining a good field of operation. His haemodynamics were stable, but IABO was inserted to prevent massive intraoperative bleeding. During the laparotomy, we identified that the stab wound entered the left liver lobe. When the knife was removed, arterial bleeding was observed and controlled by inflation of IABO; as a result, we could complete the liver suture with a good field of view. This effect might be significant

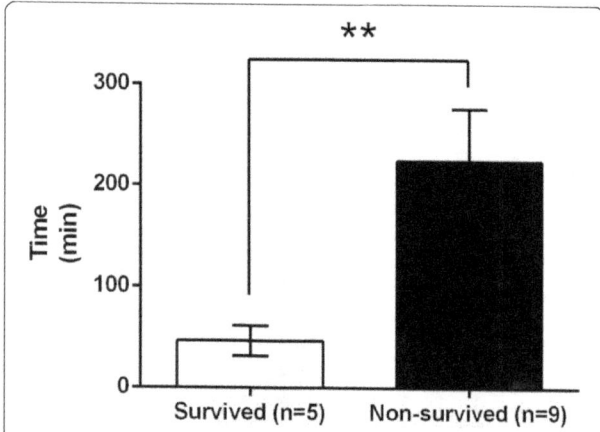

Figure 5 Comparison of total occlusion time in trauma patients who underwent intra-aortic balloon occlusion (IABO), between the survived group (n = 5) and non-survived group (n = 9). Values are reported as mean ± SE, analysed using a Mann-Whitney U test. *P < 0.05, **P < 0.01, ***P < 0.001.

for shortening the time to definitive haemostasis. Therefore, we recommend considering IABO for prevention in non-shock cases. For cases that do not present with shock immediately but may experience shock later, it may be best to detain only the sheath initially and be ready to immediately insert an IABO, when necessary.

The major complications of IABO are considered to be aortic injury, dissection, ischemia and reperfusion injury of lower part organs, and thrombosis; therefore, the contraindications include a dissecting aneurysm, significant aortic meandering or calcification, and a bleeding point located above the balloon. On the other hand, it has been reported that complications do not occur with IABO for blunt and penetrating injuries [8]. We also did not experience any aortic injury when we insert IABO blindly not use under radiography. Sovik et al reported that IABO has been used without fluoroscopy in patients with post-partum haemorrhage, and 1 of 6 patients experienced an aortic rupture necessitating surgical repair [6]. Although we also seldom use radiography, it might be helpful to prevent aortic injury. Furthermore we need carefully caution with distal organ ischemia at occlusion point. Markov et al. reported renal dysfunction and liver necrosis have been observed in a swine model at 90 minutes of IABO occlusion; however, this was not related to mortality [12]. In addition, marked splanchnic ischemia during aortic occlusion has been reported in a dog model [14]. We had only one patient with slight renal dysfunction. In this case, the total occlusion time was 37 minutes (incomplete occlusion), and the blood urea nitrogen/creatinine increased to 31.1/1.97 and was improved only by fluid infusion. Although it was not a serious complication, it was likely due to ischemia from IABO; therefore, attention should be paid to this potential complication.

However, limited data from well-organized studies are available, and empirical descriptions indicate that approximately 45 minutes is the limit. It would be helpful to have a staff to manage the balloon and try to minimize incomplete or intermittent occlusion for the maintenance of blood pressure. Moreover, the range of occlusion should be narrowed, e.g., occlusion below the bifurcation of renal arteries in case of pelvic fracture. In addition, the sheath should be as thin as possible. In Japan, a 10-Fr sheath is widely used, but a 7-Fr sheath was recently developed (RESCUE BALLOON®; Tokai Medical Products Inc., Tokyo, Japan) and used clinically.

This study has certain limitations. This study was not a randomized, controlled trial, which may have introduced bias; furthermore, the severity of the patients who survived and who were non-survived was not the same. However, as IABO tends to be used in emergency situations, it is practically difficult to perform a randomized trial. Additional multicentre studies are required to determine the effectiveness of this device.

Conclusions
Based on our results relating to the effectiveness of IABO for traumatic haemorrhagic shock, a reduction in blood transfusion volume and shorter total occlusion times (i.e., immediate definitive haemostasis) are important for survival. IABO is an effective device to treat traumatic haemorrhagic shock; however, these recommendations and awareness of potential complications are necessary for success.

Competing interests
The authors declare that they have no competing interests.

Authors' contributions
TI, YM, RF, YI, and KU participated in the treatment of patients and data collection. TI analysed the data and drafted the manuscript. NS participated in the design of the study and helped to draft the manuscript. All authors read and approved the final manuscript.

Acknowledgements
We appreciate Hiroyuki Yokota MD PhD, the professor of the Department of Emergency and Critical Care Medicine, Nippon Medical School, who generally supervised the study.
We also would like to thank the medical clerk who assisted with the data collection.

Author details
[1]Graduate School of Emergency and Critical Care Medicine, Nippon Medical School, Tokyo, Japan. [2]Department of Primary Care and Emergency Medicine, Kyoto University, Kyoto, Japan. [3]Emergency and Critical Care Center, Nippon Medical School Tama- Nagayama Hospital, Tokyo, Japan.

References
1. Ledgerwood AM. The role of thoracic aortic occlusion for massive hemoperitoneum. J Trauma-Inj Infect Crit Care. 1976;16(08):610.
2. Sankaran S, Lucas C, Walt AJ. Thoracic aortic clamping for prophylaxis against sudden cardiac arrest during laparotomy for acute massive hemoperitoneum. J Trauma. 1975;15(4):290–6.
3. Edwards WS, Salter Jr PP, Carnaggio VA. Intraluminal aortic occlusion as a possible mechanism for controlling massive intra-abdominal hemorrhage. Surg Forum. 1953;4:496–9.
4. Martinelli T, Thony F, Declety P, Sengel C, Broux C, Tonetti J, et al. Intra-aortic balloon occlusion to salvage patients with life-threatening hemorrhagic shocks from pelvic fractures. J Trauma. 2010;68(4):942–8.
5. Gupta BK, Khaneja SC, Flores L, Eastlick L, Longmore W, Shaftan GW. The role of intra-aortic balloon occlusion in penetrating abdominal trauma. J Trauma. 1989;29(6):861–5.
6. Sovik E, Stokkeland P, Storm BS, Asheim P, Bolas O. The use of aortic occlusion balloon catheter without fluoroscopy for life-threatening post-partum haemorrhage. Acta Anaesthesiol Scand. 2012;56:388–93.
7. Stannard A, Eliason JL, Rasmussen TE. Resuscitative endovascular balloon occlusion of the aorta (REBOA) as an adjunct for hemorrhagic shock. J Trauma. 2011;71(6):1869–72.
8. Brenner ML, Moore LJ, DuBose JJ, Tyson GH, McNutt MK, Albarado RP, et al. A clinical series of resuscitative endovascular balloon occlusion of the aorta for hemorrhage control and resuscitation. J Trauma Acute Care Surg. 2013;75(3):506–11.
9. White JM, Cannon JW, Stannard A, Markov NP, Spencer JR, Rasmussen TE. Endovascular balloon occlusion of the aorta is superior to resuscitative thoracotomy with aortic clamping in a porcine model of hemorrhagic shock. Surgery. 2011;150(3):400–9.
10. Morrison JJ, Percival TJ, Markov NP, Villamaria C, Scott DJ, Saches KA, et al. Aortic balloon occlusion is effective in controlling pelvic hemorrhage. J Surg Res. 2012;177(2):341–7.
11. Scott DJ, Eliason JL, Villamaria C, Morrison JJ, Houston RT, Spencer JR, et al. A novel fluoroscopy-free, resuscitative endovascular aortic balloon occlusion system in a model of hemorrhagic shock. J Trauma Acute Care Surg. 2013;75(1):122–8.
12. Markov NP, Percival TJ, Morrison JJ, Ross JD, Scott DJ, Spencer JR, et al. Physiologic tolerance of descending thoracic aortic balloon occlusion in a swine model of hemorrhagic shock. Surgery. 2013;153(6):848–56.
13. Avaro JP, Mardelle V, Roch A, Gil C, de Biasi C, Oliver M, et al. Forty-minute endovascular aortic occlusion increases survival in an experimental model of uncontrolled hemorrhagic shock caused by abdominal trauma. J Trauma. 2011;71(3):720–5. discussion 725-726.
14. Cruz Jr RJ, Poli de Figueiredo LF, Bras JL, Rocha e Silva M. Effects of intra-aortic balloon occlusion on intestinal perfusion, oxygen metabolism and gastric mucosal PCO2 during experimental hemorrhagic shock. Eur Surg Res. 2004;36(3):172–8.

27

Looking beyond discharge: clinical variables at trauma admission predict long term survival in the older severely injured patient

Miklosh Bala[1*], Jeffry L Kashuk[2], Dafna Willner[3], Dima Kaluzhni[3], Tali Bdolah-Abram[4] and Gidon Almogy[1]

Abstract

Background: Long term follow up is difficult to obtain in most trauma settings, these data are essential for assessing outcomes in the older (≥60) patient. We hypothesized that clinical data obtained during initial hospital stay could accurately predict long term survival.

Study design: Using our trauma registry and hospital database, we reviewed all trauma admissions (age ≥60, ISS > 15) to our Level 1 center over the most recent 7 years. Mechanism of injury, co-morbidities, ICU admission, and ultimate disposition were assessed for 2-7 years post-discharge. Primary outcome was defined as long term survival to the end of the last year of the study.

Results: Of 342 patients discharged following initial admission, mean age was 76.2 ± 9.7, and ISS was 21.5 ± 6.9. 119 patients (34.8%) died (mean follow up 18.8 months; range 1.1-66.2 months). For 233 survivors, mean follow-up was 50.2 months (range 24.8-83.8 months). Univariate analysis disclosed post-discharge mortality was associated with age (80.1 ± 9.64 vs. 74.2 ± 9.07), mean number of co-morbidities (1.6 ± 1.1 vs. 1.0 ± 1.2), fall as a mechanism, lower GCS upon arrival (11.85 ± 4.21 vs. 13.73 ± 2.89), intubation at the scene and discharge to an assisted living facility (p < 0.001 for all). Cox regression analysis hazard ratio showed that independent predictors of mortality on long term follow-up included: older age, fall as mechanism, lower GCS at admission and discharge to assisted living facility (all = p < 0.0001).

Conclusions: Nearly two-thirds of patients ≥60 who were severely injured survived >4 years following discharge; furthermore, admission data, including younger age, injury mechanism other than falls, higher GCS and home discharge predicted a favorable long term outcome. These findings suggest that common clinical data at initial admission can predict long term survival in the older trauma patient.

Introduction

The population of the western world is simultaneously aging and living longer. In Israel, the rate of increase of the elderly population is expected to be 2.5 times that of the general population [1]. Furthermore, as is the case in Japan, Australia, and Sweden, Israel has the highest life expectancy for males at birth in the world (79 years) [2]. Along with the prolonged life expectancy, seniors also have an improved quality of life, with increased strength and vigor, resulting in greater physical activity and mobility. Accordingly, all of these factors have resulted in a noticeable increase in the number of seniors with severe

traumatic injuries presenting to our trauma center with falls and motor vehicle crashes as the predominant mechanisms of injury [3-5].

The care and treatment of elderly trauma patients is particularly challenging to the trauma surgeon, as advanced age, extensive past medical history, and poor physiologic reserve are well-recognized risk factors for adverse outcomes following trauma [6,7]. Attempts to better characterize physiologic deficiencies in the elderly have recently been assessed via calculation of frailty indices in order to predict 6-month postoperative mortality and post-discharge institutionalization [8]. Despite increasing recognition of the unique challenges of the senior population to trauma care, little information is currently available regarding specific factors that predict morbidity and mortality in this group, including an improved

* Correspondence: rbalam@hadassah.org.il
[1]Department of Surgery and Shock Trauma Unit, Hadassah-Hebrew University Medical Center, Jerusalem, Israel

understanding of long term outcome following discharge [9,10]. Others have shown that the outcome of elderly trauma patients hospitalized in major trauma centers is better than can be predicted based on current indices and therefore, aggressive treatment may improve their chances of regaining their pre-injury status. Lastly, not only in the senior population but in all trauma patients, increasing costs of care have led to careful considerations of resource allocation and improved recognition of scenarios where care may be futile [10].

Based upon all of the above factors, our primary objective in the current study was to describe and define the long term outcome of elderly patients following severe trauma in our Israeli level 1 regional trauma center over the most recent 7 year time frame. Our secondary objective was to identify predictors of long term survival in this population.

Methods

We searched our trauma data base for all trauma patients ≥60 years of age who presented to Trauma Unit of Hadassah University Medical Center, Ein Kerem campus, Jerusalem, the regional Level I Trauma Center, with an ISS of ≥16 between January 2006 and December 2010. Discharged patients were followed after discharge either home or to institutional placement for the duration of the study time frame or until mortality. Long term follow up was recorded on survivors discharged from hospital following admission from January 2006. Exclusion criteria included patients who were pronounced dead upon arrival and patients who were transferred from other acute care hospitals.

All charts were retrospectively reviewed for demographics (age, gender, pre-existing co-morbidities, pre-existing anticoagulation medications, mechanism of injury, ISS, head abbreviated injury score [AIS], GCS at scene and upon presentation to the ED, intubation at scene or in ED, injured body regions, admission serum creatinine and INR, intensive care unit length of stay (ICU LOS), hospital LOS, surgical interventions, complications (infectious and non-infectious), and in-hospital mortality.

Any mortality within 30 days of injury was considered an in-hospital death regardless of patient location at the time of death. Time of death was extracted from the medical records which are updated regularly by the Israeli Governmental Ministry of Internal Affairs registry. Outcome variables were mortality and discharge placement. Discharge placement was defined as the patient destination after acute care in the trauma center, being home, rehabilitation center, assisted-living facility (ALF) (defined as lower level of dependence requiring professional support), or transfer to another acute care hospital. Co-morbidities were defined as noted in Table 1.

Table 1 Definition of co-morbidities identified in the study population

Cardiac disease	Known history of ischemic heart disease, previous cardiac interventions
Malignancy	Currently under oncological follow up or treatment for active oncological disease
Diabetes mellitus	Patient requiring insulin or oral hypoglycemic therapy
Neurological disease	History of cerebro-vascular accident, severe parkinsonism and/ or antiepileptic therapy
Dementia	Any case with established diagnosis of dementia
Hypertension	History of hypertension requiring medication
Chronic anticoagulation	Patients currently on anticoagulation (LMWH or Warfarin), and /or antiplatelet therapy (excluding aspirin)
Chronic renal failure	History of preexisting renal insufficiency on admission
Chronic obstructive pulmonary disease	Ongoing treatment for COPD

The absolute number of co-morbidities was calculated for patients with more than one listed illness.

Statistical analysis

For quantitative variables, data is presented as mean and standard deviation (SD). The Chi-square test as well as the Fisher's exact test was used to test the association between two qualitative variables. The Chi-square test for trends was used for qualitative ordinal variables. The Student's T test was used to compare quantitative variables between the two groups. Univariate survival analysis was performed by Kaplan-Meier (K-M) methodology with significance of the difference between survival curves determined by the log-rank test. Variables which were significant in the K-M analysis, were entered into a stepwise, (forward, likelihood ratio) Cox regression model. A logistic regression model was used to define predictors of death during the follow up period.

All tests applied were two-tailed, with p value of 0.05 or less considered statistically significant. Statistical analysis was performed using IBM SPSS Statistics (IBM Corp. Released 2011. IBM SPSS Statistics for Windows, Version 20.0. Armonk, NY: IBM Corp.)

Results
Patient population

416 patients ≥60 years of age with an ISS ≥16 met inclusion criteria with complete data, and were identified who presented to our trauma unit during the study period. Mean age was 76.9 ± 9.6 years of which 232 (55.8%) were male. Of note, 174 (41.8%) were ≥80 years of age. As expected, in-hospital mortality rate was closely associated with age. The overall death rate was

17.8% (74 / 416). In the group ≥80 years of age 23.4% (41/ 174) died, vs. 16.8% (23/137) in the 70-79 year group, and 9.5% (10/105) in the 60-69 year group (p = 0.003). Only one patient (0.2%) died following discharge but within 30 days of the trauma and was considered as in-hospital death.

Post-discharge survival

The demographic and clinical characteristics of the patients in the post discharge survival category are noted in Table 2. 342 patients were discharged from the hospital and were available for follow up. Of this group, 133 patients (38.9%) were ≥80 years of age. During the follow-up period, 119 patients (34.8%) died (non-survivor group) at a mean follow up of 18.8 months (range: 1.1-66.2 months). 223 patients (65.2%) survived at a mean follow up of 50.2 months (range: 24.8-83.8 months). On univariate analysis, older age was significantly associated with a poor long term outcome (p < 0.0001). Patients who

were involved in road traffic collisions, (pedestrians and passengers) were significantly more likely to have a favorable long term outcome compared with those whose mechanism of injury was a fall (p < 0.01). A higher head region AIS was significantly associated with a poorer outcome. Similarly, a low GCS upon admission and the need for intubation at the scene, but not in the ED, were associated with a worse outcome (p < 0.0001, and p < 0.01, respectively). Interestingly, parameters of in-hospital course, including requirement for ICU admission, blood transfusion and in-hospital complications (infectious and non-infectious) did not influence long term outcome (Table 2). Overall LOS was shorter for the survival group but this difference did not reach statistical significance. Ultimate discharge destination was significantly associated with outcome. Patients who were either discharged home or to a rehabilitation facility had a significantly improved long term outcome (p < 0.001) compared to those who were discharged to an ALF.

Table 2 Univariate analysis of long term survival

	Non-survivors (n = 119)	Survivors (n = 223)	P value
Age (mean ± SD)	80.1 ± 9.64	74.2 ± 9.07	<0.0001
Males (n, %)	66 (55.5)	121 (54.3)	NS
MOI (n, %)			
Fall	93 (78.2)	131 (58.7)	<0.001
MVA car	8 (6.7)	37 (16.6)	0.01
MVA pedestrian	11 (9.2)	46 (20.6)	<0.01
Assault	3 (2.5)	3 (1.3)	NS
Burn	2 (1.7)	2 (0.9)	NS
ISS (mean ± SD)	21.8 ± 7.6	21.8 ± 6.9	NS
Probability of survival (mean ± SD)	78.1 ± 24.65	84.4 ± 19.69	0.01
Head AIS (mean ± SD)	4.21 ± 0.765	3.86 ± 0.944	0.001
GCS upon admission (mean ± SD)	11.85 ± 4.21	13.73 ± 2.89	<0.0001
Intubation (n, %)			
At scene	11 (9.2)	5 (2.2)	<0.01
In ED	8 (6.7)	18 (8.1)	NS
Required operation (n, %)	38 (31.9)	89 (39.9)	NS
LOS (mean ± SD)	20.03 ± 19.51	16.09 ± 16.9	0.05
Admitted to ICU (n, %)	62 (52.1)	111 (49)	NS
Blood transfusion (n, %)	55 (46.2)	104 (46.6)	NS
In-hospital complications (n, %)	23 (19.3)	47 (21.1)	NS
Discharge destination (n, %)			
Rehabilitation	18 (15.1)	66 (29.6)	<0.01
Home	35 (29.4)	112 (50.2)	<0.001
Assistant living facility	65 (54.6)	38 (17.0)	<0.0001
Other hospital	1 (0.8)	7 (3.1)	NS

MOI–mechanism of injury; ED–emergency department; LOS–length of stay; ICU–intensive care unit; SD–standard deviation; MVA–motor vehicle accident; GCS–Glasgow Coma Scale; AIS–abbreviated injury score; ISS–injury severity score; NS–not significant.

Effect of co-morbidity on survival

The impacts of pre-existing co-morbidities on survival following discharge are noted in Table 3. On univariate analysis, dementia, ischemic heart disease (IHD), diabetes mellitus (DM), and hypertension (HTN) were found to be significantly associated with post discharge death (p < 0.05 for all). Of note, malignancy and COPD failed to impact survival, but the number of patients in these groups was insufficient to draw any conclusions. The mean number of co-morbidities was significantly associated with long-term mortality (p < 0.0001) (Table 3).

Analysis of post-discharge mortality

In order to analyze post-discharge mortality, patients were grouped into an 'early' group (mortality < 3 months post-injury) and a 'late' group (mortality >3 months post-injury). The pattern of injury, GCS upon arrival, and co-morbidities were not different between the groups. Early post-discharge mortality (≤90 days) occurred in 17 patients (14.3%), while 102 patients (85.7%) died >90 days following discharge (Table 4). Of note, post-discharge mortality was not affected by admission parameters, but by hospital course. Neither age nor mechanisms of injury were found to be risk factors for early post-discharge mortality following injury. Patients who required ICU admission were at increased risk for early death following discharge compared with those who died after a period ≥3 months (14/ 17 [82.4%] vs. 48/102 patients [47.1%], respectively, p < 0.01). Early versus late death was also associated with transfusion of blood products (12 /17 patients [70.6%] vs. 43/102 patients [42.2%], respectively, p = 0.04) and with the development of in-hospital complications (7/17 [41.2%] vs. 16/102

[15.7%], respectively, p = 0.02). ISS was noted to be higher for those who died early, but this difference did not reach statistical significance (mean ISS 25.1 ± 10.7, vs. 21.3 ± 6.9, respectively, p = 0.05). The pattern of injury, GCS upon arrival, and co-morbidities were not different between the groups.

Predictors of long-term survival

Univariate survival curves demonstrated that age, mechanism of injury, GCS upon admission and discharge destination were significantly associated with long-term survival (Figure 1). Multivariate analysis was performed to analyze those factors predictive of survival. Parameters which were found to be significant on univariate analysis were entered into a forward stepwise Cox regression model. As noted age, fall as mechanism of injury, GCS and renal failure upon admission and discharge destination were found to be predictors of long term survival (Table 5).

Discussion

The major finding of this study is that in the elderly population following severe trauma, long term survival can be predicted based on the pre-hospital parameters of age, mechanism of injury, and GCS on admission. In contrast, parameters in hospital care, including blood transfusion, requirement for ICU admission, surgical procedures and complications did not predict long term survival in this elderly group.

There is a paucity of data describing the long term outcome of the injured geriatric patient, accordingly, this was a primary objective of our study. Contrary to what is often assumed, we have demonstrated that long term survival subsequent to a severe trauma in the elderly population is not uncommon, for we noted that almost two-thirds of elderly patients who were discharged from the hospital were alive at a mean follow up of over 4 years.

Previous reports have analyzed the course and in-hospital outcome of elderly patients following trauma [4,11,12]. A mature trauma system performance could be assessed by the percent of severely injured patients who are discharged from the trauma center. For example, Florida trauma system analysis over a 15 year period showed significant increase in both the number of elderly injured and the severity of injury [13]. Others [14] stressed the importance of triage of the severely injured elderly patients to designated trauma centers. This resulted in significantly higher overall discharge when compared to non-trauma centers.

Not surprisingly, and in concert with others [4,15] our data demonstrated that chronological age is a predictor of post-discharge mortality. The post-discharge survival of patients ≥ 80 years is significantly worse compared to

Table 3 Univariate analysis of the effect of co-morbidities on survival

	Non-survivors (n = 119)	Survivors (n = 223)	P value
CRF	11 (9.2)	9 (4.0)	0.05
Anti-coagulant therapy	6 (5.0)	24 (10.8)	0.1
HTN	56 (47.1)	78 (35.0)	0.03
IHD	38 (31.9)	49 (22.0)	0.05
DM	35 (29.4)	39 (17.5)	0.01
COPD	1 (0.8)	2 (0.9)	NS
Dementia	18 (15.1)	1 (0.5)	<0.0001
CVA and/or neurologic disease	20 (16.8)	21 (9.4)	0.05
Malignancy	5 (4.2)	4 (1.8)	NS
≥3 co-morbidities	26 (21.9)	31 (13.9)	0.06
Mean number of co-morbidities	1.6 ± 1.1	1.0 ± 1.2	<0.0001

CRF–chronic renal failure; HTN–hypertension; IHD–ischemic heart disease; DM–diabetes mellitus; COPD–chronic obstructive pulmonary disease; CVA–cerebro-vascular accident.

Table 4 Univariate analysis of early versus late mortality

	Early death (<3 months) (n = 17)	Late death (≥3 months) (n = 102)	P value
Age (mean ± SD)	81.1 ± 6.8	79.9 ± 10.0	NS
Males (n, %)	9 (52.9)	57 (55.9)	NS
MOI (n, %)			
Fall	14 (82.4)	79 (77.5)	NS
MVA car	1 (5.9)	7(6.9)	NS
MVA pedestrian	2 (11.8)	8 (7.8)	NS
Other	0 (0)	8 (7.8)	NS
ISS (Median, range)	25 (16-25)	17 (16-25)	0.1
Probability of survival (mean ± SD)	69.9 ± 28.9	79.4 ± 23.6	0.1
Head trauma (n, %)	12 (70.6)	65 (63.7)	NS
GCS upon admission (mean ± SD)	10.9 ± 4.6	12 ± 4.1	NS
Intubation (n, %)			
At scene	2 (11.8)	9 (8.8)	NS
In ED	1 (5.9)	7 (6.9)	NS
Required operation (n, %)	8(47.1)	30 (29.4)	NS
LOS (mean ± SD)	28.8 ± 19.4	18.6 ± 19.2	<0.05
Admitted to ICU (n, %)	14 (82.4)	48 (47.1)	<0.01
Blood transfusion (n, %)	12 (70.6)	43 (42.2)	0.04
In-hospital complications (n, %)	7 (41.2)	16 (15.7)	0.02
Discharge destination (n, %)			
Rehabilitation	2 (11.8)	16 (15.7)	NS
Home	1 (5.9)	34 (33.3)	0.02
Assistant living facility	14 (82.4)	51 (50.0)	0.02
Other hospital	0 (0.0)	1 (1.0)	NS

NS–not significant; MOI–mechanism of injury; MVA–motor vehicle accidents; ED–Emergency Department; ICU–intensive care unit. Data shown as number (and percentage) and mean (±SD).

their younger counterparts. These intuitive findings could not be explained by the ISS, which was not different between the age groups. Although age related co-morbidities likely contribute to long term survival, we were surprised to note that age, rather than co-morbidities and ISS, was an independent predictor of death, particularly in the ≥80 age group.

It has been noted that in the elderly population, multi-system trauma from falls predominant with increasing age, with a corresponding decreasing frequency of motor vehicular and pedestrian related injuries [5]. Similarly, we noted that falls were the most common mechanism of injury and were associated with poor long term outcome. It has been suggested that a senior's propensity to fall may indicate poor functional capacity and higher mortality risk in this population [16].

Various studies confirm that pre-existing co-morbidities significantly increase the risk of mortality following blunt trauma in geriatric patients [17-20]. The association between DM and early death in the elderly population has been previously noted for general in-hospital admissions [21,22]. Similarly, we noted that the most common pre-existing co-morbidities in our population were HTN, followed by IHD and DM. On univariate analysis these conditions and dementia were associated with poor long term survival. However, on multivariate analysis none of these co-morbidities predicted long term survival. Interestingly, the mean number of co-morbidities was also associated with poor long term outcome.

Traumatic brain injury in geriatric patients has been recognized to result in a worse outcome when compared to younger counterparts, with a low admission GCS commonly recognized as a poor prognostic indicator [23]. Others [24] have argued that perhaps poor overall condition, rather than head injury, per se, determines outcome. We noted that a low GCS, and not head AIS, was found to be an independent predictor of post-discharge mortality. It may be argued that the general condition of the patient, and not the exact type of head injury, is what determines long term outcome [24].

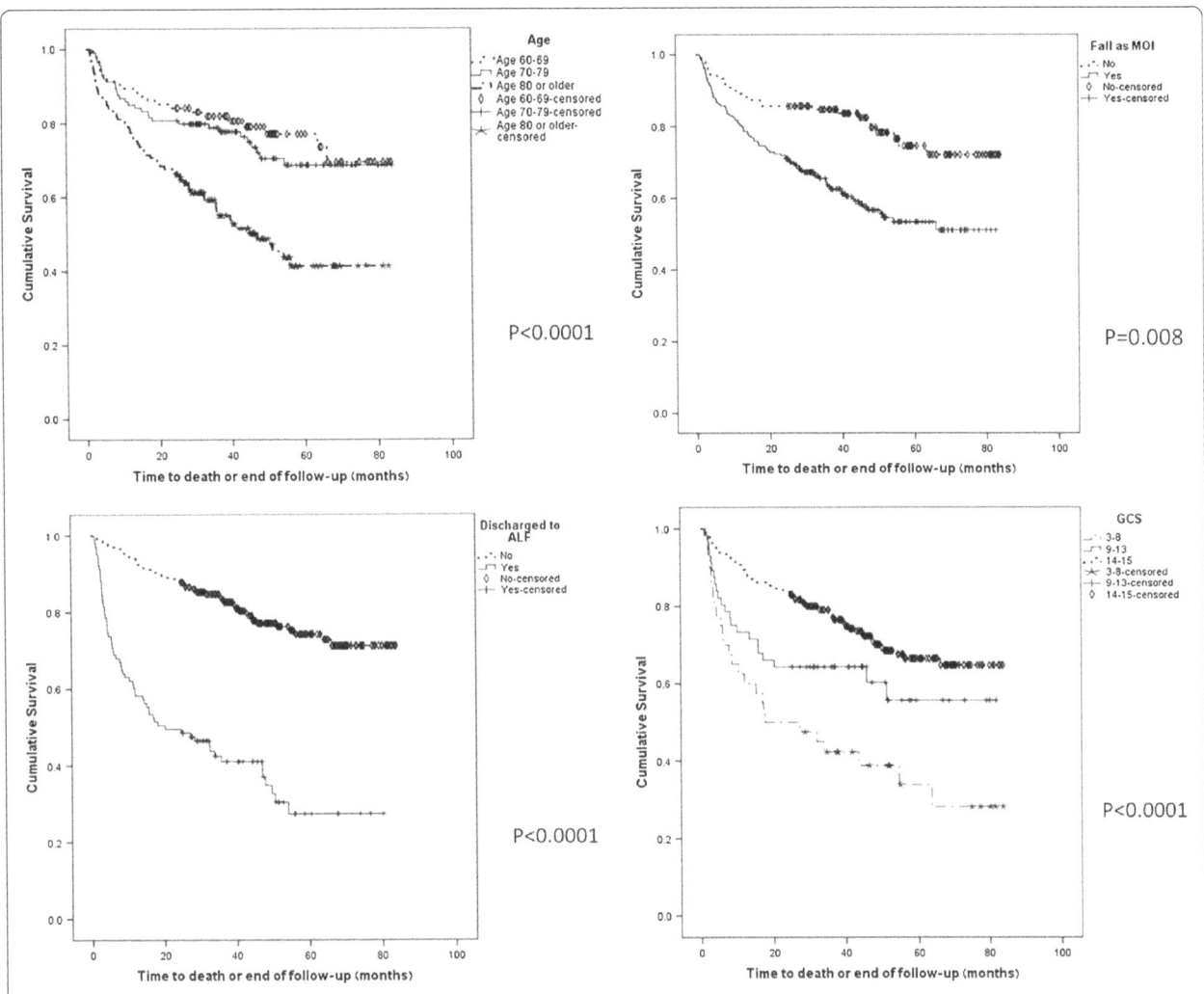

Figure 1 Cox regression model for parameters predicting early post discharge death: age >80; fall as a mechanism of injury; discharge to assisted living facility (ALF); low GCS on arrival to emergency department.

Our finding that more than half of patients in our study required ICU admission (173 patients, 50.6%) and over a third of that group required an operation confirms the fact that considerable acute care resources were utilized for the treatment of these seriously injured elderly patients.

Demographics, pre-hospital and admission parameters could not predict the likelihood of early post-discharge death (within 3 months of injury). However, in-hospital course including the need for ICU admission, blood transfusion and in-hospital complications were found to be associated with early (<3 month) post-discharge mortality. Thus, our data suggest that the characteristics of early post-discharge death may be more similar to in-hospital death than to death during long term follow up.

While our study does not contain data concerning the cost of trauma care in this population, the financial burden of end of life care has been well described [25]. Accordingly, one might surmise that recognition of

parameters that aid in predicting long term survival in these patients would avert the allocation of limited resources and funds on patients with a predicted poor outcome. Currently, in our country and in our institution, there are no limitations in hospital resource allocation for injured elderly patients, although continued concerns

Table 5 Predictors of long term survival in severely injured elderly trauma patients

	Adjusted hazard ratio	95% confidence interval	P value
Age	1.044	1.022-1.065	<0.0001
Fall as mechanism of injury	1.90	1.181-3.057	<0.01
Low GCS in ED	0.883	0.845-0.924	<0.0001
Creatinine in ED	1.003	1.000-1.005	0.03
Discharge to ALF	0.315	0.214-0.463	<0.0001

GCS–Glasgow coma scale; ED–emergency department; ALF–assisted living facility.

world-wide for the costs of care could lead to such limitations. Accordingly, we and others [13,14] believe that increased attention to the growing burden of geriatric trauma care is imperative for future trauma system design, performance improvement, and resource allocation in an effort to improve outcomes in this group.

Legner et al [26] demonstrated a 3.5 times greater mortality at 1 year for patients ≥65 years of age undergoing abdomino-pelvic surgery discharged to a skilled nursing facility compared with those discharged home. Not surprisingly, we found that discharge to an ALF (27% of patients) had a negative impact on long term outcome. This can be explained by the significant differences in physical therapy and occupational therapy options available for patients in rehabilitation programs compared with patients at ALF. Selection bias of patients in a poorer overall condition to ALF could also explain these findings.

There are a number of significant strengths and limitations of this study. Inclusion criteria were ISS >15 thus making this cohort of patients appropriate for the study of long term survival. We excluded patients who died in the hospital from the analysis of delayed long term mortality because the acute mortality from major trauma is determined largely by the severity of the initial injury. This study design allowed us to potentially separate the effects of the initial injury, but rather to use the initial data of patient admission to predict long term outcome.

The major limitation of this study is related to retrospective data analysis. In our trauma registry comorbidities are listed by reviewing previous discharge letters with the incumbent limitations of such data. Finally, data on pre-injury living status for the 148 patients who returned home is not available, and therefore, we cannot draw any definitive conclusions regarding the home status of this group.

In conclusion, we have shown that clinical and demographic factors are associated with long term, post-discharge outcome following severe trauma in geriatric patients, and we noted that almost 2/3 of elderly patients injured following a trauma were discharged from the hospital with a favorable long term outcome. We noted that common demographic and clinical parameters, including age ≥ 80, lower GCS upon arrival and fall as the mechanism of injury are clear predictors of a poor long term outcome for severely injured geriatric trauma patients.

Although most studies commonly evaluate in hospital, < 30 day mortality, our findings expands our understanding of factors contributing towards long term post-discharge survival. Given the substantial and increasing burden of the elderly sustaining traumatic injury, our findings underscore the importance of additional research to further identify risks and prognostic factors to improve

our trauma care and performance improvement, in order to ultimately impact survival in the injured elderly patient. The role of a geriatric consultation service could be crucial in their care and play an important role in the framework of a multi-disciplinary team.

Competing interests

All authors declare that they have no competing interests.

Authors' contributions

MB–literature search, study design, data collection, data analysis, data interpretation, writing, critical revision. JLK–study design, data interpretation, writing, critical revision. DW–data analysis, data interpretation, writing, critical revision. DK–data collection, data analysis. TBA–data analysis, data interpretation. GA–literature search, study design, data collection, data analysis, data interpretation, writing, critical revision. All authors read and approved the final manuscript.

Author details

^{1}Department of Surgery and Shock Trauma Unit, Hadassah-Hebrew University Medical Center, Jerusalem, Israel. ^{2}Director of Surgical Research and Academic Development, EM Care Acute Care Surgery, Dallas, Texas, USA. ^{3}Department of Anesthesiology and Intensive Care Unit, Hadassah-Hebrew University Medical Center, Jerusalem, Israel. ^{4}Department of Social Medicine, Hadassah-Hebrew University Medical Center, Jerusalem, Israel.

References

1. Habot B, Tsin S: **Geriatrics in the new millennium, Israel.** *IMAJ* 2003, **5**:319–321.
2. World Health Organization (WHO): *WHO Statistical Information System (WHOSIS).* http://www.who.int/whosis.
3. McMahon DJ, Shapiro MB, Kauder DR: **The injured elderly in the trauma intensive care unit.** *Surg Clin North Am* 2000, **80**:1005–1019.
4. Clement ND, Tennant C, Muwanga C: **Polytrauma in the elderly: predictors of the cause and time of death.** *Scand J Trauma Resusc Emerg Med* 2010, **18**:26.
5. Labib N, Nouh T, Winocour S, Deckelbaum D, Banici L, Fata P, Razek T, Khwaja K: **Severely injured geriatric population: morbidity, mortality, and risk factors.** *J Trauma* 2011, **71**:1908–1914.
6. Jacobs DG: **Special considerations in geriatric injury.** *Curr Opin Crit Care* 2003, **9**:535–539.
7. Tornetta P III, Mostafavi H, Riina J, Turen C, Reimer B, Levine R, Behrens F, Geller J, Ritter C, Homel P: **Morbidity and mortality in elderly trauma patients.** *J Trauma* 1999, **46**:702–706.
8. Robinson TN, Eiseman B, Wallace JI, Church SD, McFann KK, Pfister SM, Sharp TJ, Moss M: **Redefining geriatric preoperative assessment using frailty, disability and co-morbidity.** *Ann Surg* 2009, **250**:449–455.
9. Lehmann R, Beekley A, Casey L, Salim A, Martin M: **The impact of advanced age on trauma triage decisions and outcomes: a statewide analysis.** *Am J Surg* 2009, **197**:571–575.
10. Rogers A, Rogers F, Bradburn E, Krasne M, Lee J, Wu D, Edavettal M, Horst M: **Old and undertriaged: a lethal combination.** *Am Surg* 2012, **78**:711–715.
11. Ferrera PC, Bartfield JM, D'Andrea CC: **Outcomes of admitted geriatric trauma victims.** *Am J Emerg Med* 2000, **18**:575–580.
12. Kuhne CA, Ruchholtz S, Kaiser GM, Nast-Kolb D, Working Group on Multiple Trauma of the German Society of Trauma: **Mortality in severely injured elderly trauma patients–when does age become a risk factor?** *World J Surg* 2005, **29**:1476–1482.
13. Ciesla DJ, Tepas JJ III, Pracht EE, Langland-Orban B, Cha JY, Flint LM: **Fifteen-year trauma system performance analysis demonstrates optimal coverage for most severely injured patients and identifies a vulnerable population.** *J Am Coll Surg* 2013, **216**:687–695.
14. Pracht EE, Langland-Orban B, Flint L: **Survival advantage for elderly trauma patients treated in a designated trauma center.** *J Trauma* 2011, **71**:69–77.

15. Giannoudis PV, Harwood PJ, Court-Brown CM, Pape HC: **Severe and multple trauma in older patients; incidence and mortality.** *Injury* 2009, **40**:362–367.

16. Aschkenasy MT, Rothenhaus TC: **Trauma and falls in the elderly.** *Emerg Med Clin North Am* 2006, **24**:413–432.

17. Milzman DP, Boulanger BR, Rodriguez A, Soderstrom CA, Mitchell KA, Magnant CM: **Preexisting disease in trauma patients: a predictor of fate independent of age and injury severity score.** *J Trauma* 1992, **32**:236–243.

18. Bochicchio GV, Joshi M, Bochicchio K, Shih D, Meyer W, Scalea TM: **Incidence and impact of risk factors in critically ill trauma patients.** *World J Surg* 2006, **30**:114–118.

19. Morris JA Jr, MacKenzie EJ, Edelstein SL: **The effect of preexisting conditions on mortality in trauma patients.** *JAMA* 1990, **263**:1942–1946.

20. Taylor MD, Tracy JK, Meyer W, Pasquale M, Napolitano LM: **Trauma in the elderly: intensive care unit resource use and outcome.** *J Trauma* 2002, **53**:407–414.

21. Zekry D, Frangos E, Graf C, Michel JP, Gold G, Krause KH, Herrmann FR, Vischer UM: **Diabetes, comorbidities and increased long-term mortality in older patients admitted for geriatric inpatient care.** *Diabetes Metab* 2012, **38**:149–155.

22. Hollis S, Lecky F, Yates DW, Woodford M: **The effect of pre-existing medical conditions and age on mortality after injury.** *J Trauma* 2006, **61**:1255–1260.

23. Utomo WK, Gabbe BJ, Simpson PM, Cameron PA: **Predictors of in-hospital mortality and 6-month functional outcomes in older adults after moderate to severe traumatic brain injury.** *Injury* 2009, **40**:973–977.

24. Marquez de la Plata CD, Hart T, Hammond FM, Frol AB, Hudak A, Harper CR, O'Neil-Pirozzi TM, Whyte J, Carlile M, Diaz-Arrastia R: **Impact of age on long term recovery from traumatic brain injury.** *Arch Phys Med Rehab* 2008, **89**:896–903.

25. Grossman MD, Ofurum U, Stehly CD, Stoltzfus J: **Long-term survival after major trauma in geriatric trauma patients: the glass is half full.** *J Trauma Acute Care Surg* 2012, **72**:1181–1185.

26. Legner VJ, Massarweh NN, Symons RG, McCormick WC, Flum DR: **The significance of discharge to skilled care after abdominopelvic surgery in older adults.** *Ann Surg* 2009, **249**:250–255.

The open abdomen in trauma and non-trauma patients: WSES guidelines

Federico Coccolini[1*], Derek Roberts[2], Luca Ansaloni[1], Rao Ivatury[3], Emiliano Gamberini[4], Yoram Kluger[5], Ernest E. Moore[6], Raul Coimbra[7], Andrew W. Kirkpatrick[2], Bruno M. Pereira[8], Giulia Montori[1], Marco Ceresoli[1], Fikri M. Abu-Zidan[9], Massimo Sartelli[10], George Velmahos[11], Gustavo Pereira Fraga[8], Ari Leppaniemi[12], Matti Tolonen[12], Joseph Galante[13], Tarek Razek[14], Ron Maier[15], Miklosh Bala[16], Boris Sakakushev[17], Vladimir Khokha[18], Manu Malbrain[19], Vanni Agnoletti[4], Andrew Peitzman[20], Zaza Demetrashvili[21], Michael Sugrue[22], Salomone Di Saverio[23], Ingo Martzi[24], Kjetil Soreide[25,26], Walter Biffl[27], Paula Ferrada[3], Neil Parry[28], Philippe Montravers[29], Rita Maria Melotti[30], Francesco Salvetti[1], Tino M. Valetti[31], Thomas Scalea[32], Osvaldo Chiara[33], Stefania Cimbanassi[33], Jeffry L. Kashuk[34], Martha Larrea[35], Juan Alberto Martinez Hernandez[36], Heng-Fu Lin[37], Mircea Chirica[38], Catherine Arvieux[38], Camilla Bing[39], Tal Horer[40], Belinda De Simone[41], Peter Masiakos[42], Viktor Reva[43], Nicola DeAngelis[44], Kaoru Kike[45], Zsolt J. Balogh[46], Paola Fugazzola[1], Matteo Tomasoni[1], Rifat Latifi[47], Noel Naidoo[48], Dieter Weber[49], Lauri Handolin[50], Kenji Inaba[51], Andreas Hecker[52], Yuan Kuo-Ching[53], Carlos A. Ordoñez[54], Sandro Rizoli[55], Carlos Augusto Gomes[56], Marc De Moya[57], Imtiaz Wani[58], Alain Chichom Mefire[59], Ken Boffard[60], Lena Napolitano[61] and Fausto Catena[62]

Abstract

Damage control resuscitation may lead to postoperative intra-abdominal hypertension or abdominal compartment syndrome. These conditions may result in a vicious, self-perpetuating cycle leading to severe physiologic derangements and multiorgan failure unless interrupted by abdominal (surgical or other) decompression. Further, in some clinical situations, the abdomen cannot be closed due to the visceral edema, the inability to control the compelling source of infection or the necessity to re-explore (as a "planned second-look" laparotomy) or complete previously initiated damage control procedures or in cases of abdominal wall disruption. The open abdomen in trauma and non-trauma patients has been proposed to be effective in preventing or treating deranged physiology in patients with severe injuries or critical illness when no other perceived options exist. Its use, however, remains controversial as it is resource consuming and represents a non-anatomic situation with the potential for severe adverse effects. Its use, therefore, should only be considered in patients who would most benefit from it. Abdominal fascia-to-fascia closure should be done as soon as the patient can physiologically tolerate it. All precautions to minimize complications should be implemented.

Keywords: Open abdomen, Laparostomy, Non-trauma, Trauma, Peritonitis, Pancreatitis, Vascular emergencies, Intra-abdominal infection, Fistula, Nutrition, Re-exploration, Reintervention, Closure, Biological, Synthetic, Mesh, Technique, Timing, Guidelines

* Correspondence: federico.coccolini@gmail.com
[1]General Emergency and Trauma Surgery, Bufalini Hospital, Viale Giovanni Ghirotti, 286, 47521 Cesena, Italy
Full list of author information is available at the end of the article

Background

Damage control management (DCM) of severely injured or physiologically deranged patients is considered by many to consist of damage control resuscitation (DCR) and damage control surgery (DCS). Use of DCM in patients with deranged physiology may trigger intra-abdominal hypertension (IAH) or abdominal compartment syndrome (ACS) that may aggravate physiologic derangement or multiorgan failure (MOF) in a vicious circle unless interrupted by abdominal decompression (surgical or other) [1, 2]. Further, in other clinical situations, the abdomen cannot be closed due to visceral edema, the inability to completely control the compelling source of infection or to the necessity to re-explore (in a "planned re-look laparotomy") or to complete DCS procedures or in cases of abdominal wall damage. Although open abdomen (OA) has been proposed to be effective in preventing or treating deranged physiology in patients with severe injuries or critical illness, it must be recognized as a non-anatomic situation that has potential for severe side effects while increasing resource utilization [3].

The World Society for Emergency Surgery (WSES) accepted the definitions of IAH, ACS, and related conditions published by the World Society Abdominal Compartment Syndrome in 2013 (WSACS) [2–4] (Fig. 1).

OA management consists of intentionally leaving the abdominal fascial edges of the paired rectus abdominus muscles un-approximated (laparostomy) in order to truncate operation, prevent IAH/ACS, and facilitate re-exploration without damaging the abdominal fascia [3]. Temporary abdominal closure (TAC) refers to the method for providing protection to the abdominal viscera during the time the fascia remains open [2, 5]. Patients undergoing OA management are at risk of developing entero-atmospheric fistula (EAF) and a "frozen abdomen," intra-abdominal abscesses, and lower rates of definitive fascial closure [6, 7]. The risk-benefit ratio must be kept in mind in

using OA. It should not be performed liberally. Measures to mitigate complications are necessary. In all patients with an OA, every effort should be exerted to achieve primary fascial closure (i.e., fascia-to-fascia closure of the abdominal wall within the index hospitalization) as soon as the patient can physiologically tolerate it [3].

Purpose and use of this guideline

The guidelines are evidence-based, with the grades of recommendation, based on the evidence. These guidelines present methods for optimal management of open abdomen in trauma and non-trauma patients. They do not represent a standard of practice. They are suggested plans of care, based on best available evidence and a consensus of experts. They, however, do not exclude other approaches as being within a standard of practice. For example, they should not be used to compel adherence to a given method of medical management, which should be finally determined after taking into account conditions at the relevant medical institution (staff levels, experience, equipment, etc.) and the characteristics of the individual patient. The responsibility for the results, however, rests with the engaging practitioners and not aged therein, and not the consensus group.

Methods

A computerized search was performed in MEDLINE, EMBASE, and Scopus by an information scientist/librarian for the time range of January 1980 to August 2017. The terms open abdomen, laparostomy, injuries, trauma, peritonitis, pancreatitis, vascular, ischemia, resuscitation, adult, management, infection, intensive care unit, anastomosis, vasopressors, and follow-up in various combinations with the use of the Boolean operators "AND" and "OR" were used. No search restrictions were imposed. The dates were selected to allow comprehensive published abstracts of clinical trials, consensus conferences, comparative studies, congresses, guidelines, government publications, multicenter studies, systematic reviews, meta-analyses, large case series, original articles, and randomized controlled trials. Case reports and small case series were excluded. We also analyzed the reference lists of relevant narrative review articles identified during the search to identify any studies that may have been missed.

For each article, we subsequently applied a level of evidence (LE) using the Grading of Recommendations, Assessment, Development, and Evaluation (GRADE) system [8] (Table 1). The full GRADE process was not used, as this system is difficult to apply when scant evidence exists. A group of experts in the field of OA management, coordinated by a central coordinator, were subsequently convened in order to elicit their evidence-based opinions on certain key clinical questions relating to the OA. Through a Delphi process, the clinical questions were discussed in rounds.

IAH grade	IAP [mmHg]
Grade I	12 - 15
Grade II	16 - 20
Grade III	21 - 25
Grade IV	> 25
ACS	> 20 with new organ disfunction/failure

Fig. 1 WSACS grading of intra-abdominal hypertension (IAH) (IAP intra-abdominal pressure, ACS abdominal compartment syndrome) [4]

Table 1 GRADE system to evaluate the level of evidence and recommendation

Grade of recommendation	Clarity of risk/benefit	Quality of supporting evidence	Implications
1A			
Strong recommendation, high-quality evidence	Benefits clearly outweigh risk and burdens, or vice versa	RCTs without important limitations or overwhelming evidence from observational studies	Strong recommendation, applies to most patients in most circumstances without reservation
1B			
Strong recommendation, moderate-quality evidence	Benefits clearly outweigh risk and burdens, or vice versa	RCTs with important limitations (inconsistent results, methodological flaws, indirect analyses, or imprecise conclusions) or exceptionally strong evidence from observational studies	Strong recommendation, applies to most patients in most circumstances without reservation
1C			
Strong recommendation, low-quality or very low-quality evidence	Benefits clearly outweigh risk and burdens, or vice versa	Observational studies or case series	Strong recommendation but subject to change when higher quality evidence becomes available
2A			
Weak recommendation, high-quality evidence	Benefits closely balanced with risks and burden	RCTs without important limitations or overwhelming evidence from observational studies	Weak recommendation, best action may differ depending on the patient, treatment circumstances, or social values
2B			
Weak recommendation, moderate-quality evidence	Benefits closely balanced with risks and burden	RCTs with important limitations (inconsistent results, methodological flaws, indirect, or imprecise) or exceptionally strong evidence from observational studies	Weak recommendation, best action may differ depending on the patient, treatment circumstances, or social values
2C			
Weak recommendation, low-quality or very low-quality evidence	Uncertainty in the estimates of benefits, risks, and burden; benefits, risk, and burden may be closely balanced	Observational studies or case series	Very weak recommendation; alternative treatments may be equally reasonable and merit consideration

The central coordinator assembled the different answers derived from each round. Each version was then revised and improved through iterative evaluation. The final version about which the agreement was reached resulted in the comments and recommendations made in the present guideline. Statements have been summarized in Table 2.

Indications
Trauma patients

Persistent hypotension, acidosis (pH <7.2), hypothermia (temperature < 34°C) and coagulopathy are strong predictors of the need for abbreviated laparotomy and open abdomen in trauma patients (Grade 2A)

Risk factors for abdominal compartment syndrome such as damage control surgery, injuries requiring packing and planned reoperation, extreme visceral or retroperitoneal swelling, obesity, elevated bladder pressure when abdominal closure is attempted,

abdominal wall tissue loss and aggressive resuscitation are predictors of the necessity for open abdomen in trauma patients (Grade 2B)

Decompressive laparotomy is indicated in abdominal compartment syndrome if medical treatment has failed after repeated and reliable IAP measurements (Grade 2B)

The inability to definitively control the source of contamination or the necessity to evaluate bowel perfusion may be an indicator to leave the abdomen open in post-traumatic bowel injuries (Grade 2B)

Severely injured patients with hemodynamic instability are at higher risk of ACS for several reasons (i.e., aggressive resuscitation, ischemia-reperfusion injury, visceral or retroperitoneal swelling, recurrent bleeding, and intra-peritoneal packing) [9–12].

Table 2 Summary of statements

	Statements
Indications	
Trauma patients	Persistent hypotension, acidosis (pH <7.2), hypothermia (temperature < 34°C) and coagulopathy are strong predictors of the need for abbreviated laparotomy and open abdomen in trauma patients (Grade 2A)
	Risk factors for abdominal compartment syndrome such as damage control surgery, injuries requiring packing and planned reoperation, extreme visceral or retroperitoneal swelling, obesity, elevated bladder pressure when abdominal closure is attempted, abdominal wall tissue loss and aggressive resuscitation are predictors of the necessity for open abdomen in trauma patients (Grade 2B)
	Decompressive laparotomy is indicated in abdominal compartment syndrome if medical treatment has failed after repeated and reliable IAP measurements (Grade 2B)
	The inability to definitively control the source of contamination or the necessity to evaluate the bowel perfusion may be an indicator to leave the abdomen open in post-traumatic bowel injuries (Grade 2B)
Non-trauma patients	Decompressive laparotomy is indicated in abdominal compartment syndrome if medical treatment has failed after repeated and reliable IAP measurements (Grade 2B)
➤ Peritonitis	The open abdomen is an option for emergency surgery patients with severe peritonitis and severe sepsis/septic shock under the following circumstances: abbreviated laparotomy due to the severe physiological derangement, the need for a deferred intestinal anastomosis, a planned second look for intestinal ischemia, persistent source of peritonitis (failure of source control), or extensive visceral oedema with the concern for development of abdominal compartment syndrome (Grade 2C).
➤ Vascular emergencies	The open abdomen should be considered following management of hemorrhagic vascular catastrophes such as ruptured abdominal aortic aneurysm (Grade 1C)
	The open abdomen should be considered following surgical management of acute mesenteric ischemic insults (Grade 2C).
➤ Pancreatitis	In patients with severe acute pancreatitis unresponsive to step-up conservative management surgical decompression and open abdomen open are effective in treating abdominal compartment syndrome (Grade 2C)
	Leaving the abdomen open after surgical necrosectomy for infected pancreatic necrosis is not recommended except in those situations with high risk factors to develop abdominal compartment syndrome (Grade 1C)
Management	
Trauma and non-trauma patients	The role of Damage Control Resuscitation in OA management is fundamental and may influence outcome (Grade 2A)
ICU management	A multidisciplinary approach is encouraged, especially during the patient's ICU admission (Grade 2A)
	Intra-abdominal pressure measurement is essential in critically ill patients at risk for IAH/ACS (Grade 1B)
	Physiologic optimization is one of the determinants of early abdominal closure (Grade 2A)
	Inotropes and vasopressors administration should be tailored according to patient condition and performed surgical interventions (Grade 1A)
	Fluid balance should be carefully scrutinized (Grade 2A)
	High attention to body temperature should be given, avoiding hypothermia (Grade 2A)
	In presence of coagulopathy or high risk of bleeding the negative pressure should be down regulated balancing the therapeutic necessity of negative pressure and the hemorrhage risk (Grade 2B).
Technique for temporary abdominal closure	Negative pressure wound therapy with continuous fascial traction should be suggested as the preferred technique for temporary abdominal closure (Grade 2B).
	Temporary abdominal closure without negative pressure (e.g. Bogota bag) can be applied in low resource settings accepting a lower delayed fascial closure rate and higher intestinal fistula rate (Grade 2A).
	No definitive recommendations can be given about temporary abdominal closure with NPWT in combination with fluid instillation even if it seems to improve results in trauma patients (Not grades).
Re-exploration before definitive closure	Open abdomen re-exploration should be conducted no later than 24-48 hours after the index and any subsequent operation, with the duration from the previous operation shortening with increasing degrees of patient non-improvement and hemodynamic instability (Grade 1C).
	The abdomen should be maintained open if requirements for on-going resuscitation and/or the source of contamination persists, if a deferred intestinal anastomosis is needed, if there is the necessity for a planned second look for ischemic intestine and lastly if there are concerns about abdominal compartment syndrome development (Grade 2B).
Nutritional support	Open abdomen patients are in a hyper-metabolic condition; immediate and adequate nutritional support is mandatory (Grade 1C).
	Open abdomen techniques result in a significant nitrogen loss that must be replaced with a balanced nutrition regimen (Grade 1C).

Table 2 Summary of statements (Continued)

	Statements
	Early enteral nutrition should be started as soon as possible in presence of viable and functional gastrointestinal tract (Grade 1C).
	Enteral nutrition should be delayed in patients with an intestinal tract in discontinuity (temporarily stapled stumps), or in situations of a high output fistula with no possibility to obtain feeding access distal to the fistula or with signs of intestinal obstruction (Grade 2C)
	Oral feeding is not contraindicated and should be used where possible (Grade 2C).
Patient mobilization	To date, no recommendations can be made about early mobilization of patients with open abdomen (Not graded).
Definitive closure	
Trauma and non-trauma patients	Fascia and/or abdomen should be definitively closed as soon as possible (Grade 1C).
Open abdomen definitive closure	Early fascial and/or abdominal definitive closure should be the strategy for management of the open abdomen once any requirements for on-going resuscitation have ceased, the source control has been definitively reached, no concern regarding intestinal viability persist, no further surgical re-exploration is needed and there are no concerns for abdominal compartment syndrome (Grade 1B).
➤ Non-mesh-mediated techniques	Primary fascia closure is the ideal solution to restore the abdominal closure (2A).
	Component separation is an effective technique; however it should not be used for fascial temporary closure. It should be considered only for definitive closure (Grade 2C).
	Planned ventral hernia (skin graft or skin closure only) remains an option for the complicated open abdomen (i.e. in the presence of entero-atmospheric fistula or in cases with a protracted open abdomen due to underlying diseases) or in those settings where no other alternatives are viable (Grade 2C)
➤ Mesh-mediated techniques	The use of synthetic mesh (polypropylene, polytetrafluoruroethylene (PTFE) and polyester products) as a fascial bridge should not be recommended in definitive closure interventions after open abdomen and should be placed only in patients without other alternatives (Grade 1B).
	Biologic meshes are reliable for definitive abdominal wall reconstruction in the presence of a large wall defect, bacterial contamination, comorbidities and difficult wound healing (Grade 2B).
	Non–cross-linked biologic meshes seem to be preferred in sublay position when the linea alba can be reconstructed. (Grade 2B).
	Cross-linked biologic meshes in fascial-bridge position (no linea alba closure) maybe associated with less ventral hernia recurrence (Grade 2B).
	NPWT can be used in combination with biologic mesh to facilitate granulation and skin closure (Grade 2B).
Complications management	
Trauma and non-trauma patients	Preemptive measures to prevent entero-atmospheric fistula and frozen abdomen are imperative (i.e. early abdominal wall closure, bowel coverage with plastic sheets, omentum or skin, no direct application of synthetic prosthesis over bowel loops, no direct application of NPWT on the viscera and deep burying of intestinal anastomoses under bowel loops) (Grade 1C).
	Entero-atmospheric fistula management should be tailored according to patient conditions, fistula output and position and anatomical features (Grade 1C)
	In the presence of entero-atmospheric fistula the caloric intake and protein demands are increased; the nitrogen balance should be evaluated and corrected and protein supplemented (Grade 1C).
	Nutrition should be reviewed and optimized upon recognition of entero-atmospheric fistula (Grade 1C)
	Entero-atmospheric fistula effluent isolation is essential for proper wound healing. Separating the wound into different compartments to facilitate the collection of fistula output is of paramount importance (Grade 2A).
	In the presence of entero-atmospheric fistula in open abdomen, negative pressure wound therapy makes effluent isolation feasible and wound healing achievable (Grade 2A).
	Definitive management of entero-atmospheric fistula should be delayed to after the patient has recovered and the wound completely healed (Grade 1C).

In fact, the post-traumatic physiological derangements and the consequent DCM expose patients at risk for increased intra-abdominal pressure. Risk factors associated with ACS requiring an OA after trauma, indicating a higher need for OA, are acidosis with pH $\leq$ 7.2, lactate levels $\geq$ 5 mmol/L, base deficit (BD) $\geq$ – 6 in patients older than 55 years or $\geq$ – 15 in patients younger than 55 years, core temperature $\leq$ 34 °C, systolic pressure $\leq$

70 mmHg, estimated blood loss ≥ 4 L during the operation and/or transfusion requirement ≥ 10 U of packed red blood cells in the pre- or pre- and intraoperative settings, and severe coagulation derangements (INR/PT > 1.5 times normal, with or without a concomitant PTT > 1.5 times normal) [10, 13–17].

Other recognized risk factors for IAH should be kept into consideration: obesity, pancreatitis, hepatic failure/cirrhosis, positive end-expiratory pressure > 10 cm H$_2$0, respiratory failure, acute respiratory distress syndrome [18].

All non-surgical treatment should be implemented to prevent or reduce IAH before proceeding to surgical decompression (i.e., nasogastric and colonic decompression, prokinetic agents, adequate patient positioning and avoidance of constrictive dressings, eventual escharotomy and percutaneous decompression, adequate mechanical ventilation, analgesia, sedation and neuromuscular blockade, balanced fluid resuscitation, eventual diuretic therapy and continuous veno-venous hemofiltration/ultrafiltration, and vasoactive medications).

Moreover, failure to definitively control the source of infection at the index operation or the necessity to check bowel perfusion during DCM or abdominal wall tissue loss represents indications to OA management in traumatic abdominal injuries [3, 11].

Non-trauma patients

Decompressive laparotomy is indicated in abdominal compartment syndrome if medical treatment has failed after repeated and reliable IAP measurements (Grade 2B)

Peritonitis

The open abdomen is an option for emergency surgery patients with severe peritonitis and severe sepsis/septic shock under the following circumstances: abbreviated laparotomy due to severe physiological derangement, the need for a deferred intestinal anastomosis, a planned second look for intestinal ischemia, persistent source of peritonitis (failure of source control), or extensive visceral oedema with the concern for development of abdominal compartment syndrome (Grade 2C).

Some patients suffering from severe peritonitis may experience a disease progression to septic shock with no room for definitive surgical procedures [3, 19]. In these cases, surgical operation should be abbreviated even in advanced age [20]. In hypotensive patients requiring high-dose vasopressors or inotropes infusion intestinal continuity restoration may be deferred [21]. In incomplete source control or in the presence of visceral edema and/or decreased abdominal wall compliance primary

complete fascia closure should not be attempted because of the high risk of IAH/ACS [22]. In all these situations, the abdomen may be left open. However, there is no definitive data regarding the use of the OA in the face of severe peritonitis and therefore, caution should be exercised when using OA in these circumstances.

Vascular emergencies

The open abdomen should be considered following management of hemorrhagic vascular catastrophes such as ruptured abdominal aortic aneurysm (Grade 1C)

The open abdomen should be considered following surgical management of acute mesenteric ischemic insults (Grade 2C).

Up to 20% of patients experiencing a ruptured AAA repair develop ACS. Mortality is high (30–50%) and is almost doubled in presence of ACS [23, 24]. OA reduces the ACS incidence [25]. No definitive indications to OA exist; the relative indications to OA are massive resuscitation, deranged physiology, fascial tension at closure, use of balloon occlusion of the aorta, and blood loss > 5 L [25–27].

Advanced age is not a contraindication to DCM [20].

ACS can occur even after endovascular repair (EVAR), and the major risk factor appears to be massive resuscitation [23]. Risk of graft infection due to OA management has been demonstrated to be low [28].

The use of OA after perfusion restoration in a patient with acute mesenteric ischemia as in occlusive proximal or distal superior mesenteric artery emboli, watershed necrosis after AAA repairs (open or endovascular), and non-occlusive mesenteric ischemia (e.g., post-arrest or resuscitation from shock/arrest) should be considered in case of deranged physiology and bowel edema and necessity to perform a second look or delayed anastomosis [29–31].

Mesenteric venous thrombosis requiring laparotomy does not routinely mandate OA as often as mesenteric ischemia [32]; however, the risk of IAH/ACS imposes attention to IAP.

Pancreatitis

In patients with severe acute pancreatitis unresponsive to step-up conservative management surgical decompression and open abdomen open are effective in treating abdominal compartment syndrome (Grade 2C)

Leaving the abdomen open after surgical necrosectomy for infected pancreatic necrosis is not recommended except in those situations with high risk factors to develop abdominal compartment syndrome (Grade 1C)

MOF is the factor mainly associated with mortality in acute pancreatitis (AP) especially when infected necrosis [33–37] is present. As in many other conditions, secondary IAH/ACS may aggravate MOF in a vicious circle [38]. IAH/ACS should be prevented and treated as far as it is possible with non-surgical measures. Surgical decompression is the last but effective tool; it should not be delayed in case of ACS [4, 39]. Pancreatic necrosis may become infected after the first week [40]. The presence of organ failure, early bacteremia, and the extent of pancreatic necrosis are factors associated with infection [40]. Surgical necrosectomy should be considered when more conservative management as percutaneous drainage fails [41]. In case of necrosectomy, OA may be considered, but it is not mandatory. It should be considered only if risks for IAH/ACS exist.

Management
Trauma and non-trauma patients

ICU management

The role of Damage Control Resuscitation in OA management is fundamental and may influence outcome (Grade 2A)

A multidisciplinary approach is encouraged, especially during the patient's ICU admission (Grade 2A)

Intra-abdominal pressure measurement is essential in critically ill patients at risk for IAH/ACS (Grade 1B)

Physiologic optimization is one of the determinants of early abdominal closure (Grade 2A)

Inotropes and vasopressors administration should be tailored to patient's condition and performed surgical interventions (Grade 1A)

Fluid balance should be carefully scrutinized (Grade 2A)

High attention to body temperature should be given, avoiding hypothermia (Grade 2A)

In presence of coagulopathy or high risk of bleeding the negative pressure should be down regulated balancing the therapeutic necessity of negative pressure and the hemorrhage risk (Grade 2B).

The initial management is fundamental. DCR is part of DCM utilized in treating severely injured and severely physiologically deranged patients. It passes through some cornerstone actions as volume resuscitation, reversal of coagulopathy, correction of acidosis, and all the other pertinent resuscitative measures aiming to restore the normal physiology. The fluid status, nutrition, and respiratory mechanics should also be kept into consideration in managing OA. In fact the possibility of recurrent ACS with its related high mortality is to be posed into consideration [42–44].

Abdominal pressure should be measured in all patients at risk of developing IAH/ACS; in fact, it has been demonstrated that clinical examination is inaccurate in diagnosing IAH/ACS [45]. As a general principle, it should be measured every 12 h and every 4–6 h once ACS/IAH has been detected or if organ failure happens.

Physiology optimization is necessary to allow early abdominal closure. In fact, prolonged OA may delay extubation, increase the risk for EAF and frozen abdomen, and increase complications [46].

Multidisciplinary collaboration with all teams managing the patient is required for optimal care of OA patients.

The real extent of heat loss in OA and a temporary abdominal dressing cannot be quantified. It is well known that patient physiology is impaired by hypothermia and its related hypo-perfusion effects such as heart function depression, reduced oxygen delivery, coagulation cascade alteration, and acidosis.

In trauma patients, the "lethal triad" should be rapidly interrupted [47–53].

It is well known that mortality increases in trauma patients with significant core-body temperature drop [54].

Commercial NPWT systems significantly reduce heat loss but the non-commercial ones still maintain a reduced heat isolation capacity. For this reason, the heat loss control is of paramount importance especially in those settings where non-commercial systems are utilized.

During ICU stay, it is important to ensure analgesia over hypnosis and consider multimodal analgesia to reduce opioid infusion, trying to keep the patient "awake" but well adapted to mechanical ventilation. Moreover, protective mechanical ventilation strategies should be adopted.

Fluid balance is important as well in OA management and should be carefully scrutinized to avoid over- or under- resuscitation. Careful monitoring and maintenance of adequate urinary output could help in evaluating adequacy of resuscitation effects. Continuous monitoring of cardiac output (CO), targeting at low/normal values, is essential to avoid fluid overload and vasopressor abuse. If increasing vasopressors induce low CO, and fluid responsiveness is transient, consider to target treatments (included inotropes) to the best compromise between MAP, CO, and fluid amount. High-rate maintenance fluid infusions should be avoided. As a counterpart, whenever possible, frequent, small-volume fluid boluses should be preferred. Hypertonic crystalloid and colloid-based resuscitation seem to decrease the risk of iatrogenic, induce resuscitation, and increase IAP [55]. Daily patient weights may help in evaluating fluid retention.

Inotrope infusion should be balanced keeping in mind the patients' condition, the performed surgical procedures, and the necessity to prevent further complications due to their overuse [56, 57].

Volumetric-based monitoring technologies can be very useful in hemodynamic evaluation during DCR phases in critically ill patients. In fact, the elevated intra-abdominal and intra-thoracic pressure can impair the real value of the measurements obtained with traditional pressure-based parameters such as pulmonary artery occlusion pressure and central venous pressure [58–60]. The alteration of these parameters can potentially lead to wrong decisions as regards the correct fluid status and as a consequence the necessary amount of fluid to be administered. This balance is essential also to optimize the surgical success of primary fascial closure [12, 61, 62].

Technique for temporary abdominal closure

Negative pressure wound therapy with continuous fascial traction should be suggested as the preferred technique for temporary abdominal closure (Grade 2B).

Temporary abdominal closure without negative pressure (e.g. Bogota bag) can be applied in low resource settings accepting a lower delayed fascial closure rate and higher intestinal fistula rate (Grade 2A).

No definitive recommendations can be given about temporary abdominal closure with NPWT in combination with fluid instillation even if it seems to improve results in trauma patients (Not graded).

Several strategies to maintain the OA have been described. They result in different delayed fascial closure rate and EAF risk. In general, negative pressure associated to a dynamic component (mesh-mediated fascial traction or dynamic sutures) allows to reach the best results in terms of delayed fascial closure, but dynamic sutures result more often in fistula [3]. Negative pressure without a dynamic component (Barker's VAC or commercial products) results in a moderate delayed fascial closure rate and a fistula rate similar to mesh closure without negative pressure [3].

Recent data from the International Register of Open Abdomen (IROA study) showed that different techniques of OA resulted in different results according to the treated disease [63] (trauma and severe peritonitis) and if treated with or without negative pressure in terms of abdominal

closure and mortality rate. The results favored the non-negative pressure systems in trauma and negative pressure temporary closure in severe peritonitis patients [46]. Also, recent contradictory data from a single-center RCT showed that NPWT and fluid instillation seemed to improve outcomes in trauma patients in terms of early and primary closure [64].

Another important issue in OA management is the necessity to balance the antimicrobial therapy in relation to positive cultures of intra-abdominal fluids. Two options are generally followed without any strong literature evidence: treating all the cultured organisms (with high proportions of staphylococci, candida, and MDR Gram-negative bacilli including *Pseudomonas*) or a "wait and see" strategy. WSES suggests to follow guidelines for intra-abdominal infections [65].

Re-exploration before definitive closure

Open abdomen re-exploration should be conducted no later than 24-48 hours after the index and any subsequent operation, with the duration from the previous operation shortening with increasing degrees of patient non--improvement and hemodynamic instability (Grade 1C).

The abdomen should be maintained open if requirements for on-going resuscitation and/or the source of contamination persists, if a deferred intestinal anastomosis is needed, if there is the necessity for a planned second look for ischemic intestine and lastly if there are concerns about abdominal compartment syndrome development (Grade 2B).

Indications to re-explore an OA may vary between trauma and non-trauma patients. In general, the patient's non-improvement possibly is due to an intra-abdominal reason. No definitive data regarding the timing of re-operation in OA patients exist [6, 66]. It is generally recommended that OA patients should be re-explored 24–72 h after the initial or any subsequent surgical intervention [2, 67, 68]. Some data regarding trauma patients showed that the time of re-exploration reduces the primary fascial closure rate of 1.1% for each hour after the first 24 h after the index operation [69]. Moreover, increased complication rate was observed in patients having the first re-operation after 48 h [3, 69].

In non-trauma patients, the indication to re-explore the abdominal cavity are less definite and usually are due to the necessity to continue DCM, to the impossibility to definitively control the source of infection or to the necessity to re-asses the bowel vascularization or lastly, to concerns regarding the possibility of ACS [2, 3, 20, 70].

Even though there is some evidence that OA may be justified in severely injured or physiologically deranged patients with the aim to manipulate the systemic immune response and ameliorate the bio mediator burden, no definitive statement can be made [3, 71–75].

Nutritional support

Open abdomen patients are in a hyper-metabolic condition; immediate and adequate nutritional support is mandatory (Grade 1C).

Open abdomen techniques result in a significant nitrogen loss that must be replaced with a balanced nutrition regimen (Grade 1C).

Early enteral nutrition should be started as soon as possible in the presence of viable and functional gastrointestinal tract (Grade 1C).

Enteral nutrition should be delayed in patients with an intestinal tract in discontinuity (temporarily closed loops), or in situations of a high output fistula with no possibility to obtain feeding access distal to the fistula or with signs of intestinal obstruction (Grade 2C)

Oral feeding is not contraindicated and should be used where possible (Grade 2C).

Malnutrition is a risk factor for poor outcomes [76]. Critically ill patients with OA are in a hyper-catabolic state with an estimated nitrogen loss of almost 2 g/L of abdominal fluid output. Abdominal fluid evacuation is to be measured in order to adjust nutritional integrations [77]. In case of EAF, nitrogen loss greatly increases. Parenteral nutrition should be started as soon as possible. Once the resuscitation is almost complete and the GI tract is viable, enteral nutrition (EN) should be started. Relative contraindication to EN is a viable bowel shorter than 75 cm [78].

Polymeric formula supplying a daily intake of 20- to 30-kcal/kg non-protein calories with 1.5- to 2.5-g/kg proteins is usually sufficient to maintain a positive nitrogen balance.

EN starting within the first 24–48 h improves wound healing and fascial closure rate, decreases catabolism, reduces pneumonia and fistula rate, preserves GI tract integrity, and finally reduces complications, length of hospital stay, and costs [79–81]. Compared to prolonged total parenteral nutrition, early EN decreases septic complications especially in abdominal trauma and traumatic brain injuries [3, 79, 82, 83].

Patient mobilization

No recommendations can be made about early mobilization of patients with open abdomen (Not graded).

No definite evidence exists regarding the optimal timing for mobilization of patients with OA [84]. Prolonged bed rest is associated with a significant increase in morbidity. Mobilization occurring within the first 2-5 days of ICU admission is defined "early" [85] and it is associated with positive effects on outcomes [86–90].

OA patients with NPWT may be "early" mobilized by active or passive transfer thanks to the provisional abdominal wall function supplied by NPWT systems [3].

Definitive closure
Open abdomen definitive closure

Fascia and/or abdomen should be definitively closed as soon as possible (Grade 1C).

Early fascial and/or abdominal definitive closure should be the strategy for management of the open abdomen once any requirements for on-going resuscitation have ceased, the source control has been definitively reached, no concern regarding intestinal viability persist, no further surgical re-exploration is needed and there are no concerns for abdominal compartment syndrome (Grade 1B).

The priority in order to reduce mortality, complications, and length of stay linked to the OA should be the early definitive abdominal closure [10, 91, 92]. Major factors influencing early definitive closure are postoperative ICU management and the TAC technique [93]. Early fascial closure is commonly defined as occurring within 4–7 days from the index operation [21]. In contrast to trauma patients, those affected by abdominal sepsis usually experience a lower rate of early fascial closure [94] even though continuous fascial traction seems to increase this rate [95]. Fascial closure should be attempted as soon as the source of infection is controlled [96].

Solutions to definitively close an open abdomen
In case of prolonged OA, fascia retraction and large abdominal wall defects requiring complex abdominal wall reconstruction may occur. In contaminated fields, the complication risk in abdominal wall definitive closure is increased [92, 97–99].

Techniques used to definitively close the abdomen are principally divided into non-mesh and mesh mediated.

Non-mesh-mediated closure techniques

Primary fascia closure is the ideal solution to restore the abdominal closure (2A).

Component separation is an effective technique; however it should not be used for fascial temporary closure. It should be considered only for definitive closure (Grade 2C).

Planned ventral hernia (skin graft or skin closure only) remains an option for the complicated open abdomen (i.e. in the presence of entero-atmospheric fistula or in cases with a protracted open abdomen due to underlying diseases) or in those settings where no other alternatives are viable (Grade 2C)

Abdominal component separation should be considered an elective procedure for ventral hernia repair [100]. In fact, it should not be used during the OA management but reserved to the definitive closure interventions. At a delayed time point, very good results reaching up to 75% of fascial closure rate have been reported [101]. The separation of components can be approached anteriorly or posteriorly [102, 103].

Planned ventral hernia represents a valid alternative to cover abdominal viscera and to prevent EAF. In fact, in cases of persistent contamination, several comorbidities or in severely ill patients, with or without sufficient skin to cover the abdominal wall defect, delaying the eventual synthetic prosthetic reconstruction may be a safer option. The decision either to close the skin or to perform vascularized flaps, pedicled flaps in small-/mid-sized defects, or free flaps such as tensor fasciae latae for extensive thoraco-abdominal defects is usually taken, considering the wound conditions, the dimension of the skin defect, and the center facilities [13].

Mesh-mediated closure techniques

The use of synthetic mesh (polypropylene, polytetrafluoruroethylene (PTFE) and polyester products) as a fascial bridge should not be recommended in definitive closure interventions after open abdomen and should be placed only in patients without other alternatives (Grade 1B).

Biologic meshes are reliable for definitive abdominal wall reconstruction in the presence of a large wall defect, bacterial contamination, comorbidities and difficult wound healing (Grade 2B).

Non–cross-linked biologic meshes seem to be preferred in sublay position when the linea alba can be reconstructed. (Grade 2B).

Cross-linked biologic meshes in fascial-bridge position (no linea alba closure) maybe associated with less ventral hernia recurrence (Grade 2B).

NPWT can be used in combination with biologic mesh to facilitate granulation and skin closure (Grade 2B).

Several data exist regarding the abdominal wall closure after OA [104, 105]. Non-absorbable synthetic materials (i.e., polypropylene mesh) in a bridging position (i.e., no linea alba closure), where no native tissue protect viscera, may induce several local side effects (adhesions, erosions, and fistula formation) [106–111]. Synthetic meshes in contaminated fields are not recommended by guidelines in emergency abdominal wall reconstruction [112].

Biological prostheses (BP) were designed to perform as permanent surgical prosthesis in abdominal wall repair, minimizing mesh-related complications. Non-cross-linked biologic mesh is easily integrated, with reduced fibrotic reaction and lesser infection and removal rate [113].

BP can be used as a bridge for large abdominal wall defects [114–127]; however, the long-term outcome of a bridging non-cross-linked BP is laxity of the abdominal wall and a high rate of recurrent ventral hernia [113]. As a consequence, non-cross-linked BP should be used in a sublay position (i.e., with linea alba closure) and cross-linked ones should be preferred when the fascial bridge is needed [128–130]. BP could also tolerate adjunctive NPWT to facilitate wound healing, granulation, and skin closure [131–133].

Complication management

Preemptive measures to prevent entero-atmospheric fistula and frozen abdomen are imperative (i.e. early abdominal wall closure, bowel coverage with plastic sheets, omentum or skin, no direct application of synthetic prosthesis over bowel loops, no direct application of NPWT on the viscera and deep burying of intestinal anastomoses under bowel loops) (Grade 1C).

Entero-atmospheric fistula management should be tailored according to patient condition, fistula output and position and anatomical features (Grade 1C).

In the presence of entero-atmospheric fistula the caloric intake and protein demands are increased; the nitrogen balance should be evaluated and corrected and protein supplemented (Grade 1C).

Nutrition should be reviewed and optimized upon recognition of entero-atmospheric fistula (Grade 1C).

Entero-atmospheric fistula effluent isolation is essential for proper wound healing. Separating the wound into different compartments to facilitate the collection of fistula output is of paramount importance (Grade 2A).

In the presence of entero-atmospheric fistula in open abdomen, negative pressure wound therapy makes effluent isolation feasible and wound healing achievable (Grade 2A).

Definitive management of entero-atmospheric fistula should be delayed to after the patient has recovered and the wound completely healed (Grade 1C).

Risk factors for frozen abdomen and EAF in OA are delayed abdominal closure, non-protection of bowel loops during OA, presence of bowel injury and repairs or anastomosis, colon resection during DCS, the large fluid resuscitation volume (> 5 L/24 h), the presence of intra-abdominal sepsis/abscess, and the use of polypropylene mesh directly over the bowel [66, 134–139]. All risk factors often linked as a "vicious cycle" may contribute to the development of frozen abdomen and EAF. Complications increase mortality, length of stays, and costs [140]. Some preemptive measures to prevent this complication are early abdominal wall closure, bowel coverage with plastic sheets, omentum or skin, no direct application of synthetic prosthesis on bowel, no direct application of NPWT on the viscera, and intestinal anastomosis deep buring under bowel loops [73, 141, 142]. EAF can be classified based on the output: low (< 200 mL/day), moderate (200–500 mL/day), and high (> 500 mL/day) [143]; usually, the greater the output, the higher the difficulty in managing the EAF [144, 145]. In EAF management, the definition of characteristics and anatomical features are extremely important in planning the best treatment [146]. The intra-abdominal situation can be classified according to the WSACS classification (Fig. 2) [147]. Nutrition plays a pivotal role in EAF management. While early EN improves outcomes [81, 148–151], it may increase EAF output even if it seems not to impair final outcomes [152, 153]. Spontaneous closure of an EAF is quite impossible; for this reason, the treatment should try to isolate the fistula effluent to allow granulation tissue formation around [3]. Many different effective techniques have been described with no definitive results [138, 144, 145, 154–157]. NPWT in all its variants is effective and the most accepted technique [3]. It often allows EAF isolation, adequate wound management, re-epithelization, and eventual subsequent skin graft with the final conversion of the EAF into a sort of enterostomy. EAF definitive treatment (i.e., fistula closure and abdominal wall reconstruction) should be postponed at least of 6 months and only after the patient and the wound healed completely [3].

Conclusions

Open abdomen in trauma and non-trauma patients is dramatically effective in facing the deranged

BJORK CLSSIFICATION 2009		BJORK CLASSIFICATION 2016	
GRADE	**DESCRIPTION**	**GRADE**	**DESCRIPTION**
1 A	Clean OA without adherence between bowel and abdominal wall or fixity	1 A	Clean OA without adherence between bowel and abdominal wall or fixity
B	Contaminated OA without adherence/fixity	B	Contaminated OA without adherence/fixity
		C	Enteric leak, no fixation
2 A	Clean OA developing adherence/fixity	2 A	Clean OA developing adherence/fixity
B	Contaminated OA developing adherence/fixity	B	Contaminated OA developing adherence/fixity
		C	Enteric leak, developing fixation
3 A	OA complicated by fistula formation	3 A	Clean, frozen abdomen
		B	Contaminated, frozen abdomen
4	Frozen OA with adherent/fixed bowel; unable to close surgically; with or without fistula	4	Established enteroatmospheric fistula, frozen abdomen

Fig. 2 Open Abdomen classification according to Björck et al. [147]

physiology of severe injuries or critical illness when no other perceived options exist. Its use remains very controversial and is a matter of great debate, as it is a non-anatomic situation with potential severe side effects and increased resource utilization. Moreover, the lack of definitive data demands carefully tailoring its use to each single patient, taking care to not over-use it. Abdominal closure attempt should be done as soon as the patient can physiologically tolerate it. All possible precautions should be implemented to minimize complications. Results improve proportionate to the clinicians' team's experience with the intricacies of open abdomen management.

Abbreviations

AAST: American Association for the Surgery of Trauma; ACS: Abdominal compartment syndrome; AP: Acute pancreatitis; CO: Cardiac output; DCM: Damage control management; DCR: Damage control resuscitation; DCS: Damage control surgery; EAF: Entero-atmospheric fistula; EN: Enteral nutrition; EVAR: Endovascular repair; GRADE: Grading of Recommendations Assessment, Development and Evaluation; IAH: Intra-abdominal hypertension; IAP: Intra-abdominal pressure; INR: International normalized ratio; MAP: Mean arterial pressure; MOF: Multiple organ failure; NPWT: Negative pressure wound therapy; OA: Open abdomen procedure; PTFE: Polytetrafluoruroethylene; rAAA: Ruptured abdominal aortic aneurysm; RCT: Randomized controlled trial; TAC: Temporal abdominal closure; TEG: Thromboelastography; TPN: Parenteral nutrition; WSACS: World Society Abdominal Compartment Syndrome; WSES: World Society of Emergency Surgery

Acknowledgements

Special thanks to Ms. Franca Boschini (Bibliographer, Medical Library, Papa Giovanni XXIII Hospital, Bergamo, Italy) for the precious bibliographical work.

Funding

None

Authors' contributions

FCo, DR, LA, RI, EG, YK, EEM, RC, AWK, BMP, GM, MCe, FMA-Z, MSa, GV, GPF, AL, MTol, JG, TR, RM, MB, BS, VK, MM, VA, AP, ZD, MSu, SDS, IM, KS, WB, PFe, NP, PMo, RMM, FS, TMV, TS, OC, SC, JLK, ML, JAMH, HFL, MCh, CA, CB, TH, BDS, PMa, VR, NDA, KK, ZJB, PFu, MTom, RL, NN, DW, LH, KI, AH, YKC, CAO, SR, CAG, MDM, IW, ACM, KB, LN, and FCa contributed to the manuscript conception and draft, critically revised the manuscript, contributed with the important scientific knowledge, and gave final approval of the manuscript.

Competing interests

The authors declare that they have no competing interests.

Author details

[1]General Emergency and Trauma Surgery, Bufalini Hospital, Viale Giovanni Ghirotti, 286, 47521 Cesena, Italy. [2]Department of Surgery, Foothills Medical Centre, Calgary, Canada. [3]Virginia Commonwealth University, Richmond, VA, USA. [4]ICU Department, Bufalini Hospital, Cesena, Italy. [5]Division of General Surgery, Rambam Health Care Campus, Haifa, Israel. [6]Trauma Surgery, Denver Health, Denver, CO, USA. [7]Department of Surgery, UC San Diego Health System, San Diego, USA. [8]Faculdade de Ciências Médicas (FCM)–Unicamp Campinas, Campinas, SP, Brazil. [9]Department of Surgery, College of Medicine and Health Sciences, UAE University, Al-Ain, United Arab Emirates. [10]Department of Surgery, Macerata Hospital, Macerata, Italy. [11]Department of Trauma, Emergency Surgery and Surgical Critical Care, Massachusetts General Hospital, Boston, MA, USA. [12]Second Department of Surgery, Meilahti Hospital, Helsinki, Finland. [13]Trauma and Acute Care Surgery and Surgical Critical Care Trauma, Department of Surgery, University of California, Davis, USA. [14]General and Emergency Surgery, McGill University Health Centre, Montréal, QC, Canada. [15]Department of Surgery, Harborview Medical Centre, Seattle, USA. [16]General Surgery Department, Hadassah Medical Centre, Jerusalem, Israel. [17]First Clinic of General Surgery, University Hospital/UMBAL/St George Plovdiv, Plovdiv, Bulgaria. [18]General Surgery, Mozir Hospital, Mozir City, Belarus. [19]ICU and High Care Burn Unit, Ziekenhius Netwerk Antwerpen, Antwerpen, Belgium. [20]Department of Surgery, Trauma and Surgical Services, University of Pittsburgh School of Medicine, Pittsburgh, USA. [21]Department of Surgery, Tbilisi State Medical University, Kipshidze Central University Hospital, Tbilisi, Georgia. [22]General Surgery Department, Letterkenny Hospital, Letterkenny, Ireland. [23]Addenbrooke's Hospital, Cambridge, UK. [24]Klinik für Unfall-, Hand- und Wiederherstellungschirurgie Universitätsklinikum Goethe-Universität Frankfurt, Frankfurt, Germany. [25]Department of Clinical Medicine, University of Bergen, Bergen, Norway. [26]Department of Gastrointestinal Surgery, Stavanger University Hospital, Stavanger, Norway. [27]Acute Care Surgery, The Queen's Medical Center, Honolulu, HI, USA. [28]General and Trauma Surgery Department, London Health Sciences Centre, Victoria Hospital, London, ON, Canada. [29]Département d'Anesthésie-Réanimation, CHU Bichat Claude-Bernard-HUPNVS, Assistance Publique-Hôpitaux de Paris, University Denis Diderot, Paris, France. [30]ICU Department, Sant'Orsola-Malpighi University Hospital, Bologna, Italy. [31]ICU Department, Papa Giovanni XXIII Hospital, Bergamo, Italy. [32]Surgery Department, University of Maryland School of Medicine, Baltimore, MD, USA. [33]Emergency and Trauma Surgery Department, Niguarda Hospital, Milano, Italy. [34]General Surgery Department, Assuta Medical Centers, Tel Aviv, Israel. [35]General Surgery, "General Calixto García", Habana Medicine University, Havana, Cuba. [36]General Surgery, Medical Faculty "General Calixto Garcia", Habana Medicine University, Havana, Cuba. [37]Division of Trauma, Department of Surgery, Far-Eastern Memorial Hospital, New Taipei City, Taiwan, Republic of China. [38]Clin. Univ. de Chirurgie Digestive et de l'Urgence, CHUGA-CHU Grenoble Alpes UGA-Université Grenoble Alpes, Grenoble, France. [39]General and Emergency Surgery Department, Empoli Hospital, Empoli, Italy. [40]Department of Cardiothoracic and Vascular Surgery, Örebro University Hospital and Örebro University, Orebro, Sweden. [41]General Surgery, Perpignan Hospital, Perpignan, France. [42]Pediatric Trauma Service, Massachusetts General Hospital, Boston, MA, USA. [43]General and Emergency Surgery, Sergei Kirov Military Academy, Saint Petersburg, Russia. [44]Unit of Digestive Surgery, HPB Surgery and Liver Transplant, Henri Mondor Hospital, Créteil, France. [45]Department of Primary Care and Emergency Medicine, Kyoto University Graduate School of Medicine, Kyoto, Japan. [46]Department of Traumatology, John Hunter Hospital and University of Newcastle, Newcastle, NSW, Australia. [47]General Surgery Department, Westchester Medical Center, Westchester, NY, USA. [48]Department of Surgery, University of KwaZulu-Natal, Durban, South Africa. [49]Department of General Surgery, Royal Perth Hospital, The University of Western Australia & The University of Newcastle, Perth, Australia. [50]Trauma Unit, Helsinki University Hospital, Helsinki, Finland. [51]Division of Trauma and Critical Care, LAC+USC Medical Center, University of Southern California, California, Los Angeles, USA. [52]General and Thoracic Surgery, Giessen Hospital, Giessen, Germany. [53]Acute Care Surgery and Traumatology, Taipei Medical University Hospital, Taipei City, Taiwan, Republic of China. [54]Trauma and Acute Care Surgery, Fundacion Valle del Lili, Cali, Colombia. [55]Trauma and Acute Care Service, St Michael's Hospital, Toronto, ON, Canada. [56]Hospital Universitário Terezinha de Jesus, Faculdade de Ciências Médicas e da Saúde de Juiz de Fora (SUPREMA), Juiz de Fora, Brazil. [57]Trauma, Acute Care Surgery, Medical College of Wisconsin/Froedtert Trauma Center, Milwaukee, WI, USA. [58]Department of Surgery, Sheri-Kashmir Institute of Medical Sciences, Srinagar, India. [59]Department of Surgery and Obs/Gyn, Faculty of Health Sciences, University of Buea, Buea, Cameroon. [60]Milpark Hospital Academic Trauma Center, University of the Witwatersrand, Johannesburg, South Africa. [61]Acute Care Surgery, Department of Surgery, University of Michigan Health System, Ann Arbor, MI, USA. [62]Emergency and Trauma Surgery, Parma Maggiore Hospital, Parma, Italy.

References

1. Bailey J, Shapiro MJ. Abdominal compartment syndrome. Crit Care. 2000;4:23–9.
2. Sartelli M, Abu-Zidan FM, Ansaloni L, Bala M, Beltrán MA, Biffl WL, et al. The role of the open abdomen procedure in managing severe abdominal sepsis: WSES position paper. World J Emerg Surg. 2015;10:35.
3. Coccolini F, Montori G, Ceresoli M, Catena F, Moore EE, Ivatury R, et al. The role of open abdomen in non-trauma patient: WSES Consensus Paper. World J Emerg Surg. 2017;12:39.
4. Kirkpatrick AW, Roberts DJ, De Waele J, Jaeschke R, Malbrain MLNG, De Keulenaer B, et al. Intra-abdominal hypertension and the abdominal compartment syndrome: updated consensus definitions and clinical practice guidelines from the World Society of the Abdominal Compartment Syndrome. Intensive Care Med. 2013;39:1190–206.
5. Leppäniemi AK. Laparotomy: why and when? Crit Care. 2010;14:216.
6. Coccolini F, Biffl W, Catena F, Ceresoli M, Chiara O, Cimbanassi S, et al. The open abdomen, indications, management and definitive closure. World J Emerg Surg. 2015;10:32.
7. Sartelli M, Catena F, Ansaloni L, Coccolini F, Corbella D, Moore EE, et al. Complicated intra-abdominal infections worldwide: the definitive data of the CIAOW study. World J Emerg Surg. 2014;9:37.
8. Oxford centre for evidence-based medicine - levels of evidence (March 2009) - CEBM [Internet]. Available from: http://www.cebm.net/oxford-centre-evidence-based-medicine-levels-evidence-march-2009/
9. Dubose JJ, Scalea TM, Holcomb JB, Shrestha B, Okoye O, Inaba K, et al. Open abdominal management after damage-control laparotomy for trauma: a prospective observational American Association for the Surgery of Trauma multicenter study. J Trauma Acute Care Surg. 2013;74:113-20-2.
10. Regner JL, Kobayashi L, Coimbra R. Surgical strategies for management of the open abdomen. World J Surg. 2012;36:497–510.
11. Diaz JJ, Cullinane DC, Dutton WD, Jerome R, Bagdonas R, Bilaniuk JW, et al. The management of the open abdomen in trauma and emergency general surgery: part 1-damage control. J Trauma. 2010;68:1425–38.
12. Teixeira PGR, Salim A, Inaba K, Brown C, Browder T, Margulies D, et al. A prospective look at the current state of open abdomens. Am Surg. 2008;74:891–7.
13. Chiara O, Cimbanassi S, Biffl W, Leppaniemi A, Henry S, Scalea TM, et al. International consensus conference on open abdomen in trauma. J Trauma Acute Care Surg. 2016;80:173–83.
14. Girard E, Abba J, Boussat B, Trilling B, Mancini A, Bouzat P, Létoublon C, Chirica M, Arvieux C. Damage control surgery for non-traumatic abdominal emergencies. World J Surg. 2017 Sep 25. https://doi.org/10.1007/s00268-017-4262-6. [Epub ahead of print].
15. Roberts DJ, Bobrovitz N, Zygun D a, Ball CG, Kirkpatrick a W, Faris PD, et al. Indications for use of damage control surgery and damage control interventions in civilian trauma patients: a scoping review. J Trauma Acute Care Surg. 2015;78:1187–96.
16. Roberts DJ, Bobrovitz N, Zygun DA, Ball CG, Kirkpatrick AW, Faris PD, et al. Indications for use of damage control surgery in civilian trauma patients: a content analysis and expert appropriateness rating study. Ann Surg. 2016;263:1018–27.
17. Roberts DJ, Zygun DA, Faris PD, Ball CG, Kirkpatrick AW, Stelfox HT, et al. Opinions of practicing surgeons on the appropriateness of published indications for use of damage control surgery in trauma patients: an international cross-sectional survey. J Am Coll Surg. 2016;223:515–29.
18. Holodinsky JK, Roberts DJ, Ball CG, Blaser AR, Starkopf J, Zygun DA, et al. Risk factors for intra-abdominal hypertension and abdominal compartment syndrome among adult intensive care unit patients: a systematic review and meta-analysis. Crit Care. 2013;17:R249.
19. Moore LJ, Moore FA. Epidemiology of sepsis in surgical patients. Surg Clin North Am. 2012;92:1425–43.
20. Weber DG, Bendinelli C, Balogh ZJ. Damage control surgery for abdominal emergencies. Br J Surg. 2014;101:e109–18.
21. Ordóñez CA, Sánchez ÁI, Pineda JA, Badiel M, Mesa R, Cardona U, et al. Deferred primary anastomosis versus diversion in patients with severe secondary peritonitis managed with staged laparotomies. World J Surg. 2010;34:169–76.
22. Plantefeve G, Hellmann R, Pajot O, Thirion M, Bleichner G, Mentec H. Abdominal compartment syndrome and intraabdominal sepsis: two of the same kind? Acta Clin Belg. 2007;62:162–7.
23. Rubenstein C, Bietz G, Davenport DL, Winkler M, Endean ED. Abdominal compartment syndrome associated with endovascular and open repair of ruptured abdominal aortic aneurysms. J Vasc Surg. 2015;61:648–54.
24. Reite A, Soreide K, Ellingsen CL, Kvaløy JT, Vetrhus M. Epidemiology of ruptured abdominal aortic aneurysms in a well-defined Norwegian population with trends in incidence, intervention rate, and mortality. J Vasc Surg. 2015;61:1168–74.
25. Ersryd S, Djavani-Gidlund K, Wanhainen A, Björck M. Abdominal compartment syndrome after surgery for abdominal aortic aneurysm: a nationwide population based study. Eur J Vasc Endovasc Surg. 2016;52:158–65.
26. Björck M. Management of the tense abdomen or difficult abdominal closure after operation for ruptured abdominal aortic aneurysms. Semin Vasc Surg. 2012;25:35–8.
27. Bala M, Kashuk J, Moore EE, Kluger Y, Biffl W, Gomes CA, et al. Acute mesenteric ischemia: guidelines of the World Society of Emergency Surgery. World J Emerg Surg. 2017;12:38.
28. Acosta S, Wanhainen A, Bjorck M. Temporary abdominal closure after abdominal aortic aneurysm repair: a systematic review of contemporary observational studies. Eur J Vasc Endovasc Surg. 2016;51:371–8.
29. Kougias P, Lau D, El Sayed HF, Zhou W, Huynh TT, Lin PH. Determinants of mortality and treatment outcome following surgical interventions for acute mesenteric ischemia. J Vasc Surg Off Publ Soc Vasc Surg [and] Int Soc Cardiovasc Surgery, North Am Chapter. 2007;46:467–74.
30. Tilsed JVT, Casamassima A, Kurihara H, Mariani D, Martinez I, Pereira J, et al. ESTES guidelines: acute mesenteric ischaemia. Eur J Trauma Emerg Surg. 2016;42:253–70.
31. Bruns BR, Ahmad SA, O'Meara L, Tesoriero R, Lauerman M, Klyushnenkova E, et al. Nontrauma open abdomens: a prospective observational study. J Trauma Acute Care Surg. 2016;80:631–6.
32. Schermerhorn ML, Giles KA, Hamdan AD, Wyers MC, Pomposelli FB. Mesenteric revascularization: management and outcomes in the United States, 1988-2006. J Vasc Surg. NIH Public Access. 2009;50:341–348.e1.
33. Banks PA, Bollen TL, Dervenis C, Gooszen HG, Johnson CD, Sarr MG, et al. Classification of acute pancreatitis—2012: revision of the Atlanta classification and definitions by international consensus. Gut. 2013;62:102–11.
34. Halonen KI, Pettilä V, Leppäniemi AK, Kemppainen E a, Puolakkainen P a, Haapiainen RK. Multiple organ dysfunction associated with severe acute pancreatitis. Crit Care Med. 2002;30:1274–9.
35. Buter A, Imrie CW, Carter CR, Evans S, McKay CJ. Dynamic nature of early organ dysfunction determines outcome in acute pancreatitis. Br J Surg. 2002;89:298–302.
36. Mofidi R, Duff MD, Wigmore SJ, Madhavan KK, Garden OJ, Parks RW. Association between early systemic inflammatory response, severity of multiorgan dysfunction and death in acute pancreatitis. Br J Surg. 2006;93:738–44.
37. Petrov MS, Shanbhag S, Chakraborty M, Phillips ARJ, Windsor JA. Organ failure and infection of pancreatic necrosis as determinants of mortality in patients with acute pancreatitis. Gastroenterology. 2010;139:813–20.
38. De Waele JJ, Leppäniemi AK. Intra-abdominal hypertension in acute pancreatitis. World J Surg. 2009;33:1128–33.
39. Mentula P, Hienonen P, Kemppainen E, Puolakkainen P, Leppäniemi A. Surgical decompression for abdominal compartment syndrome in severe acute pancreatitis. Arch Surg. 2010;145:764–9.
40. Besselink MG, Van Santvoort HC, Boermeester MA, Nieuweohuijs VB, Van Goor H, Dejong CHC, et al. Timing and impact of infections in acute pancreatitis. Br J Surg. 2009;96:267–73.
41. van Santvoort HC, Besselink MG, Bakker OJ, Hofker HS, Boermeester M a, Dejong CH, et al. A step-up approach or open necrosectomy for necrotizing pancreatitis. N Engl J Med. 2010;362:1491–502.
42. Balogh Z, Moore FA, Moore EE, Biffl WL. Secondary abdominal compartment syndrome: a potential threat for all trauma clinicians. Injury. 2007;38:272–9.
43. Biffl WL, Moore EE, Burch JM, Offner PJ, Franciose RJ, Johnson JL. Secondary abdominal compartment syndrome is a highly lethal event. Am J Surg. 2001;182:645–8.
44. Holcomb JB, Tilley BC, Baraniuk S, Fox EE, Wade CE, Podbielski JM, et al. Transfusion of plasma, platelets, and red blood cells in a 1:1:1 vs a 1:1:2 ration and mortality in patients with severe trauma. JAMA. 2015;313:471–82.
45. Sugrue M, Bauman A, Jones F, Bishop G, Flabouris A, Parr M, et al. Clinical examination is an inaccurate predictor of intraabdominal pressure. World J Surg. 2002;26:1428–31.

46. Coccolini F, Montori G, Ceresoli M, Catena F, Ivatury R, Sugrue M, et al. IROA: International Register of Open Abdomen, preliminary results. World J Emerg Surg. 2017;12:10.

47. Rotondo MF, Zonies DH. The damage control sequence and underlying logic. Surg Clin North Am. 1997;77:761–77.

48. Sagraves SG, Toschlog EA, Rotondo MF. Damage control surgery—the intensivist's role. J Intensive Care Med. 2006;21:5–16.

49. Chabot E, Nirula R. Open abdomen critical care management principles: resuscitation, fluid balance, nutrition, and ventilator management. Trauma Surg Acute Care Open. BMJ Specialist Journals. 2017;2:e000063.

50. Rohrer MJ, Natale AM. Effect of hypothermia on the coagulation cascade. Crit Care Med. 1992;20:1402–5.

51. Davenport R, Khan S. Management of major trauma haemorrhage: treatment priorities and controversies. Br J Haematol. 2011;155:537–48.

52. Abramson D, Scalea TM, Hitchcock R, Trooskin SZ, Henry SM, Greenspan J. Lactate clearance and survival following injury. J Trauma. 1993;35:584-8-9.

53. Davenport R. Pathogenesis of acute traumatic coagulopathy. Transfusion. 2013;53:23S–7S.

54. Jurkovich GJ, Greiser WB, Luterman A, Curreri PW. Hypothermia in trauma victims: an ominous predictor of survival. J Trauma. 1987;27:1019–24.

55. Harvin JA, Mims MM, Duchesne JC, Cox CS, Wade CE, Holcomb JB, et al. Chasing 100%: the use of hypertonic saline to improve early, primary fascial closure after damage control laparotomy. J Trauma Acute Care Surg. 2013;74:426-30-2.

56. van Rooijen SJ, Huisman D, Stuijvenberg M, Stens J, Roumen RMH, Daams F, et al. Intraoperative modifiable risk factors of colorectal anastomotic leakage: why surgeons and anesthesiologists should act together. Int J Surg. 2016;36:183–200.

57. Fischer PE, Nunn AM, Wormer BA, Christmas AB, Gibeault LA, Green JM, et al. Vasopressor use after initial damage control laparotomy increases risk for anastomotic disruption in the management of destructive colon injuries. Am J Surg. 2013;206:900–3.

58. Cheatham ML, Safcsak K, Block EF, Nelson LD. Preload assessment in patients with an open abdomen. J Trauma. 1999;46:16–22.

59. Ghneim MH, Regner JL, Jupiter DC, Kang F, Bonner GL, Bready MS, et al. Goal directed fluid resuscitation decreases time for lactate clearance and facilitates early fascial closure in damage control surgery. Am J Surg. 2013;206:995-9-1000.

60. Finfer S, Bellomo R, Boyce N, French J, Myburgh J, Norton R, et al. A comparison of albumin and saline for fluid resuscitation in the intensive care unit. N Engl J Med. 2004;350:2247–56.

61. Huang Q, Zhao R, Yue C, Wang W, Zhao Y, Ren J, et al. Fluid volume overload negatively influences delayed primary facial closure in open abdomen management. J Surg Res. 2014;187:122–7.

62. Patel NY, Cogbill TH, Kallies KJ, Mathiason MA. Temporary abdominal closure: long-term outcomes. J Trauma. 2011;70:769–74.

63. Coccolini F, Catena F, Montori G, Ceresoli M, Manfredi R, Nita GE, et al. IROA: the International Register of Open Abdomen.: an international effort to better understand the open abdomen: call for participants. World J Emerg Surg. 2015;10:37.

64. Smith JW, Matheson PJ, Franklin GA, Harbrecht BG, Richardson JD, Garrison RN. Randomized controlled trial evaluating the efficacy of peritoneal resuscitation in the management of trauma patients undergoing damage control surgery. J Am Coll Surg. 2017;224:396–404.

65. Sartelli M, Chichom-Mefire A, Labricciosa FM, Hardcastle T, Abu-Zidan FM, Adesunkanmi AK, et al. The management of intra-abdominal infections from a global perspective: 2017 WSES guidelines for management of intra-abdominal infections. World J Emerg Surg. 2017;12:29.

66. Atema JJ, Gans SL, Boermeester MA. Systematic review and meta-analysis of the open abdomen and temporary abdominal closure techniques in non-trauma patients. World J Surg. 2015;39:912–25.

67. Karmali S, Evans D, Laupland KB, Findlay C, Ball CG, Bergeron E, et al. To close or not to close, that is one of the questions? Perceptions of Trauma Association of Canada surgical members on the management of the open abdomen. J Trauma. 2006;60:287–93.

68. Kirkpatrick AW, Laupland KB, Karmali S, Bergeron E, Stewart TC, Findlay C, et al. Spill your guts! Perceptions of Trauma Association of Canada member surgeons regarding the open abdomen and the abdominal compartment syndrome. J Trauma. 2006;60:279–86.

69. Pommerening MJ, Dubose JJ, Zielinski MD, Phelan HA, Scalea TM, Inaba K, et al. Time to first take-back operation predicts successful primary fascial closure in patients undergoing damage control laparotomy. Surg (United States). 2014;156:431–8.

70. Singer M, Deutschman CS, Seymour CW, Shankar-Hari M, Annane D, Bauer M, et al. The third international consensus definitions for sepsis and septic shock (sepsis-3). JAMA. 2016;315:801–10.

71. Emr B, Sadowsky D, Azhar N, Gatto LA, An G, Nieman GF, et al. Removal of inflammatory ascites is associated with dynamic modification of local and systemic inflammation along with prevention of acute lung injury: in vivo and in silico studies. Shock. 2014;41:317–23.

72. Kubiak BD, Albert SP, Gatto L a, Snyder KP, Maier KG, Vieau CJ, et al. Peritoneal negative pressure therapy prevents multiple organ injury in a chronic porcine sepsis and ischemia/reperfusion model. Shock. 2010;34:525–34.

73. Cheatham ML, Demetriades D, Fabian TC, Kaplan MJ, Miles WS, Schreiber MA, et al. Prospective study examining clinical outcomes associated with a negative pressure wound therapy system and Barker's vacuum packing technique. World J Surg. 2013;37:2018–30.

74. Kirkpatrick AW, Roberts DJ, Faris PD, Ball CG, Kubes P, Tiruta C, et al. Active negative pressure peritoneal therapy after abbreviated laparotomy: the intraperitoneal vacuum randomized controlled trial. Ann Surg. 2015;262:38–46.

75. Wang J, Kubes P. A reservoir of mature cavity macrophages that can rapidly invade visceral organs to affect tissue repair. Cell. 2016;165:668–78.

76. Giner M, Laviano A, Meguid MM, Gleason JR. In 1995 a correlation between malnutrition and poor outcome in critically ill patients still exists. Nutrition. 1996;12:23–9.

77. Cheatham ML, Safcsak K, Brzezinski SJ, Lube MW. Nitrogen balance, protein loss, and the open abdomen. Crit Care Med. 2007;35:127–31.

78. Majercik S, Kinikini M, White T. Enteroatmospheric fistula: from soup to nuts. Nutr Clin Pract. 2012;27:507–12.

79. Collier B, Guillamondegui O, Cotton B, Donahue R, Conrad A, Groh K, et al. Feeding the open abdomen. JPEN J Parenter Enteral Nutr. 2007;31:410–5.

80. Cothren CC, Moore EE, Ciesla DJ, Johnson JL, Moore JB, Haenel JB, et al. Postinjury abdominal compartment syndrome does not preclude early enteral feeding after definitive closure. Am J Surg. 2004;188:653–8.

81. Dissanaike S, Pham T, Shalhub S, Warner K, Hennessy L, Moore EE, et al. Effect of immediate enteral feeding on trauma patients with an open abdomen: protection from nosocomial infections. J Am Coll Surg. 2008; 207:690–7.

82. Marik PE, Zaloga GP. Meta-analysis of parenteral nutrition versus enteral nutrition in patients with acute pancreatitis. BMJ. 2004;328:1407–10.

83. McClave SA, Heyland DK. The physiologic response and associated clinical benefits from provision of early enteral nutrition. Nutr Clin Pract. 2009;24:305–15.

84. Open Abdomen Advisory Panel, Campbell A, Chang M, Fabian T, Franz M, Kaplan M, et al. Management of the open abdomen: from initial operation to definitive closure. Am Surg. 2009;75:S1–22.

85. Hodgson CL, Berney S, Harrold M, Saxena M. Clinical review: early patient mobilization in the ICU. Crit Care. 2013;17:207.

86. Truong A, Fan E, Brower R, Needham D. Bench-to-bedside review: mobilizing patients in the intensive care unit—from pathophysiology to clinical trials. Crit Care. 2009;13:216.

87. Pavy-Le Traon A, Heer M, Narici MV, Rittweger J, Vernikos J. From space to Earth: advances in human physiology from 20 years of bed rest studies (1986-2006). Eur J Appl Physiol. 2007;101:143–94.

88. Herridge MS. Building consensus on ICU-acquired weakness. Intensive Care Med. 2009;35:1–3.

89. Cuthbertson BH, Roughton S, Jenkinson D, Maclennan G, Vale L. Quality of life in the five years after intensive care: a cohort study. Crit Care. 2010;14:R6.

90. Burtin C, Clerckx B, Robbeets C, Ferdinande P, Langer D, Troosters T, et al. Early exercise in critically ill patients enhances short-term functional recovery. Crit Care Med. 2009;37:2499–505.

91. Demetriades D, Salim A. Management of the open abdomen. Surg Clin North Am. 2014;94:131–53.

92. Choi JJ, Palaniappa NC, Dallas KB, Rudich TB, Colon MJ, Divino CM. Use of mesh during ventral hernia repair in clean-contaminated and contaminated cases: outcomes of 33,832 cases. Ann Surg. 2012;255:176–80.

93. Godat L, Kobayashi L, Costantini T, Coimbra R. Abdominal damage control surgery and reconstruction: world society of emergency surgery position paper. World J Emerg Surg. 2013;8:53.

94. Paul JS, Ridolfi TJ. A case study in intra-abdominal sepsis. Surg Clin North Am. 2012;92:1661–77.

95. Tolonen M, Mentula P, Sallinen V, Rasilainen S, Bäcklund M, Leppäniemi A. Open abdomen with vacuum-assisted wound closure and mesh-mediated fascial traction in patients with complicated diffuse secondary peritonitis. J Trauma Acute Care Surg. 2017;82:1100–5.

96. Lambertz A, Mihatsch C, Röth A, Kalverkamp S, Eickhoff R, Neumann UP, et al. Fascial closure after open abdomen: initial indication and early revisions are decisive factors—a retrospective cohort study. Int J Surg. 2015;13:12–6.

97. Rasilainen SK, Juhani MP, Kalevi LA. Microbial colonization of open abdomen in critically ill surgical patients. World J Emerg Surg. 2015;10:25.

98. Leber GE, Garb JL, Alexander a I, Reed WP. Long-term complications associated with prosthetic repair of incisional hernias. Arch Surg. 1998;133:378–82.

99. Mathes SJ, Steinwald PM, Foster RD, Hoffman WY, Anthony JP. Complex abdominal wall reconstruction: a comparison of flap and mesh closure. Ann Surg. 2000;232:586–96.

100. Ramirez OM, Ruas E, Dellon AL. "Components separation" method for closure of abdominal-wall defects: an anatomic and clinical study. Plast Reconstr Surg. 1990;86:519–26.

101. Rasilainen SK, Mentula PJ, Leppäniemi AK. Components separation technique is feasible for assisting delayed primary fascial closure of open abdomen. Scand J Surg. 2016;105:17–21.

102. de Vries Reilingh TS, van Goor H, Charbon JA, Rosman C, Hesselink EJ, van der Wilt GJ, et al. Repair of giant midline abdominal wall hernias: "components separation technique" versus prosthetic repair : interim analysis of a randomized controlled trial. World J Surg. Springer. 2007;31:756–63.

103. Yegiyants S, Tam M, Lee DJ, Abbas MA. Outcome of components separation for contaminated complex abdominal wall defects. Hernia. 2012;16:41–5.

104. Sharrock AE, Barker T, Yuen HM, Rickard R, Tai N. Management and closure of the open abdomen after damage control laparotomy for trauma. A systematic review and meta-analysis. Injury Elsevier Ltd. 2015;47:296–306.

105. Atema JJ, de Vries FEE, Boermeester MA. Systematic review and meta-analysis of the repair of potentially contaminated and contaminated abdominal wall defects. Am J Surg Elsevier Inc. 2016;212:982–95.

106. Dinsmore RC, Calton WC, Harvey SB, Blaney MW. Prevention of adhesions to polypropylene mesh in a traumatized bowel model. J Am Coll Surg. 2000; 191:131–6.

107. van't Riet M, de Vos van Steenwijk PJ, Bonthuis F, Marquet RL, Steyerberg EW, Jeekel J, et al. Prevention of adhesion to prosthetic mesh: comparison of different barriers using an incisional hernia model. Ann Surg. 2003;237:123–8.

108. Konstantinovic ML, Lagae P, Zheng F, Verbeken EK, De Ridder D, Deprest JA. Comparison of host response to polypropylene and non-cross-linked porcine small intestine serosal-derived collagen implants in a rat model. BJOG An Int J Obstet Gynaecol. 2005;112:1554–60.

109. Fansler RF, Taheri P, Cullinane C, Sabates B, Flint LM. Polypropylene mesh closure of the complicated abdominal wound. Am J Surg. 1995;170:15–8.

110. Voyles CR, Richardson JD, Bland KI, Tobin GR, Flint LM, Polk HC. Emergency abdominal wall reconstruction with polypropylene mesh: short-term benefits versus long-term complications. Ann Surg. 1981;194:219–23.

111. Brown GL, Richardson JD, Malangoni MA, Tobin GR, Ackerman D, Polk HC. Comparison of prosthetic materials for abdominal wall reconstruction in the presence of contamination and infection. Ann Surg. 1985;201:705–11.

112. Sartelli M, Coccolini F, van Ramshorst GH, Campanelli G, Mandalà V, Ansaloni L, et al. WSES guidelines for emergency repair of complicated abdominal wall hernias. World J Emerg Surg. 2013;8:50.

113. Cornwell KG, Landsman A, James KS. Extracellular matrix biomaterials for soft tissue repair. Clin Podiatr Med Surg. 2009;26:507–23.

114. Badylak SF. Xenogeneic extracellular matrix as a scaffold for tissue reconstruction. Transpl Immunol. 2004;12:367–77.

115. Winters JC. InteXen tissue processing and laboratory study. Int Urogynecol J Pelvic Floor Dysfunct. 2006;17:S34–8.

116. Petter-Puchner AH, Dietz UA. Biological implants in abdominal wall repair. Br J Surg. 2013;100:987–8.

117. Montori G, Coccolini F, Manfredi R, Ceresoli M, Campanati L, Magnone S, et al. One year experience of swine dermal non-crosslinked collagen prostheses for abdominal wall repairs in elective and emergency surgery. World J Emerg Surg. 2015;10:28–35.

118. Primus FE, Harris HW. A critical review of biologic mesh use in ventral hernia repairs under contaminated conditions. Hernia. 2013;17:21–30.

119. Gurrado A, Franco IF, Lissidini G, Greco G, De Fazio M, Pasculli A, et al. Impact of pericardium bovine patch (Tutomesh®) on incisional hernia treatment in contaminated or potentially contaminated fields: retrospective comparative study. Hernia. 2015;19:259–66.

120. de Moya MA, Dunham M, Inaba K, Bahouth H, Alam HB, Sultan B, et al. Long-term outcome of acellular dermal matrix when used for large traumatic open abdomen. J Trauma Inj Infect Crit Care. 2008;65:349–53.

121. Ginting N, Tremblay L, Kortbeek JB. Surgisis® in the management of the complex abdominal wall in trauma: a case series and review of the literature. Injury. 2010;41:970–3.

122. Patton JH, Berry S, Kralovich KA. Use of human acellular dermal matrix in complex and contaminated abdominal wall reconstructions. Am J Surg. 2007;193:360–3.

123. Maurice SM, Skeete DA. Use of human acellular dermal matrix for abdominal wall reconstructions. Am J Surg. 2009;197:35–42.

124. Lin HJ, Spoerke N, Deveney C, Martindale R. Reconstruction of complex abdominal wall hernias using acellular human dermal matrix: a single institution experience. Am J Surg. 2009;197:599–603.

125. Diaz JJ, Conquest AM, Ferzoco SJ, Vargo D, Miller P, Wu Y-C, et al. Multi-institutional experience using human acellular dermal matrix for ventral hernia repair in a compromised surgical field. Arch Surg. 2009;144:209–15.

126. Lee EI, Chike-Obi CJ, Gonzalez P, Garza R, Leong M, Subramanian A, et al. Abdominal wall repair using human acellular dermal matrix: a follow-up study. Am J Surg. 2009;198:650–7.

127. Pomahac B, Aflaki P. Use of a non-cross-linked porcine dermal scaffold in abdominal wall reconstruction. Am J Surg. Elsevier Inc. 2010;199:22–7.

128. Chand B, Indeck M, Needleman B, Finnegan M, Van Sickle KR, Ystgaard B, et al. A retrospective study evaluating the use of Permacol™ surgical implant in incisional and ventral hernia repair. Int J Surg. Elsevier Ltd. 2014;12:296–303.

129. Holihan JL, Nguyen DH, Nguyen MT, Mo J, Kao LS, Liang MK. Mesh location in open ventral hernia repair: a systematic review and network meta-analysis. World J Surg. 2016;40:89–99.

130. Eriksson A, Rosenberg J, Bisgaard T. Surgical treatment for giant incisional hernia: a qualitative systematic review. Hernia. 2014;18:31–8.

131. Caviggioli F, Klinger FM, Lisa A, Maione L, Forcellini D, Vinci V, et al. Matching biological mesh and negative pressure wound therapy in reconstructing an open abdomen defect. Case Rep Med. Hindawi Publishing Corporation. 2014;2014:235930.

132. Dietz UA, Wichelmann C, Wunder C, Kauczok J, Spor L, Strauß A, et al. Early repair of open abdomen with a tailored two-component mesh and conditioning vacuum packing: a safe alternative to the planned giant ventral hernia. Hernia. 2012;16:451–60.

133. Rasilainen SK, Mentula PJ, Leppäniemi AK. Vacuum and mesh-mediated fascial traction for primary closure of the open abdomen in critically ill surgical patients. Br J Surg. 2012;99:1725–32.

134. Richter S, Dold S, Doberauer JP, Mai P, Schuld J. Negative pressure wound therapy for the treatment of the open abdomen and incidence of enteral fistulas: a retrospective bicentre analysis. Gastroenterol Res Pract. 2013;2013:6–11.

135. Bradley MJ, Dubose JJ, Scalea TM, Holcomb JB, Shrestha B, Okoye O, et al. Independent predictors of enteric fistula and abdominal sepsis after damage control laparotomy: results from the prospective AAST Open Abdomen registry. JAMA Surg. 2013;148:947–54.

136. Martinez JL, Luque-De-Leon E, Mier J, Blanco-Benavides R, Robledo F. Systematic management of postoperative enterocutaneous fistulas: factors related to outcomes. World J Surg. 2008;32:436–43.

137. Tavusbay C, Genc H, Cin N, Kar H, Kamer E, Atahan K, et al. Use of a vacuum-assisted closure system for the management of enteroatmospheric fistulae. Surg Today. Springer Japan. 2015;45:1102–11.

138. D'Hondt M, Devriendt D, Van Rooy F, Vansteenkiste F, D'Hoore A, Penninckx F, et al. Treatment of small-bowel fistulae in the open abdomen with topical negative-pressure therapy. Am J Surg. Elsevier Inc. 2011;202:e20–4.

139. Marinis A, Gkiokas G, Argyra E, Fragulidis G, Polymeneas G, Voros D. "Enteroatmospheric fistulae"—gastrointestinal openings in the open abdomen: a review and recent proposal of a surgical technique. Scand J Surg. 2013;102:61–8.

140. Teixeira PGR, Inaba K, Dubose J, Salim A, Brown C, Rhee P, et al. Enterocutaneous fistula complicating trauma laparotomy: a major resource burden. Am Surg. 2009;75:30–2.

141. Schecter WP, Ivatury RR, Rotondo MF, Hirshberg A. Open abdomen after trauma and abdominal sepsis: a strategy for management. J Am Coll Surg. 2006;203:390–6.

142. Carlson GL, Patrick H, Amin AI, McPherson G, MacLennan G, Afolabi E, et al. Management of the open abdomen. Ann Surg. 2013;257:1154–9.

143. Schecter WP, Hirshberg A, Chang DS, Harris HW, Napolitano LM, Wexner SD, et al. Enteric fistulas: principles of management. J Am Coll Surg. Elsevier Inc. 2009;209:484–91.

144. Di Saverio S, Tarasconi A, Inaba K, Navsaria P, Coccolini F, Costa Navarro D, et al. Open abdomen with concomitant enteroatmospheric fistula: attempt

to rationalize the approach to a surgical nightmare and proposal of a clinical algorithm. J Am Coll Surg. 2015;220:e23–33.

145. Di Saverio S, Tarasconi A, Walczak DA, Cirocchi R, Mandrioli M, Birindelli A, et al. Classification, prevention and management of entero-atmospheric fistula: a state-of-the-art review. Langenbeck's Arch Surg. 2016;401:1–13.

146. Polk TM, Schwab CW. Metabolic and nutritional support of the enterocutaneous fistula patient: a three-phase approach. World J Surg. 2012;36:524–33.

147. Björck M, Kirkpatrick AW, Cheatham M, Kaplan M, Leppäniemi A, de Waele JJ. Amended classification of the open abdomen. Scand J Surg. 2016;105:5–10.

148. Moore FA, Feliciano DV, Andrassy RJ, McArdle AH, Booth FV, Morgenstein-Wagner TB, et al. Early enteral feeding, compared with parenteral, reduces postoperative septic complications. The results of a meta-analysis. Ann Surg. Lippincott, Williams, and Wilkins. 1992;216:172–83.

149. Byrnes MC, Reicks P, Irwin E. Early enteral nutrition can be successfully implemented in trauma patients with an "open abdomen". Am J Surg. 2010;199:359–63.

150. Chung CK, Whitney R, Thompson CM, Pham TN, Maier RV, O'Keefe GE. Experience with an enteral-based nutritional support regimen in critically ill trauma patients. J Am Coll Surg. 2013;217:1108–17.

151. Parent BA, Mandell SP, Maier RV, Minei J, Sperry J, Moore EE. Safety of minimizing preoperative starvation in critically ill and intubated trauma patients. J Trauma Acute Care Surg. 2016;80:957–63.

152. Reinisch A, Liese J, Woeste G, Bechstein W, Habbe N. A retrospective, observational study of enteral nutrition in patients with enteroatmospheric fistulas. Ostomy Wound Manage. 2016;62:36–47.

153. Yin J, Wang J, Yao D, Zhang S, Mao Q, Kong W, et al. Is it feasible to implement enteral nutrition in patients with enteroatmospheric fistulae? A single-center experience. Nutr Clin Pract. 2014;29:656–61.

154. Navsaria PH, Bunting M, Omoshoro-Jones J, Nicol AJ, Kahn D. Temporary closure of open abdominal wounds by the modified sandwich-vacuum pack technique. Br J Surg. 2003;90:718–22.

155. Al-Khoury G, Kaufman D, Hirshberg A. Improved control of exposed fistula in the open abdomen. J Am Coll Surg. 2008;206:397–8.

156. Layton B, DuBose J, Nichols S, Connaughton J, Jones T, Pratt J. Pacifying the open abdomen with concomitant intestinal fistula: a novel approach. Am J Surg. Elsevier Inc. 2010;199:e48–50.

157. Rekstad LC, Wasmuth HH, Ystgaard B, Stornes T, Seternes A. Topical negative-pressure therapy for small bowel leakage in a frozen abdomen: a technical report. J Trauma Acute Care Surg. 2013;75:487–91.

29

Alcohol-related hospitalizations of adult motorcycle riders

Hang-Tsung Liu[1], Chi-Cheng Liang[1], Cheng-Shyuan Rau[2], Shiun-Yuan Hsu[1] and Ching-Hua Hsieh[1*]

Abstract

Objective: To provide an overview of the demographic characteristics of adult motorcycle riders with alcohol-related hospitalizations.

Methods: Data obtained from the Trauma Registry System were retrospectively reviewed for trauma admissions at a level I trauma center between January 1, 2009 and December 31, 2013. Out of 16,548 registered patients, detailed information was retrieved regarding 1,430 (8.64%) adult motorcycle riders who underwent a blood alcohol concentration (BAC) test. A BAC level of 50 mg/dL was defined as the cut-off value for alcohol intoxication.

Results: In this study, alcohol consumption was more frequently noted among male motorcycle riders, those aged 30–49 years, those who had arrived at the hospital in the evening or during the night, and those who did not wear a helmet. Alcohol consumption was associated with a lower percentage of sustained severe injury (injury severity score ≥25) and lower frequencies of specific body injuries, including cerebral contusion (0.6; 95% confidence interval [CI] = 0.42–0.80), lung contusion (0.5; 95% CI = 0.24–0.90), lumbar vertebral fracture (0.1; 95% CI = 0.01–0.80), humeral fracture (0.5; 95% CI = 0.27–0.90), and radial fracture (0.6; 95% CI = 0.40–0.89). In addition, alcohol-intoxicated motorcycle riders who wore helmets had significantly lower frequencies of cranial fracture (0.4; 95% CI = 0.29–0.67), epidural hematoma (0.5; 95% CI = 0.29–0.79), subdural hematoma (0.4; 95% CI = 0.28–0.64), subarachnoid hemorrhage (0.5; 95% CI = 0.32–0.72), and cerebral contusion (0.4; 95% CI = 0.25–0.78).

Conclusions: Motorcycle riders who consumed alcohol presented different characteristics and bodily injury patterns relative to sober patients, suggesting the importance of helmet use to decrease head injuries in alcohol-intoxicated riders.

Keywords: Trauma, Blood alcohol concentration (BAC), Injury severity score (ISS), Motorcycle, Helmet

Background

Motorcyclists are extremely vulnerable road participants who are exposed to severe and often fatal injuries. They are reportedly 8 times more likely to be injured per vehicle mile and 35 times more likely to die in a motor vehicle traffic crash than are automobile passengers [1]. These findings are of particular concern because the average age of motorcyclists is increasing [2]. In Taiwan, motorcyclists comprise a major portion of the trauma population; nearly 60% of all driving fatalities involve motorcycles [3]. Therefore, the identification of high-risk injury patterns may be beneficial in terms of improving

* Correspondence: m93chinghua@gmail.com
[1]Department of Trauma Surgery, Kaohsiung Chang Gung Memorial Hospital and Chang Gung University College of Medicine, No. 123, Ta-Pei Road, Niao-Song District, Kaohsiung City 833, Taiwan

the care and final outcomes of trauma patients admitted to hospitals [4].

Risky drinking has been consistently and strongly associated with higher frequencies of emergency department visits and hospitalizations [5,6]. In trauma patients, alcohol intoxication may lead to a higher preclinical mortality, impact of speed differences, and injury severity [7]. At lower blood alcohol concentration (BAC) levels, motorcyclists are more often involved in crashes than are car drivers [8]. Nearly 60% and 40% of car and motorcycle driver fatalities, respectively, involved alcohol consumption [9], which even at doses as low as 10–40 mg/dL can impair driving performance [10]. Furthermore, the risk of involvement in a fatal accident increases exponentially with the driver's BAC level [11].

However, Mann et al. explained that higher BAC levels might lead to less severe injuries without impacting mortality or the length of hospital stay (LOS) [12]. The odds ratio (OR) of collision between motorcyclists and unexpected pedestrians in an urban scenario increased 3-fold at a BAC of 0.02% relative to sobriety [13]. Furthermore, hazard perception ability, measured by responses to a peripheral detection task, was impaired following alcohol consumption [13]. Riding performance and hazard perception ability were shown to be impaired at a BAC of 0.05% [13]. Considering that almost all motorcycles are forbidden on highways in Taiwan and other Asian cities and that most traffic accidents occur in relatively crowded streets and at low velocities in these cities, the impact of alcohol intoxication on motorcycle injuries in Taiwan differs from that observed in Western countries and should be reevaluated. Therefore, the purpose of this epidemiologic study was to investigate the injury patterns, severity, and mortality of adult patients hospitalized for alcohol-related injuries sustained in motorcycle accidents at a level I trauma center in southern Taiwan.

Methods

Study design

The study was conducted at Kaohsiung Chang Gung Memorial Hospital, a 2400-bed facility and level I regional trauma center that provides care to trauma patients primarily from the southern region of Taiwan. The Chang Gung Medical Foundation Institutional Review Board approved this study prior to its commencement (approval number 103-3628B). A retrospective study was designed to review all patients whose data were entered into the Trauma Registry System between January 1, 2009 and December 31, 2013. Out of 16,548 registered patients, 1,430 (8.64%) adult motorcycle riders and passengers (both referred to as riders hereafter) underwent a BAC test. Patients who did not undergo the BAC test were excluded from the study. A BAC level of 50 mg/dL, the legal limit for drivers in Taiwan, was defined as the cut-off value. Therefore, patients with a BAC level ≥50 mg/dL at the time of arrival at the hospital were considered intoxicated and were included in the study for further analysis. Detailed patient information was retrieved from the Trauma Registry System of our institution and included the following variables: age, gender, vital signs upon admission, arrival time at the hospital, injury mechanism, BAC levels upon arrival, Glasgow coma scale (GCS), abbreviated injury scale (AIS) of each body region, injury severity score (ISS), new injury severity score (NISS), trauma-injury severity score (TRISS), associated injuries, LOS, length of intensive care unit stay (LICUS), and in-hospital mortality rate. The first GCS score recorded in the emergency department was used in the analysis to minimize the effect of alcohol metabolism over time. Data collected regarding the populations of motorcycle riders with a positive BAC (n = 601, 42.0%) were compared to

data from those with a negative BAC (n = 829, 58.0%) using SPSS v.20 statistical software (IBM Corporation, Armonk, NY, USA), and Pearson's chi-squared test, Fisher's exact test, or the independent Student's t-test was used as appropriate. All results are presented as means ± standard errors. A p-value <0.05 was considered statistically significant.

Results

The mean ages of patients with positive and negative BAC levels were 39.2 ± 11.7 years and 39.5 ± 14.1 years, respectively (Table 1). After age stratification (by decade), a positive BAC was more frequently observed among patients aged 30–49 years and a negative BAC was more frequently observed among those aged 20–29 years and ≥50 years. A positive BAC was significantly associated with gender and the time of arrival at the hospital. Of the 601 patients with a positive BAC, 89.4% (n = 537) were men and 10.6% (n = 64) were women. Of the 829 patients with a negative BAC, 64.7% (n = 536) were men and 35.3% (n = 293) were women. Most patients with a

Table 1 Demographics and characteristics of adult motorcycle riders with positive and negative blood alcohol concentration

Variables	BAC+, n (%)	BAC-, n (%)	p
	N = 601	N = 829	
Age (years)	39.2 ±11.7	39.5 ±14.1	0.000
Age category			
20-29 years	148 (24.6%)	278 (33.5%)	0.000
30-39 years	169 (28.1%)	142 (17.1%)	0.000
40-49 years	153 (25.5%)	147 (17.7%)	0.000
50-59 years	102 (17.0%)	190 (22.9%)	0.006
≥60 years	29 (4.8%)	72 (8.7%)	0.005
Gender			0.000
Male	537 (89.4%)	536 (64.7%)	
Female	64 (10.6%)	293 (35.3%)	
Time			
7:00-17:00	112 (18.6%)	384 (46.3%)	0.000
17:00-23:00	252 (41.9%)	280 (33.8%)	0.002
23:00-7:00	237 (39.4%)	165 (19.9%)	0.000
Helmet			
Drivers(+)	411 (68.4%)	648 (78.2%)	0.000
Drivers(-)	145 (24.1%)	108 (13.0%)	0.000
Passengers(+)	13 (2.2%)	25 (3.0%)	0.322
Passengers(-)	10 (1.7%)	7 (0.8%)	0.158
Unknown	22 (3.7%)	41 (4.9%)	0.242
BAC level (mg/dL)			
Mean	193.1 ±72.6	6.4 ±6.6	0.000
Range	50-443.1	0-49.8	

positive BAC arrived at the hospital in the evening (17:00–23:00) and during the night (23:00–7:00); most patients with a negative BAC arrived during the daytime (7:00–17:00). When patients were analyzed with respect to helmet use, for which data were recorded for 96.3% of patients with a positive BAC and 95.1% of patients with a negative BAC, the percentage of drivers who wore a helmet was significantly higher among those with a negative BAC than among those with a positive BAC (78.2% vs. 68.4%; p = 0.000). In addition, the percentage of riders who had not worn a helmet was significantly higher among drivers with a positive BAC than among those with a negative BAC (24.1% vs. 13.0%; p = 0.000). In contrast, no significant difference regarding helmet use was observed between motorcycle passengers with positive and negative BAC levels. The mean BAC levels of injured adult motorcycle riders admitted to the trauma center with negative and positive BAC levels were 6.4 mg/dL (range: 0–49.8 mg/dL) and 193.1 mg/dL (range: 50–443.1 mg/dL), respectively. The mean BAC level among patients with a positive BAC was nearly 4 times the legal limit permitted for drivers in Taiwan.

As shown in Table 2, the GCS score was significantly lower among patients with a positive BAC than among those with a negative BAC (12.1 ± 3.9 vs. 12.9 ± 3.6; p = 0.003); however, the difference was <1 point. The incidence of unclear consciousness (GCS score ≤8) was

significantly higher among patients with a positive BAC than among those with a negative BAC (20.3% vs. 16.2%; p = 0.004). The percentage of patients with a GCS score of 9–12 was also significantly higher among patients with a positive BAC than among those with a negative BAC (15.8% vs. 10.0%; p = 0.001). In contrast, the percentage of patients with a GCS score ≥13 was significantly higher among those with a negative BAC than among those with a positive BAC (73.8% vs. 63.9%; p = 0.000). According to the AIS, patients with a positive BAC had a higher rate of facial injury than did those with a negative BAC ((45.6% vs. 39.7%; p = 0.026). The frequencies of injuries to the head/neck, thorax, abdomen, and extremities did not significantly differ between these 2 groups. Alcohol consumption was associated with a lower ISS (12.9 ± 9.3 vs. 14.1 ± 10.0; p = 0.059) and NISS (15.4 ± 11.1 vs. 16.5 ± 11.9; p = 0.052) than was sobriety, although these difference were not significant. However, no differences were observed between the positive and negative BAC groups in terms of the TRISS (0.933 ± 0.155 and 0.931 ± 0.157, respectively; p = 0.910) or in-hospital mortality rate (3.2% and 4.9%, respectively; p = 0.097). When the patients were stratified according to the ISS (i.e., <16, 16–24, and ≥25), an ISS ≥25 was more common among patients with a negative BAC than among those with a positive BAC (15.3% vs. 10.1%; p = 0.004).

Alcohol use was not associated with the LOS in patients with a positive or negative BAC (12.0 days and 13.2 days,

Table 2 Glasgow coma scale and injury-related characteristics of adult motorcycle riders with positive and negative blood alcohol concentration

Variables	BAC + N = 601	BAC-N = 829	p
GCS	12.1±3.9	12.9 ±3.6	0.003
GCS, n (%)			
≤8	122 (20.3%)	134 (16.2%)	0.004
9-12	95 (15.8%)	83 (10.0%)	0.001
≥13	384 (63.9%)	612 (73.8%)	0.000
AIS, n (%)			
Head/Neck	352 (58.6%)	492 (59.3%)	0.767
Face	274 (45.6%)	329 (39.7%)	0.026
Thorax	123 (20.5%)	164 (19.8%)	0.750
Abdomen	69 (11.5%)	98 (11.8%)	0.843
Extremity	353 (58.7%)	504 (60.8%)	0.432
ISS	12.9 ±9.3	14.1 ±10.0	0.059
<16	387 (64.4%)	503 (60.7%)	0.152
16-24	153 (25.5%)	199 (24.0%)	0.529
≥25	61 (10.1%)	127 (15.3%)	0.004
NISS	15.4 ±11.1	16.5 ±11.9	0.052
TRISS	0.933 ±0.155	0.931 ±0.157	0.910
Mortality, n (%)	19 (3.2%)	41 (4.9%)	0.097

Table 3 Hospital and ICU length of stay (LOS) and mortality rates in patients stratified by the injury severity score

Variables	ISS	BAC + N = 601	BAC-N = 829	p
LOS		12.0 ±11.3	13.2 ±14.4	0.183
n (%)	<16	387 (64.4%)	503 (60.7%)	0.152
	16-24	153 (25.5%)	199 (24.0%)	0.529
	≥25	61 (10.1%)	127 (15.3%)	0.004
days	<16	9.5 ±9.1	9.9 ±7.7	0.176
	16-24	14.7±11.7	15.2 ±12.6	0.816
	≥25	21.4 ±15.9	23.7 ±26.7	0.085
LICUS		221 (36.8%)	339 (40.9%)	0.115
n (%)	<16	59 (26.7%)	93 (27.4%)	0.848
	16-24	106 (48.0%)	139 (41.0%)	0.105
	≥25	56 (25.3%)	107 (31.6%)	0.113
days	<16	4.4 ±3.9	5.0 ±3.5	0.973
	16-24	5.7 ±4.8	6.3 ±5.7	0.497
	≥25	9.9 ±8.3	13.0 ±15.7	0.029
Mortality				
n (%)	<16	3 (0.8%)	3 (0.6%)	0.747
	16-24	5 (3.3%)	6 (3.0%)	0.892
	≥25	11 (18.0%)	32 (25.2%)	0.274

Table 4 Associated injuries of the adult motorcycle riders with positive and negative blood alcohol concentration

Variable	BAC + N = 601	BAC- N = 829	Odds ratio (95% CI)	p
Head trauma, n(%)				
Neurologic deficit	13 (2.2)	21 (2.5)	0.9 (0.42-1.71)	0.650
Cranial fracture	130 (21.6)	149 (18.0)	1.3 (0.97-1.64)	0.085
Epidural hematoma (EDH)	82 (13.6)	109 (13.1)	1.0 (0.77-1.42)	0.786
Subdural hematoma (SDH)	126 (21.0)	185 (22.3)	0.9 (0.72-1.19)	0.541
Subarachnoid hemorrhage (SAH)	142 (23.6)	231 (27.9)	0.8 (0.63-1.02)	0.072
Intracerebral hematoma (ICH)	34 (5.7)	54 (6.5)	0.9 (0.55-1.34)	0.506
Cerebral contusion	60 (10.0)	134 (16.2)	0.6 (0.42-0.80)	0.001
Cervical vertebral fracture	9 (1.5)	13 (1.6)	1.0 (0.41-2.25)	0.915
Maxillofacial trauma, n(%)				
Maxillary fracture	110 (18.3)	125 (15.1)	1.3 (0.95-1.67)	0.104
Mandibular fracture	50 (8.3)	53 (6.4)	1.3 (0.89-1.99)	0.164
Orbital fracture	39 (6.5)	38 (4.6)	1.4 (0.91-2.29)	0.115
Nasal fracture	20 (3.3)	22 (2.7)	1.3 (0.68-2.34)	0.456
Thoracic trauma, n(%)				
Rib fracture	86 (14.3)	99 (11.9)	1.2 (0.90-1.68)	0.188
Hemothorax	16 (2.7)	22 (2.7)	1.0 (0.52-1.93)	0.992
Pneumothorax	18 (3.0)	28 (3.4)	0.9 (0.48-1.61)	0.686
Hemopneumothorax	12 (2.0)	25 (3.0)	0.7 (0.33-1.32)	0.231
Lung contusion	12 (2.0)	35 (4.2)	0.5 (0.24-0.90)	0.020
Thoracic vertebral fracture	5 (0.8)	7 (0.8)	1.0 (0.31-3.12)	0.980
Abdominal trauma, n(%)				
Intra-abdominal injury	13 (2.2)	27 (3.3)	0.7 (0.34-1.28)	0.216
Hepatic injury	35 (5.8)	50 (6.0)	1.0 (0.62-1.50)	0.870
Splenic injury	16 (2.7)	21 (2.5)	1.1 (0.54-2.03)	0.879
Retroperitoneal injury	2 (0.3)	4 (0.5)	0.7 (0.13-3.77)	0.665
Renal injury	6 (1.0)	9 (1.1)	0.9 (0.33-2.60)	0.873
Urinary bladder injury	2 (0.3)	1 (0.1)	2.8 (0.25-30.56)	0.387
Lumbar vertebral fracture	1 (0.2)	13 (1.6)	0.1 (0.01-0.80)	0.008
Extremity trauma, n(%)				
Scapular fracture	25 (4.2)	19 (2.3)	1.9 (1.01-3.39)	0.044
Clavicle fracture	96 (16.0)	105 (12.7)	1.3 (0.97-1.77)	0.076
Humeral fracture	15 (2.5)	41 (4.9)	0.5 (0.27-0.90)	0.018
Radial fracture	37 (6.2)	82 (9.9)	0.6 (0.40-0.89)	0.012
Ulnar fracture	25 (4.2)	43 (5.2)	0.8 (0.48-1.31)	0.368
Metacarpal fracture	15 (2.5)	21 (2.5)	1.0 (0.50-1.93)	0.965
Pelvic fracture	20 (3.3)	34 (4.1)	0.8 (0.46-1.41)	0.449
Femoral fracture	57 (9.5)	87 (10.5)	0.9 (0.63-1.27)	0.531
Patella fracture	21 (3.5)	27 (3.3)	1.1 (0.60-1.92)	0.806
Tibia fracture	57 (9.5)	78 (9.4)	1.0 (0.71-1.44)	0.962
Fibular fracture	31 (5.2)	52 (6.3)	0.8 (0.51-1.28)	0.374
Calcaneal fracture	17 (2.8)	26 (3.1)	0.9 (0.48-1.67)	0.737
Metatarsal fracture	6 (1.0)	18 (2.2)	0.5 (0.18-1.15)	0.088

respectively; p = 0.183) regardless of their ISS (i.e., <16, 16–24, and ≥25; Table 3). In addition, alcohol use was not associated with the percentage of patients admitted to the ICU in the positive or negative BAC group (36.8% vs. 40.9%, respectively; p = 0.115); however, in the subgroup of patients with an ISS of ≥25, patients with a negative BAC had a longer LICUS than did those with a positive BAC ((13.0 days vs. 9.9 days; p = 0.029). No difference in the LICUS was observed between these 2 groups for the ISS <16 and 16–24 categories. To summarize, there were more patients with a negative BAC and ISS ≥25, and these patients had a longer LICUS. In addition, no significant difference was observed in mortality between the positive and negative BAC groups, regardless of injury severity.

Injuries associated with motorcycle accidents are shown in Table 4. Significantly lower ORs were observed among adult motorcycle riders with a positive BAC who experienced cerebral contusion (0.6; 95% confidence interval [CI] = 0.42–0.80; p = 0.001), lung contusion (0.5; 95% CI = 0.24–0.90; p = 0.020), lumbar vertebral fracture (0.1; 95% CI = 0.01–0.80; p = 0.008), humeral fracture (0.5; 95% CI = 0.27–0.90; p = 0.018), and radial fracture (0.6; 95% CI = 0.40–0.89; p = 0.012; Figure 1).

In subsequent analyses, we focused on accidents associated with helmet use among motorcycle riders with a positive BAC (Table 5). We found that 424 patients did and 155 patients did not wear a helmet in these alcohol-related motorcycle accidents. Motorcycle riders who had worn a helmet had significantly lower ORs for cranial fracture (0.4; 95% CI = 0.29–0.67; p = 0.000), epidural hematoma (0.5; 95% CI = 0.29–0.79; p = 0.003), subdural hematoma (0.4; 95% CI = 0.28–0.64; p = 0.000), subarachnoid hemorrhage (0.5; 95% CI = 0.32–0.72; p = 0.000), and cerebral contusion (0.4; 95% CI = 0.25–0.78; p = 0.004; Figure 2) than those who had not worn a helmet.

Discussion

In this study, we analyzed the demographics and characteristics of alcohol-related motorcycle injuries in a population of adult patients at a level I trauma center. As expected, a positive BAC was more frequently noted among male patients, those aged 30–49 years, those who arrived at the hospital in the evening or during the night, and those who did not wear a helmet. In addition, patients who consumed alcohol before their injury were more likely to suffer a facial injury and have a lower initial GCS as determined upon presentation at the emergency department.

Motorcycle riders with a positive BAC had less severe injuries (ISS ≥25) than did riders with a negative BAC. In addition, alcohol-intoxicated motorcycle riders had decreased ORs for cerebral contusion, lung contusion, lumbar vertebral fracture, humeral fracture, and radial fracture when compared with sober patients. However, this does not mean that alcohol consumption protects patients from sustaining severe injuries. Although the legal BAC limits differ from country to country, motorcycle riders are typically subjected to the same limits as car drivers [13]; however, the level of skill required to ride a motorcycle or drive a motor vehicle under the influence of the same alcohol concentration should also be considered. Alcohol-related accidents differ distinctly from non-alcohol-related crashes, and inattention is the strongest contributing factor to these accidents [14]. Motorcycle riding performance and hazard perception were shown to be impaired at a BAC of 0.05% [13]. Riders who consume alcohol are more likely to lose control of the motorcycle by driving off the road, be involved in a single vehicle accident, violate traffic control signals, and be involved in non-intersection collisions [14]. Although the relationship between a low BAC and riding performance is reported to be complex, evident

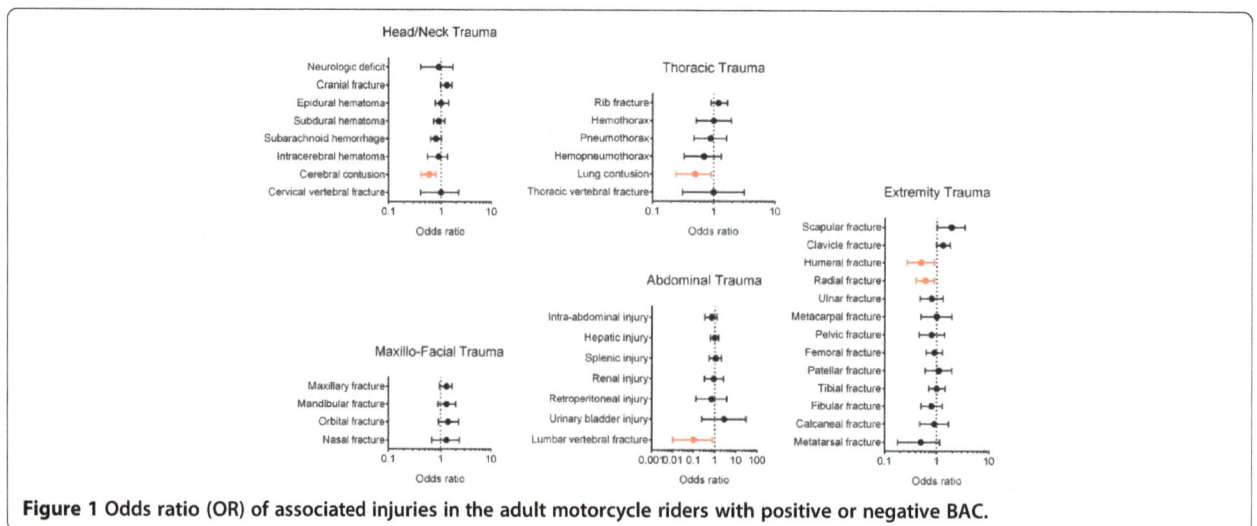

Figure 1 Odds ratio (OR) of associated injuries in the adult motorcycle riders with positive or negative BAC.

Table 5 Associated injuries of the alcohol-intoxicated adult motorcycle riders with or without helmet-wearing

Variables	Helmet + N = 424	Helmet-N = 155	Odds ratio (95% CI)	p
Head/Neck trauma, n(%)				
Neurologic deficit	9 (2.1%)	4 (2.6%)	0.8 (0.25-2.70)	0.742
Cranial fracture	73 (17.2%)	50 (32.3%)	0.4 (0.29-0.67)	0.000
Epidural hematoma (EDH)	47 (11.1%)	32 (20.6%)	0.5 (0.29-0.79)	0.003
Subdural hematoma (SDH)	71 (16.7%)	50 (32.3%)	0.4 (0.28-0.64)	0.000
Subarachnoid hemorrhage (SAH)	84 (19.8%)	53 (34.2%)	0.5 (0.32-0.72)	0.000
Intracerebral hematoma (ICH)	21 (5.0%)	10 (6.5%)	0.8 (0.35-1.64)	0.478
Cerebral contusion	32 (7.5%)	24 (15.5%)	0.4 (0.25-0.78)	0.004
Cervical vertebral fracture	6 (1.4%)	3 (1.9%)	0.7 (0.18-2.94)	0.654
Maxillofacial trauma, n(%)				
Maxillary fracture	73 (17.2%)	34 (21.9%)	0.7 (0.47-1.17)	0.195
Mandibular fracture	34 (8.0%)	13 (8.4%)	1.0 (0.49-1.86)	0.886
Orbital fracture	28 (6.6%)	10 (6.5%)	1.0 (0.49-2.16)	0.948
Nasal fracture	13 (3.1%)	5 (3.2%)	0.9 (0.33-2.71)	0.922
Thoracic trauma, n(%)				
Rib fracture	66 (15.6%)	16 (10.3%)	1.6 (0.90-2.86)	0.109
Hemothorax	11 (2.6%)	4 (2.6%)	1.0 (0.32-3.21)	0.993
Pneumothorax	11 (2.6%)	5 (3.2%)	0.8 (0.27-2.34)	0.682
Hemopneumothorax	9 (2.1%)	2 (1.3%)	1.7 (0.35-7.77)	0.516
Lung contusion	6 (1.4%)	6 (3.9%)	0.4 (0.11-1.12)	0.066
Thoracic vertebral fracture	3 (0.7%)	2 (1.3%)	0.5 (0.09-3.29)	0.502

impairment of some riding performance measures has been observed at a BAC of 0.02% but no effects, even positive ones, were demonstrated for other riding performance measures [13]. In this study, the mean BAC among patients with a positive BAC was nearly 4 times the legal limit permitted for driving in Taiwan, indicating that the riding performance in these patients was obviously impaired relative to patients with a negative BAC. Therefore, motorcycle riders who consume alcohol may tend to be involved in accidents in crowded cities and have a lower percentage of severe injury and lower frequency of specific body injuries when compared with sober motorcycle riders.

Alcohol consumption is among the most important personal risk factors for serious and fatal injuries and contributes to approximately one-third of all deaths due to alcohol-intoxicated trauma accidents [15]. Alcohol intoxication has also been described as resulting in increased mortality during the clinical course [15,16]. Motorcycle riders have an estimated 3-fold higher fatality risk at a BAC of 0.03% (95% CI = 2.8–3.5) and a 20-fold higher fatality risk at a BAC of 0.08% (95% CI = 15.0–27.3), compared with sober riders [17]. An age >60 years, lack of a helmet, driving after alcohol consumption, and driving without a valid license have been determined as factors influencing the high frequency and risk of motorcycle death [3]. Head trauma was found to be the most frequent and severe injury type among motorcycle accident cases in which alcohol consumption was the most significant factor [18]. Traumatic brain injury (67%) and hypovolemic shock (38%) have been reported as the most frequent causes of death in such cases [18]. The present study

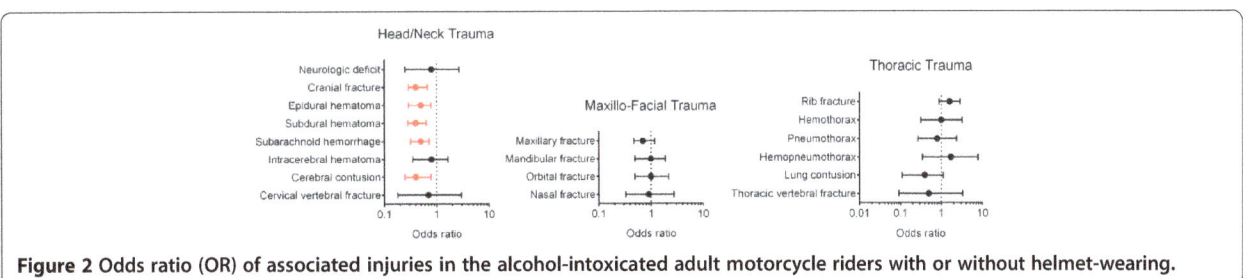

Figure 2 Odds ratio (OR) of associated injuries in the alcohol-intoxicated adult motorcycle riders with or without helmet-wearing.

further revealed that a significant percentage of alcohol-intoxicated motorcycle riders did not wear a helmet, leaving them at an increased risk of head region injury. Although the serum ethanol level has been shown to be associated independently with either increased [19,20] or decreased mortality in patients with traumatic brain injuries [21,22], some authors have reported that the risk of fatality among patients with a brain injury was significantly reduced if the patients were intoxicated (BAC ≥200 mg/dL) before the injury [23]. In the present study, the mortality rates of patients with positive and negative BAC levels did not significantly differ, regardless of the ISS (i.e., <16, 16–24, and ≥25). Our study observation was similar to that of a previous report in which the mortality risk was not higher in patients with a positive BAC [23].

Although there a mandatory law for the motorcycle rider to wear a helmet in Taiwan, the motorcyclists or passengers who are intoxicated and uninsured are less likely to wear a helmet [24]. In Los Angeles, motorcyclists who consumed alcohol were half as likely to wear a helmet, compared with nondrinkers [25]. Similar results were also observed in the present study, in which sober motorcycle drivers were significantly more likely to wear a helmet than were alcohol-intoxicated drivers. However, the helmet status did not significantly differ among motorcycle passengers. The effectiveness of helmets for reducing the risk of crash-related severe head injury in motorcyclists is well established [26]. In addition, an increased risk of adverse facial injury outcomes were observed for riders with non-fixed helmets relative to those with fixed helmets (adjusted OR = 2.10; 95% CI = 1.41–3.13) [26]. According to our analyses regarding helmet status among motorcycle riders with a positive BAC, alcohol-intoxicated riders who wore a helmet had a significantly lower OR for sustaining a cranial fracture, epidural hematoma, subdural hematoma, subarachnoid hemorrhage, or cerebral contusion. Although several preventive measures exist, wearing a helmet has particularly been shown to protect against head injuries and can be cost-effective if proposed as a regulated bylaw for motorcyclists [27-29]. In an analysis of 858,741 traffic deaths in the United States during a 20-year period, the mortality rates attributed to each of the following risk factors decreased by the corresponding percentages: no motorcycle helmet, 74%; alcohol, 53%; not wearing a seat belt, 49%; and lack of an air bag, 17% [30]. Therefore, education and prevention strategies may provide benefits by targeting high-risk populations [24].

The limitations of this study include the use of a retrospective design and the lack of data regarding the circumstances of the injury mechanism and the decision-making in dealing with the associated injuries [31]. The lack of data regarding the motorcycle speed during accidents, type of motorcycle, type of helmet material, and use of any other protective materials prevented an analysis of motorcycle-related hospitalization according to exposure-based risks. Furthermore, although rare in Taiwan, the combination of psychoactive drug and alcohol use may further increase the risk of an accident. BAC measurements are the most commonly used method to determine whether trauma patients have consumed alcohol, and all drivers involved in traffic accidents are legally compelled to undergo a test to estimate their BAC; however, a few patients may have refused to undergo an actual BAC test after alcohol consumption was confirmed using a breathalyzer. Accordingly, these patients might have been included in an incorrect analytical category because the breathalyzer results had not been noted in the medical records; however, in our experience, such cases are rare.

Conclusion

In summary, alcohol consumption was more frequently noted among male motorcycle riders, those aged 30–49 years, those who arrived at the hospital in the evening or during the night, and those who did not wear a helmet. Patients who had consumed alcohol had a lower likelihood of sustaining a severe injury (ISS ≥25) and a lower frequency of specific body injuries. In addition, alcohol-intoxicated motorcycle riders who wore helmets had significantly lower frequencies of cranial fracture, epidural hematoma, subdural hematoma, subarachnoid hemorrhage, and cerebral contusion.

Competing interests
The authors declare that they have no competing interests.

Authors' contributions
HTL wrote the manuscript; SYH and CSR conducted the study analysis and edited the tables; CCL and CHH designed the study, contributed to the data analysis and interpretation, and drafted the manuscript. All authors read and approved the final manuscript.

Funding
This research was supported by a grant from Chang Gung Memorial Hospital (CDRPG8C0031).

Author details
[1]Department of Trauma Surgery, Kaohsiung Chang Gung Memorial Hospital and Chang Gung University College of Medicine, No. 123, Ta-Pei Road, Niao-Song District, Kaohsiung City 833, Taiwan. [2]Department of Neurosurgery, Kaohsiung Chang Gung Memorial Hospital and Chang Gung University College of Medicine, No. 123, Ta-Pei Road, Niao-Song District, Kaohsiung City 833, Taiwan.

References
1. Weiss H, Agimi Y, Steiner C. Youth motorcycle-related brain injury by state helmet law type: United States, 2005-2007. Pediatrics. 2010;126(6):1149–55.
2. Brown JB, Bankey PE, Gorczyca JT, Cheng JD, Stassen NA, Gestring ML. The aging road warrior: national trend toward older riders impacts outcome after motorcycle injury. Am Surg. 2010;76(3):279–86.
3. Jou RC, Yeh TH, Chen RS. Risk factors in motorcyclist fatalities in Taiwan. Traffic Inj Prev. 2012;13(2):155–62.
4. Rogers SC, Campbell BT, Saleheen H, Borrup K, Lapidus G. Using trauma registry data to guide injury prevention program activities. J Trauma. 2010;69(4 Suppl):S209–213.

5. Moore EE. Alcohol and trauma: the perfect storm. J Trauma. 2005;59(3):S53–56. discussion S67-75.

6. McCaig LF, Nawar EW. National Hospital Ambulatory Medical Care Survey: 2004 emergency department summary. Advance data. 2006;(372):1–29.

7. Stubig T, Petri M, Zeckey C, Brand S, Muller C, Otte D, et al. Alcohol intoxication in road traffic accidents leads to higher impact speed difference, higher ISS and MAIS, and higher preclinical mortality. Alcohol (Fayetteville, NY). 2012;46(7):681–6.

8. Sun SW, Kahn DM, Swan KG. Lowering the legal blood alcohol level for motorcyclists. Accid Anal Prev. 1998;30(1):133–6.

9. Huang WS, Lai CH. Survival risk factors for fatal injured car and motorcycle drivers in single alcohol-related and alcohol-unrelated vehicle crashes. J Safety Res. 2011;42(2):93–9.

10. Ogden EJ, Moskowitz H. Effects of alcohol and other drugs on driver performance. Traffic Inj Prev. 2004;5(3):185–98.

11. Zador PL, Krawchuk SA, Voas RB. Alcohol-related relative risk of driver fatalities and driver involvement in fatal crashes in relation to driver age and gender: an update using 1996 data. J Stud Alcohol. 2000;61(3):387–95.

12. Mann B, Desapriya E, Fujiwara T, Pike I. Is blood alcohol level a good predictor for injury severity outcomes in motor vehicle crash victims? Emerg Med Int. 2011;2011:616323.

13. Filtness AJ, Rudin-Brown CM, Mulvihill CM, Lenne MG. Impairment of simulated motorcycle riding performance under low dose alcohol. Accid Anal Prev. 2013;50:608–15.

14. Kasantikul V, Ouellet JV, Smith T, Sirathranont J, Panichabhongse V. The role of alcohol in Thailand motorcycle crashes. Accid Anal Prev. 2005;37(2):357–66.

15. Zeckey C, Dannecker S, Hildebrand F, Mommsen P, Scherer R, Probst C, et al. Alcohol and multiple trauma: is there an influence on the outcome? Alcohol (Fayetteville, NY). 2011;45(3):245–51.

16. Tulloh BR, Collopy BT. Positive correlation between blood alcohol level and ISS in road trauma. Injury. 1994;25(8):539–43.

17. Keall MD, Clark B, Rudin-Brown CM. A preliminary estimation of motorcyclist fatal injury risk by BAC level relative to car/van drivers. Traffic Inj Prev. 2013;14(1):7–12.

18. Carrasco CE, Godinho M, Berti de Azevedo Barros M, Rizoli S, Fraga GP. Fatal motorcycle crashes: a serious public health problem in Brazil. WJES. 2012;7(1):S5.

19. Pories SE, Gamelli RL, Vacek P, Goodwin G, Shinozaki T, Harris F. Intoxication and injury. J Trauma. 1992;32(1):60–4.

20. Luna GK, Maier RV, Sowder L, Copass MK, Oreskovich MR. The influence of ethanol intoxication on outcome of injured motorcyclists. J Trauma. 1984;24(8):695–700.

21. Salim A, Ley EJ, Cryer HG, Margulies DR, Ramicone E, Tillou A. Positive serum ethanol level and mortality in moderate to severe traumatic brain injury. Arch Surg. 2009;144(9):865–71.

22. Talving P, Plurad D, Barmparas G, Dubose J, Inaba K, Lam L, et al. Isolated severe traumatic brain injuries: association of blood alcohol levels with the severity of injuries and outcomes. J Trauma. 2010;68(2):357–62.

23. Hsieh CH, Su LT, Wang YC, Fu CY, Lo HC, Lin CH. Does alcohol intoxication protect patients from severe injury and reduce hospital mortality? The association of alcohol consumption with the severity of injury and survival in trauma patients. Am Surg. 2013;79(12):1289–94.

24. Brown CV, Hejl K, Bui E, Tips G, Coopwood B. Risk factors for riding and crashing a motorcycle unhelmeted. J Emerg Med. 2011;41(4):441–6.

25. Ouellet JV. Helmet use and risk compensation in motorcycle accidents. Traffic Inj Prev. 2011;12(1):71–81.

26. Ramli R, Oxley J, Hillard P, Mohd Sadullah AF, McClure R. The effect of motorcycle helmet type, components and fixation status on facial injury in Klang Valley, Malaysia: a case control study. BMC Emerg Med. 2014;14(1):17.

27. Hundley JC, Kilgo PD, Miller PR, Chang MC, Hensberry RA, Meredith JW, et al. Non-helmeted motorcyclists: a burden to society? A study using the National Trauma Data Bank. J Trauma. 2004;57(5):944–9.

28. MacLeod JB, Digiacomo JC, Tinkoff G. An evidence-based review: helmet efficacy to reduce head injury and mortality in motorcycle crashes: EAST practice management guidelines. J Trauma. 2010;69(5):1101–11.

29. Schneider WH, Savolainen PT, Van Boxel D, Beverley R. Examination of factors determining fault in two-vehicle motorcycle crashes. Accid Anal Prev. 2012;45:669 76.

30

The value of Serum BNP for diagnosis of intracranial injury in minor head trauma

Ali Demir[1]*, Cemil Kavalci[2]*, Muhittin Serkan Yilmaz[1], Fevzi Yilmaz[1], Tamer Durdu[1], Mehmet Ali Ceyhan[1], Fatih Alagoz[1] and Cihat Yel[1]

Abstract

Objective: Head injury is the main cause of death among individuals younger than 45 years old. Cranial Computerized tomography (CT) is commonly used for diagnosis of head injury. Brain Natriuretic Peptide (BNP) is a peptide originally isolated from brain ventricles. The main aim of this study is to investigate BNP as an indicator of head injury among patients presenting to emergency department (ED) with minor head trauma.

Methods: This was a prospective study conducted at the emergency department of the Numune Training and Research Hospital. A total of 162 patients who presented to the ED with minor head injury were enrolled. The patients were categorized into 2 groups as the cranial CT-negative and positive groups. The normality of the data was tested using One Sample Kolmogorov Smirnov test. Mann–Whitney U test was used to compare 2 independent groups while the Kruskal-Wallis test was utilized for comparison of more than 2 groups. A p-value of <0.05 was considered to be significant.

Results: Ninety-six (59.3%) patients were male and 66 (40.7%) were female. The cranial CT-negative group had a median BNP level of 14.5 pg/ml while the cranial CT-positive group had a median BNP level of 13 pg/ml. There was no statistically significant difference between these two groups for serum BNP levels (p > 0.05).

Conclusion: This study suggested that serum BNP level wasn't used in defined of intracranial injury.

Keywords: Emergency, Head trauma, Brain natriuretic peptide

Introduction

Head traumas and traumatic cerebral injuries constitute a major etiological factor for mortality and long-term morbidity especially in adolescents, young adulthood, and elderly [1]. Motor vehicle accidents, falls from a height, assaults, and gunshot injuries are the most common causes of head injuries. Of all head injuries, 80% are minor, 10% are moderate, and 10% are major injuries [1,2]. Cranial Computerized tomography (CT) is often ordered during emergency management of patients with head trauma. Unfortunately, CT is an expensive examination, not available in everywhere and puts patients at risk for long-term risks of radiation.

Previous studies have reported that some serum markers including neuron specific enolase (NSE), S100b, Tau protein, and malonyl dialdehyde (MDA) are increased in head trauma patients [3-6]. BNP, a natriuretic peptide consisting of 32 amino acids, is an important biomarker in establishing cardiovascular disorders including congestive heart failure and ischemic cardiomyopathy. It is commonly used both for determination of presence and degree of left ventricular systolic and diastolic dysfunction. It is also a predictor of prognosis after myocardial infarction [7,8]. In addition to its cardiovascular applications, some previous reports have also suggested that it can be used in head trauma [7-13].

The present study aimed to investigate whether BNP measurement can establish head injury in patients presenting to the emergency department with minor head trauma. If the answer is yes, excess CTs could be avoided which will reduce unnecessary costs and patients' radiation exposure.

* Correspondence: ademir@ekolay.net; cemkavalci@yahoo.com
[1]Emergency Department, Numune Training and Research Hospital, Ankara 06370, Turkey
[2]Emergency Department, Baskent University Faculty of Medicine, Ankara 06450, Turkey

Materials and method

This was a prospective, case–control study conducted at the emergency department of the Numune Training and Research Hospital. It included a total of 162 patients with head trauma admitting to the emergency department who met the study inclusion criteria. The inclusion and exclusion criteria are listed on Table 1.

Demographic features of the study participants, trauma mechanisms, concurrent injuries, time elapsed after trauma, GCS scores, findings on physical examination, cranial CT results were also recorded. Trauma severity was assessed using GCS.

The study population was grouped into 2 groups as cranial CT-negative group (Group 1) that had normal head CT findings and linear fracture, and cranial CT-positive group (Group 2) that had intracranial abnormalities including brain edema, epidural or subdural hematoma, subarachnoid or intraparenchymal hemorrhage, cerebral contusion, or a depressed skull fracture. Cranial CT reports were retrieved from the hospital automation system.

The study patients underwent a head CT as necessary and serum BNP measurement with Abbot Architect kit (normal range of 0–100 pg/ml) at admission.

Clinical and demographic features of the patients were stored in a computer database. Serum BNP levels were compared between both groups. Statistical analyses were performed using SPSS 15.0 software package. Mean ± SD, median, interquartile range, and percentage values were calculated for demographic and clinical features of the study participants. Median and interquartile range values were calculated for BNP levels. Categorical variables were compared with χ^2 test. The normality of the study data was tested by means of One Sample Kolmogorov Smirnov test. As a result of the analysis, non-parametric tests were used in the analysis. As such, Mann–Whitney U test was used for comparison of two independent continuous groups, while Kruskal-Wallis test was used for multiple continuous groups. Spearman's test used to investigation a association between Serum BNP levels and elapsed time after the event. A significance level of $p < 0.05$ was accepted for all statistical tests.

Approval by the ethics committee

This study was approved by the Local Ethics Committee of the Numune Training and Research Hospital.

Results

The present study was completed at the ED of the Numune Training and Research Hospital during summer months of 2013. A total of 162 patients meeting the inclusion criteria were enrolled. Group 1 and 2 included 148 and 14 patients, respectively.

Demographic and clinical data

Ninety-six (59.3%) patients were male and 66 (40.7%) were female. Demographic and clinical findings are showed in Table 2.

The most common symptoms were headache (87%), vomiting (13%), amnesia (3.7%), unconsciousness (5%), and somnolence (3%). The most common signs on physical examination were scalp laceration (44.4%), scalp hematoma (38.8%), and raccoon eye (0.6%). Findings of head CT are given on Table 3. One hundred and thirty-four (82.7%) patients were discharged from the hospital and 28 (17.3%) were hospitalized.

BNP

Median serum BNP level was 14.5 (33) pg/ml in Group 1 and 13 (139) pg/ml in Group 2. There was no not significantly different with respect to median BNP levels between two groups (p > 0.05). Median BNP level was 10 (21) pg/ml in males and 28.50 (56) pg/ml in females. There was a significant difference between both genders with regard to median BNP levels (Z = −4.29, p < 0.05).

The patients were divided in to 2 groups. Group 1 consisted of patients with admitted to our department within 0–12 hours after events whereas group 2 consisted of patients with admitted to our department within

Table 1 The criteria for inclusion or exclusion of patients to the study

Criteria for inclusion to the study	Criteria for exclusion from the study
To be admitted to the emergency department because of a head trauma.	To be younger than 18 years old.
To be older than 18 years old.	To refuse to participate the study.
To give his/her consent to participate in study.	Having a known neurological disease.
	Having a known cardiac insufficiency.

Table 2 Demographic characteristics of the patients

	Group 1	Group 2	p
Age (average, years)	49.18 ± 20.5	42.93 ± 22.1	p > 0.05*
Gender (n)			
Male	84	12	p < 0.05**
Female	64	2	
Trauma mechanism (n)			
Motor vehicle accident	32	1	p > 0.05**
Pedestrian	9	1	
Falling	61	7	
Violent assaults	46	5	
Accompanying trauma	9	3	p < 0.05**
Bnp levels (median, IQR) (pg/ml)	14.5 (33)	13 (139)	p > 0.05*

*Mann-Witney U test, ** χ^2 test.

Table 3 Cranial CT findings of the patients

Finding	Number (n)	Percentage (%)	GCS (n) (14/15)
Normal	146	90.1	8/138
Linear fracture	1	0.6	0/1
Cerebral edema	1	0.6	0/1
Subarachnoid hemorrhage	4	2.5	0/4
Compression fracture	2	1.2	0/2
Parenchymal haemorrhage	1	0.6	0/1
Contusio cerebri	2	1.2	0/2

13–24 hours after events. There was a no significant difference between both two groups with regard to median BNP levels (Z = −1.52, p > 0.05). There was no correlation between serum BNP levels and elapsed time after the event (r = 0.125, p > 0.05). Serum BNP levels according to trauma severity are given on Table 4. There was no correlation between serum BNP levels and trauma severity (r = −0.037, p > 0.05).

Our patients in group 2 were hospitalized in neurosurgery service. They were discharged after treatment.

Discussion

Only a few studies have reported increased serum BNP levels in patients with head trauma [7-10]. Costa et al. reported that serum BNP levels did not increase in patients with head injury and it had no correlation with cerebral salt-wasting syndrome [12]. Kavalci et al. reported that serum BNP might be useful in evaluation of head trauma [13]. Cevik et al. demonstrated that BNP levels exceeding 10 pg/ml were associated with an intracranial abnormality in patients with head injury [7]. Sviri et al. showed that serum BNP levels increased immediately following head injury [8]. Similarly, Lu et al. reported that BNP levels increased in patients with head trauma [9]. Cevik et al. showed that serum BNP levels significantly differed between patients with and without head trauma [7]. In contrast, we did not detect any significant difference between the 2 groups. We believe that this re-

Table 4 BNP levels by various trauma mechanism and trauma severity

Trauma mechanism	BNP (pg/ml)	p value
Motor vehicle accident	15 (25)	p > 0.05*
Pedestrian	10 (53)	
Falling	22.5(56)	
Violent assaults	11(22)	
Glasgow coma score		
14 (n = 8)	10.5(27)	p > 0.05**
15 (n = 154)	14.5(34)	

*Kruskall-Wallis test, **Mann–Whitney U test.

sulted from a low patient number in Group 2. We suggest that further studies with larger sample size may establish a relationship between serum BNP and head trauma.

Neither, Çevik et al. nor Kavalci et al. showed a significant correlation between trauma mechanism and serum BNP. We also found a similar result. BNP appears to be released into bloodstream in all kinds of head trauma.

Çevik et al. reported a significant relevance between delay in admission and BNP levels. They showed that a positive correlation exists between admission time and BNP levels [7]. Kavalci et al. showed that there was no significant correlation between the serum BNP levels and admission time [13]. Our results are support to Kavalci et al.

GCS is commonly used for assessment of neurological status of head trauma patients. There is a general agreement on the predictive power of GCS in patients with mild and serious head trauma, although there are various approach considerations with respect to radiological evaluation of minor head trauma cases. Thus, studies aiming to establish the indications of CT scanning of the head region or criteria for hospital admission by using some biochemical markers and clinical features [3-5]. Some reports suggested that the severity of head trauma and serum BNP levels are not significantly correlated [7,10,13]. Wu et al., in contrast, reported that serum BNP levels increased to a greater extent in patients with more severe head trauma [11]. We found no significant correlation between head trauma severity and serum BNP levels. However, all of our patients with minor head trauma group. This subject should be further clarified with adequate studies.

In a study by Çevik et al. serum BNP levels were significantly higher in patients with an intracranial lesion compared to those who did not. Cevik et al. proposed that serum BNP levels can be used as a surrogate marker of head trauma [7]. In contrast, Stewart et al. and Kavalci et al. suggested that this biomarker has no any appreciable value for this indication [10]. Since our results were in line with equality of BNP elevation in both patient groups, they support the results of the studies conducted by Stewart et al. and Kavalci et al.

Conclusion

Our results suggested that serum BNP was not an adequate marker for determination of an intracranial pathology in patients with minor head trauma. As to date conflicting results have been reported, further studies with larger sample size should be followed in order to establish a possible link between serum BNP and minor head trauma.

Limitation of the study

Since the number of patients in the present study is too low, the power of the study fell short to draw any meaningful conclusion. Moreover, the patient number in Group 2 was even lower (14 patients). Despite these limitations, our study demonstrated that there was no significant difference between Group 1 and 2 although all patients in the study had demonstrable intracranial lesions. Another limitation, We didn't perform a serial BNP measurements because it is expensive.

Competing interests
The authors declare that they have no competing interests.

Authors' contributions
The quantitative analysis was planned by CK, EDA, AD. Study data were analyzed by CK and interpreted by FY, MAC. The first version of the manuscript was drafted by AD, MSY, BMS. All authors contributed to the edition and revision of the manuscript and the final version of the article was reviewed and approved by all authors.

References
1. Ingebrigtsen T, Romner B, Kock-Jensen C: **Scandinavian guidelines for initial management of minimal, mild, and moderate head injuries. The scandinavian neurotrauma committee.** *J Trauma* 2000, **48:**760–766.
2. Dietrich AM, Bowman MJ, Ginn-Pease ME, Kosnik E, King DR: **Pediatric head injuries: can clinical factors reliably predict an abnormality on computed tomography?** *Ann Emerg Med* 1993, **22:**1535–1540.
3. Poli-de-Figueiredo LF, Biberthaler P, Simao Filho C, Hauser C, Mutschler W, Jochum M: **Measurement of S-100B for risk classification of victims sustaining minor head injury-first pilot study in Brazil.** *Clinics* 2006, **61:**41–46.
4. Woertgen C, Rothoerl RD, Metz C, Brawanski A: **Comparison of clinical, radiologic, and serum marker as prognostic factors after severe head injury.** *J Trauma* 1999, **47:**1126–1130.
5. Kavalci C, Durukan P, İlhan N, Güzel A: **The value of serum MDA for the diagnosis of intracranial injury.** *Trakya Univ Tip Fak Derg* 2008, **25:**209–213.
6. Guzel A, Karasalihoglu S, Aylanç H, Temizöz O, Hiçdönmez T: **Validity of serum tau protein levels in pediatric patients with minor head trauma.** *Am J Emerg Med* 2010, **28:**399–403.
7. Çevik Y, Durukan P, Erol FS, Yıldız M, İlhan N, Serhatlıoğlu S: **Diagnostic value of bedside brain natriuretic peptide measurement in patients with head trauma.** *JAEM* 2010, **9:**21–25.
8. Sviri GE, Soustiel JF, Zaaroor M: **Alteration in brain natriuretic peptide (BNP) plasma concentration following severe traumatic brain injury.** *Acta Neurochir* 2006, **148:**529–533.
9. Lu DC, Binder DK, Chien B, Maisel A, Manley GT: **Cerebral salt wasting and elevated brain natriuretic peptide levels after traumatic brain injury: 2 case reports.** *Surg Neurol* 2008, **69:**226–229.
10. Stewart D, Waxman K, Brown A, Schuster R, Schuster L, Hvingelby EM, *et al*: **B type natriuretic peptide levels May Be elevated in the critically injured trauma patient without congestive heart failure.** *J Trauma* 2007, **63:**747–750750.
11. Wu X, Sha H, Sun Y, Gao L, Liu H, Yuan Q, *et al*: **N-terminal pro-B-type natriuretic peptide in patients with isolated traumatic brain injury: a prospective cohort study.** *J Trauma* 2011, **71:**820–825.
12. Costa KN, Nakamura HM, Cruz LR, Miranda LS, Santos-Neto RC, Cosme Sde L, Casulari LA: **Hyponatremia and brain injury: absence of alterations of serum brain natriuretic peptide and vasopressin.** *Arq Neuropsiquiatr* 2009, **67:**1037–1044.
13. Kavalci C, Akdur G, Yemenici S, Sayhan MB: **The value of serum BNP for the diagnosis of intracranial injury in head trauma.** *Tr J Emerg Med* 2012, **12:**112–116. doi:10.5505/1304.7361.2012.26576.

31

Obese patients who fall have less injury severity but a longer hospital stay than normal-weight patients

Jung-Fang Chuang[1†], Cheng-Shyuan Rau[2†], Hang-Tsung Liu[1], Shao-Chun Wu[3], Yi-Chun Chen[1], Shiun-Yuan Hsu[1], Hsiao-Yun Hsieh[1] and Ching-Hua Hsieh[1*]

Abstract

Background: The effects of obesity on injury severity and outcome have been studied in trauma patients but not in those who have experienced a fall. The aim of this study was to compare injury patterns, injury severities, mortality rates, and in-hospital or intensive care unit (ICU) length of stay (LOS) between obese and normal-weight patients following a fall.

Methods: Detailed data were retrieved for 273 fall-related hospitalized obese adult patients with a body mass index (BMI) ≥30 kg/m^2 and 2357 normal-weight patients with a BMI <25 kg/m^2 but ≥18.5 kg/m^2 from the Trauma Registry System of a Level I trauma center between January 1, 2009, and December 31, 2013. We used the Pearson's chi-squared test, Fisher's exact test, the Mann Whitney U test, and independent Student's t-test to analyze differences between the two groups.

Results: Analysis of AIS scores and AIS severity scaling from 1 to 5 revealed no significant differences in trauma regions between obese and normal-weight patients. When stratified by injury severity (Injury Severity Score [ISS] of <16, 16–24, or ≥25), more obese patients had an ISS of <16 compared to normal-weight patients (90.5 % vs. 86.0 %, respectively; $p = 0.041$), while more normal-weight patients had an ISS between 16 and 24 (11.0 % vs. 6.6 %, respectively; $p = 0.025$). Obese patients who had experienced a fall had a significantly lower ISS (median (range): 9 (1–45) vs. 9 (1–50), respectively; $p = 0.015$) but longer in-hospital LOS than did normal-weight patients (10.1 days vs. 8.9 days, respectively; $p = 0.049$). Even after taking account of possible differences in comorbidity and ISS, the obese patients have an average 1.54 day longer LOS than that of normal-weight patients. However, no significant differences were found between obese and normal-weight patients in terms of the New Injury Severity Score (NISS), Trauma-Injury Severity Score (TRISS), mortality, percentage of patients admitted to the ICU, or LOS in the ICU.

Conclusion: Obese patients who had experienced a fall did not have different injured body regions than did normal-weight patients. However, they had a lower ISS but a longer in-hospital LOS than did normal-weight patients.

Keywords: Fall, Obesity, Injury severity score, Mortality, In-hospital length of stay

* Correspondence: m93chinghua@gmail.com
†Equal contributors
[1]Department of Trauma Surgery, Kaohsiung Chang Gung Memorial Hospital and Chang Gung University College of Medicine, No.123, Ta-Pei Road, Niao-Sung District, Kaohsiung City 833, Taiwan
Full list of author information is available at the end of the article

Background

Falls are a leading cause of injury and a significant public health issue [1–3]. The incidence of falls that lead to emergency unit admission is growing with the increased size and rapid growth of the geriatric population [4, 5]. In addition, obesity is a worldwide health problem leading to a range of health consequences [6, 7]. While obesity is known to increase the risk for a variety of medical conditions including hypertension, diabetes mellitus, cardiac disease, and pulmonary thromboembolism [8], the effect of obesity on the injury pattern and outcome of trauma patients after a fall remains unclear. Evidence was found that the effect of weight on the risk of falling appeared to be linear; greater obesity was related to greater risk of falling [9–11]. Compared with normal-weight respondents, the odds ratios (OR) for risk of falling were 1.12 (95 % confidence interval [CI] = 1.01–1.24) for obesity Class 1 (BMI 30.0–34.9 kg/m^2), 1.26 (95 % CI = 1.05–1.51) for obesity Class 2 (BMI 35.0–39.9 kg/m^2), and 1.50 (95 % CI = 1.21–1.86) for obesity Class 3 (BMI ≥ 40.0 kg/m^2) [9]. In addition, obesity was associated with a 25 % higher risk (95 % CI = 1.11–1.41; $p < 0.0003$) of having fallen in the previous 12 months compared to non-obese individuals [12].

Identification of the high-risk injury patterns and better understanding of the epidemiology and outcome of fall injury in obese patients are important in order to cope with a rising number of obese patients. Therefore, this study was designed to investigate the injury characteristics, injury patterns, injury severities, and mortality rates of adult obese patients admitted and treated for fall-related injury in southern Taiwan over a five-year period at a level I trauma center.

Methods

Ethics statement

Approval for this study was obtained from the hospital's institutional review board (IRB) before its initiation (approval number 103-7110B). Given its observational nature, the requirement for written informed consent from each patient was waived by the IRB.

Study design

This retrospective study was designed to review all 16,548 hospitalized and registered patients added to the Trauma Registry System from January 1, 2009, to December 31, 2013, and select cases that met the following inclusion criteria: (1) age ≥ 18 years, (2) BMI ≥ 30 kg/m^2 for obese patients and BMI < 25 but ≥ 18.5 kg/m^2 for normal-weight patients according to the World Health Organization definition [13, 14], and (3) admittance due to a fall accident. The patients who had sustained fall injuries from all fall heights (<1 m, 1–6 m, >6 m) were included, but those who had attempted suicide in the fall or who had non-validated BMI values or incomplete data were excluded.

To compare the injury patterns, mechanisms, severity, and mortality of obese patients with those of normal-weight patients, detailed data were retrieved on age, sex, vital signs in the emergency department (ED), injury mechanism, fall height (<1 m, 1–6 m, >6 m), transportation, injury time, Glasgow Coma Scale (GCS) upon arrival at the ED, Abbreviated Injury Scale (AIS) severity score for each body region, Injury Severity Score (ISS), New Injury Severity Score (NISS), Trauma-Injury Severity Score (TRISS), in-hospital length of stay (LOS), LOS in the ICU, and in-hospital mortality. In addition, the pre-existed comorbidities and chronic dieseases including diabetes mellitus (DM), hypertension (HTN), coronary artery diseases (CAD), congestive heart failure (CHF), cerebrovascular accident (CVA), and end-stage renal disease (ESRD) were identified. A blood alcohol concentration (BAC) of 50 mg/dL at the time of arrival at the hospital was defined as the cut-off value according to the legal limit for drivers in Taiwan. The primary outcomes were injury severity scores (i.e., GCS, AIS, ISS, NISS, and TRISS), and the secondary outcomes were LOS, ICU LOS, and in-hospital mortality.

The ORs of the injured regions and associated conditions sustained by obese and normal-weight patients were calculated with 95 % CIs. Data collected regarding the obese and normal-weight population of patients who had experienced a fall were compared using SPSS v.20 statistical software (IBM, Armonk, NY, USA). Pearson's chi-squared tests, Fisher's exact tests, and independent Student's t-tests were used to analyze data as applicable. The Mann Whitney U test was used to compare the AIS severity scaling from 1 to 5 in each injury region. Ordinal data, like ISS and NISS, is presented as median (range). Data were further analyzed by a multiple linear regression adjusted for the effect of confounding variables (ie, comorbidity and ISS) to show the main effects of obesity on LOS in hospital. All other results are presented as the mean ± standard error.

Results

Injury characteristics

Among the 2630 adult patients with fall accidents, 273 (10.4 %) were obese (BMI ≥ 30 kg/m^2), and 2357 (89.6 %) were of normal weight (25 > BMI ≥ 18.5 kg/m^2) (Table 1). No statistically significant difference regarding sex was found between the obese and normal-weight patients. The mean ages of the obese and normal-weight patients were 60.6 ± 16.8 and 65.7 ± 17.1 years, respectively (p <0.001). There were significant higher incidence rates of the pre-existed comorbidities and chronic diseases including DM, HTN, and CAD in the obese patients. The majority of patients in both groups fell from a height < 1 m, implying that the majority of the patients

Table 1 Demographics of the obese and normal-weight patients with a fall injury

Variables	Obese BMI ≥ 30 n = 273	Normal 25 > BMI ≥ 18.5 n = 2357	Odds ratio (95 %)	P
Gender				
Male	114(41.8)	1080(45.8)	0.8(0.66–1.09)	0.202
Female	159(58.2)	1277(54.2)	1.2(0.92–1.52)	0.202
Age	60.6 ± 16.8	65.7 ± 17.1	—	<0.001
Comorbidity				
DM	98(35.9)	497(21.1)	2.1(1.61–2.74)	<0.001
HTN	153(56.0)	995(42.2)	1.7(1.36–2.25)	<0.001
CAD	26(9.5)	137(5.8)	1.7(1.10–2.65)	0.016
CHF	8(2.9)	51(2.2)	1.4(0.64–2.91)	0.418
CVA	25(9.2)	216(9.2)	1.0(0.65–1.54)	0.997
ESRD	0(0.0)	7(0.3)	—	1.000
Height of fall				
< 1 m	213(78.0)	1859(78.9)	1.0(0.70–1.29)	0.745
1–6 m	59(21.6)	471(20.0)	1.1(0.81–1.50)	0.525
> 6 m	1(0.4)	27(1.1)	0.3(0.04–2.34)	0.354
Alcohol > 50, n(%)	4(1.5)	51(2.2)	0.7(0.24–1.88)	0.445
GCS	14.6 ± 1.7	14.4 ± 2.0	—	0.104
≤ 8	8(2.9)	80(3.4)	0.9(0.41–1.80)	0.687
9–12	6(2.2)	88(3.7)	0.6(0.25–1.34)	0.196
≥ 13	259(94.9)	2189(92.9)	1.4(0.81–2.49)	0.218
AIS, n(%)				
Head/Neck	48(17.6)	537(22.8)	0.7(0.52–1.00)	0.050
Face	12(4.4)	154(6.5)	0.7(0.36–1.20)	0.169
Thorax	20(7.3)	174(7.4)	1.0(0.61–1.60)	0.973
Abdomen	16(5.9)	131(5.6)	1.1(0.62–1.81)	0.837
Extremity	217(79.5)	1792(76.0)	1.2(0.90–1.66)	0.203
ISS, median(range)	9(1–45)	9(1–50)	—	0.015
< 16	247(90.5)	2027(86.0)	1.5(1.02–2.36)	0.041
16–24	18(6.6)	259(11.0)	0.6(0.35–0.94)	0.025
≥ 25	8(2.9)	71(3.0)	1.0(0.46–2.04)	0.940
NISS, median(range)	9(1–66)	9(1–75)	—	0.070
TRISS	0.960 ± 0.112	0.958 ± 0.085	—	0.645
Mortality, n(%)	7(2.6)	55(2.3)	1.1(0.50–2.44)	0.812
Height of fall				
< 1 m	4(1.5)	44(1.9)	0.8(0.28–2.19)	0.639
1–6 m	3(1.1)	11(0.5)	2.4(0.66–8.55)	0.171
LOS (days)	10.1 ± 10.3	8.9 ± 8.9	—	0.049
Controlled by Comorbidity & ISS	—	—	1.01(1.01–1.03)	0.004
ICU				
Patients, n(%)	33(12.1)	375(15.9)	0.7(0.50–1.06)	0.099
< 16	15(5.5)	145(6.2)	0.9(0.51–1.53)	0.667
16–24	11(4.0)	167(7.1)	0.6(0.30–1.03)	0.057

Table 1 Demographics of the obese and normal-weight patients with a fall injury *(Continued)*

≥ 25	7(2.6)	63(2.7)	1.0(0.43–2.11)	0.916
LOS in ICU (days)	8.2 ± 8.8	7.8 ± 9.6	—	0.833
< 16	6.6 ± 6.7	6.3 ± 8.7	—	0.908
16-24	7.5 ± 6.6	7.7 ± 10.0	—	0.963
≥ 25	11.9 ± 12.5	13.3 ± 13.4	—	0.782
AIS ≥3 sites, n(%)	6(0.2)	78(3.3)	0.7(0.28–1.52)	0.323
Mortality	0(0.0)	0(0.0)	—	—
LOS (days)	16.2 ± 10.2	14.8 ± 12.2	—	0.784
ICU Patients, n(%)	3(50.0)	36(46.2)	1.2(0.22–6.14)	1.000
LOS in ICU (days)	11.3 ± 9.1	7.1 ± 6.4	—	0.293

sustained a ground-level fall occurring upon walking or with movement; however, this difference in patient number stratified by fall height (<1 m, 1–6 m, >6 m) was not statistically significant.

Injury severity

No significant differences were found between obese and normal-weight patients in GCS scores (14.6 ± 1.7 *vs.* 14.4 ± 2.0, respectively; $p = 0.104$) and the distribution of the proportion of patients at different levels of consciousness (GCS ≤8, 9–12, or ≥13) (Table 1). Analysis of AIS scores revealed no significant differences in trauma regions between obese and normal-weight patients. Comparison of the composition of AIS severity scaling from 1 to 5 in each region between obese and normal-weight patients also did not show a significant difference (Table 2). A significant difference in ISS was found between obese and normal-weight patients (median (range): 9 (1–45) *vs.* 9 (1–50), respectively; $p = 0.015$). When stratified by injury severity (ISS of <16, 16–24, or ≥25), more obese than normal-weight patients had an ISS < 16 (90.5 % vs. 86.0 %, respectively; $p = 0.041$), while more normal-weight than obese patients had an ISS between 16 and 24 (11.0 % vs. 6.6 %, respectively; $p = 0.025$). However, no significant difference were found for NISS (median (range): 9 (1–66) *vs.* 9 (1–75), respectively; $p = 0.070$), TRISS (0.960 ± 0.112 *vs.* 0.958 ± 0.085, respectively; $p = 0.645$), or in-hospital mortality (2.6 % vs. 2.3 %, respectively; $p = 0.645$). We found that obese patients had a significantly longer average in-hospital LOS than did normal-weight patients (10.1 vs. 8.9 days, respectively; $p = 0.049$). Because the detected significant higher incidence rates of DM, HTN, and CAD in the obese patients or a higher ISS may be positively correlated to a longer hospital stay, therefore, we performed a multiple linear regression analysis to investigate the effect of obesity, DM, HTN, CAD, and ISS on LOS (days) of these patients. The analysis of variance table (Table 3) indicates that the relationship between obesity and LOS is significant ($p = 0.005$), LOS in obesity tends to be 1.54 day

Table 2 Explanatory variables by a multiple regression analysis to investigate the effect of obesity, comorbidity, and ISS on LOS of these patients

Variables	Obese BMI ≥ 30 n(%)	Normal 25 > BMI ≥ 18.5 n(%)	Mann–Whitney U Test P
Head/Neck	48	537	0.210
AIS 1	2(29.2)	112(20.9)	
AIS 2	4(8.3)	44(8.2)	
AIS 3	10(20.8)	104(19.4)	
AIS 4	15(31.3)	225(41.9)	
AIS 5	5(10.4)	52(9.7)	
Face	12	154	0.550
AIS 1	4(33.3)	71(46.1)	
AIS 2	8(66.7)	83(53.9)	
Thorax	20	176	0.804
AIS 1	4(20.0)	19(10.8)	
AIS 2	5(25.0)	56(31.8)	
AIS 3	5(25.0)	77(43.8)	
AIS 4	6(30.0)	22(12.5)	
AIS 5	0(0.0)	2(1.1)	
Abdomen	17	131	0.413
AIS 1	4(23.5)	6(4.6)	
AIS 2	7(41.2)	83(63.4)	
AIS 3	6(35.3)	40(30.5)	
AIS 4	0(0.0)	2(1.5)	
Extremity	217	1792	0.073
AIS 1	9(4.2)	43(2.4)	
AIS 2	86(39.6)	633(35.3)	
AIS 3	121(55.8)	1114(62.2)	
AIS 4	0(0.0)	2(0.1)	
AIS 5	1(0.5)	0(0.0)	

Table 3 Comparison of the composition of AIS severity scaling from 1 to 5 in each region between obese and normal-weight patients

Variable	Parameter estimate	Standard error	95 % CI for parameter	P-value
Intercept	2.600	0.362	(1.891–3.310)	0.000
Obesity	1.543	0.544	(0.477–2.610)	0.005
DM	0.990	0.418	(0.170–1.809)	0.018
HTN	0.485	0.354	(−0.209–1.178)	0.171
CAD	0.962	0.690	(−0.392–2.315)	0.164
ISS	0.642	0.032	(0.579–0.705)	0.000

The multiple linear regression equation is given by: LOS (days) = 2.60 + 1.54*(obesity) + 0.99*(DM) + 0.49*(HTN) + 0.96*(CAD) + ISS*0.64, depending on obesity (o = normal weight, 1 = obesity), DM (0 = no DM, 1 = DM), HTN (0 = no HTN, 1 = HTN), CAD (0 = no CAD, 1 = CAD), and ISS (scores) of these patients

longer, on average, than that of normal-weight patients, even after taking account of possible differences in comorbidity and ISS. In addition, the relationship between ISS and LOS is highly significant ($p < 0.0005$), with a one score increase in ISS being associated with an average increase of 0.64 day LOS, after adjusting for obesity and comorbidity. However, no differences were noted in the proportion of obese and normal-weight patients admitted to the ICU as well as LOS in the ICU after stratification into either group of injury severity (ISS of <16, 16–24, or ≥25). In addition, among those who had sustained 3 or more body area injury (AIS ≥3 sites), there were no difference in obese and normal-weight patients admitted to the ICU, LOS in the ICU and in the hospital, and the mortality.

Physiological response & procedures performed at the ED
Upon arrival at the ED, no significant differences were found for GCS of <13, systolic blood pressure (SBP) of <90 mmHg, heart rate of >100 beats/min, or respiratory rates of <10 or >29. Furthermore, no significant differences were found in the odds for requiring procedures, including cardiopulmonary resuscitation, intubation, chest tube insertion, and blood transfusion, at the ED (Table 4).

Discussion
In a retrospective review of all blunt trauma patients admitted to the ICU at a Level I trauma center, prior study demonstrated that there was no difference between obese and lean patients in the type of traumatic brain injury [15]. Another study demonstrated similar injury patterns of fewer head but more chest and lower extremity injuries [16]. It has also been reported that obese trauma patients sustained more pelvic, rib, and lower extremity fractures but fewer liver injuries, mandibular fractures, and cerebral injuries than those nonobese trauma patients [17]. Based on our analysis of the AIS scores, obese patients presented no significant difference of injuries to body region from normal-weight patients. Comparison of the composition of AIS severity scaling from 1 to 5 in each region also did not show a significant difference between obese and normal-weight patients.

Longer hospitalizations of obese patients result in increased morbidity and are associated with impaired mobility, higher incidence of respiratory complications, more venous thromboembolic events, and higher nosocomial infection rates [18]. For example, obesity resulted in nearly twofold-increased odds for developing cardiac and pulmonary complications after a hip fracture as well

Table 4 Physiological response and procedures performed upon arrival at the ED

Variables	Obese BMI ≥ 30 n = 273	Normal 25 > BMI ≥ 18.5 n = 2357	Odds ratio (95 %)	P
Physiology at ER, n(%)				
GCS < 13	14(5.1)	168(7.1)	0.7(0.40–1.23)	0.218
SBP < 90 mmHg	3(1.1)	26(1.1)	1.0(0.30–3.31)	1.000
Heart rate > 100 beats/min	52(19.0)	357(15.1)	1.3(0.96–1.82)	0.092
Respiratory rate < 10 or >29	0(0.0)	6(0.3)	—	1.000
Procedures at ER, n(%)				
Cardiopulmonary resuscitation	0(0.0)	1(0.0)	—	1.000
Intubation	3(1.1)	34(1.4)	0.8(0.23–2.49)	1.000
Chest tube insertion	2(0.7)	23(1.0)	0.7(0.18–3.19)	1.000
Blood transfusion	8(2.9)	56(2.4)	1.2(0.59–2.63)	0.574

as significantly increasing the odds of developing infectious complications (OR 3.8; 95 % CI 1.9–7.6, $p < 0.001$) [19]. It has been reported that the mean duration of orthopedic surgery in morbidly obese patients was 30 % longer than in non-obese patients [20]. Moreover, medically stable obese patients were found to be almost twice as likely to experience delayed fracture fixation due to preference of the surgeon [20]. In addition, obesity in critically ill patients is significantly related to a prolonged duration of mechanical ventilation and intensive care unit length of stay [21, 22]. In this study, although obese patients had a significant lower ISS than normal-weight patients who had experienced a fall, the obese patients had a significantly longer in-hospital LOS than did normal-weight patients. Even after taking account of possible differences in comorbidity and ISS, the obese patients have an average 1.54 day longer LOS than that of normal-weight patients.

Limitation of this study involves the use of a retrospective design with its inherent selection bias and the lack of available data on the circumstances of the mechanisms of injury. In addition, the patients dead on hospital arrival or accident scene are not included into the Trauma Registry Database, thus creating a selection bias. Moreover, some well-established risk factors, including prior falls, inappropriate use of medications, gait or balance problems, and functional limitations, were not documented and analyzed in this study. Finally, this study is only descriptive and, therefore, unable to assess the effects of any particular treatment intervention; it could only rely on the assumption that assessment and management are uniform between obese and normal-weight populations.

Conclusion

The obese adult patients presented with similar injury to the body region following a fall in comparison with normal-weight patients. The obese patients had significantly lower ISS but significantly longer in-hospital LOS than did normal-weight patients. However, mortality, the percentage of patients admitted to the ICU, and LOS in the ICU exhibited no statistically significant differences between obese and normal-weight patients.

Level of evidence

Epidemiological study, level III.

Competing interests

The authors declare that they have no competing interests.

Authors' contributions

JFC revised the manuscript; CSR drafted the manuscript; HTL wrote the manuscript; SCW, YCC, and SYH performed the analysis and edited the tables; HYH revised and proofread the manuscript; CHH designed the study, contributed to the data analysis and interpretation, and drafted the manuscript. All authors read and approved the final manuscript.

Author details
^{1}Department of Trauma Surgery, Kaohsiung Chang Gung Memorial Hospital and Chang Gung University College of Medicine, No.123, Ta-Pei Road, Niao-Sung District, Kaohsiung City 833, Taiwan. ^{2}Department of Neurosurgery, Kaohsiung Chang Gung Memorial Hospital and Chang Gung University College of Medicine, Kaohsiung, Taiwan. ^{3}Department of Anesthesiology, Kaohsiung Chang Gung Memorial Hospital and Chang Gung University College of Medicine, Kaohsiung, Taiwan.

References
1. Ambrose AF, Paul G, Hausdorff JM. Risk factors for falls among older adults: a review of the literature. Maturitas. 2013;75(1):51–61.
2. Rosen T, Mack KA, Noonan RK. Slipping and tripping: fall injuries in adults associated with rugs and carpets. J Inj Violence Res. 2013;5(1):61–9.
3. Hester AL, Wei F. Falls in the community: state of the science. Clin Interv Aging. 2013;8:675–9.
4. Meschial WC, Soares DF, Oliveira NL, Nespollo AM, Silva WA, Santil FL. Elderly victims of falls seen by prehospital care: gender differences. Rev Bras Epidemiol. 2014;17(1):3–16.
5. Wendelboe AM, Landen MG. Increased fall-related mortality rates in New Mexico, 1999–2005. Public Health Rep. 2011;126(6):861–7.
6. Pi-Sunyer FX. The obesity epidemic: pathophysiology and consequences of obesity. Obes Res. 2002;10 Suppl 2:97s–104.
7. Wang Y, Lobstein T. Worldwide trends in childhood overweight and obesity. Int J Pediatr Obes. 2006;1(1):11–25.
8. Rosenfeld HE, Tsokos M, Byard RW. The association between body mass index and pulmonary thromboembolism in an autopsy population. J Forensic Sci. 2012;57(5):1336–8.
9. Himes CL, Reynolds SL. Effect of obesity on falls, injury, and disability. J Am Geriatr Soc. 2012;60(1):124–9.
10. Mitchell RJ, Lord SR, Harvey LA, Close JC. Associations between obesity and overweight and fall risk, health status and quality of life in older people. Aust N Z J Public Health. 2014;38(1):13–8.
11. Finkelstein EA, Chen H, Prabhu M, Trogdon JG, Corso PS. The relationship between obesity and injuries among U.S. adults. Am J Health Promot. 2007;21(5):460–8.
12. Mitchell RJ, Lord SR, Harvey LA, Close JC. Obesity and falls in older people: mediating effects of disease, sedentary behavior, mood, pain and medication use. Arch Gerontol Geriatr. 2015;60(1):52–8.
13. Physical status: the use and interpretation of anthropometry. Report of a WHO Expert Committee. World Health Organ Tech Rep Ser. 1995;854:1–452.
14. Obesity: preventing and managing the global epidemic. Report of a WHO consultation. World Health Organ Tech Rep Ser. 2000;894:i-xii, 1–253.
15. Brown CV, Rhee P, Neville AL, Sangthong B, Salim A, Demetriades D. Obesity and traumatic brain injury. J Trauma. 2006;61(3):572–6.
16. Brown CV, Neville AL, Rhee P, Salim A, Velmahos GC, Demetriades D. The impact of obesity on the outcomes of 1,153 critically injured blunt trauma patients. J Trauma. 2005;59(5):1048–51. discussion 1051.
17. Boulanger BR, Milzman D, Mitchell K, Rodriguez A. Body habitus as a predictor of injury pattern after blunt trauma. J Trauma. 1992;33(2):228–32.
18. Goulenok C, Monchi M, Chiche JD, Mira JP, Dhainaut JF, Cariou A. Influence of overweight on ICU mortality: a prospective study. Chest. 2004;125(4):1441–5.
19. Belmont Jr PJ, Garcia EJ, Romano D, Bader JO, Nelson KJ, Schoenfeld AJ. Risk factors for complications and in-hospital mortality following hip fractures: a study using the National Trauma Data Bank. Arch Orthop Trauma Surg. 2014;134(5):597–604.
20. Childs BR, Nahm NJ, Dolenc AJ, Vallier HA. Obesity is associated with more complications and longer hospital stays after orthopaedic trauma. J Orthop Trauma. 2015;29(11):504–9.
21. Akinnusi ME, Pineda LA, El Solh AA. Effect of obesity on intensive care morbidity and mortality: a meta-analysis. Crit Care Med. 2008;36(1):151–8.
22. Mica L, Keel M, Trentz O. The impact of body mass index on the physiology of patients with polytrauma. J Crit Care. 2012;27(6):722–6.

32

Goal-directed transfusion protocol via thrombelastography in patients with abdominal trauma

Jianyi Yin[1†], Zhenguo Zhao[2†], Yousheng Li[1*], Jian Wang[1], Danhua Yao[1], Shaoyi Zhang[1], Wenkui Yu[1], Ning Li[1] and Jieshou Li[1]

Abstract

Introduction: The optimal transfusion protocol remains unknown in the trauma setting. This retrospective cohort study aimed to determine if goal-directed transfusion protocol based on standard thrombelastography (TEG) is feasible and beneficial in patients with abdominal trauma.

Methods: Sixty adult patients with abdominal trauma who received 2 or more units of red blood cell transfusion within 24 hours of admission were studied. Patients managed with goal-directed transfusion protocol via TEG (goal-directed group) were compared to patients admitted before utilization of the protocol (control group).

Results: There were 29 patients in the goal-directed group and 31 in the control group. Baseline parameters were similar except for higher admission systolic blood pressure in the goal-directed group than the control group (121.8 ± 23.1 mmHg vs 102.7 ± 26.5 mmHg, $p < 0.01$). At 24 h, patients in the goal-directed group had shorter aPTT compared to patients in the control group (39.2 ± 16.3 s vs 58.6 ± 36.6 s, $p = 0.044$). Administration of total blood products at 24 h appeared to be fewer in the goal-directed group than the control group (10.2 [7.0-43.1]U vs 14.8 [8.3-37.6]U, $p = 0.28$), but this was not statistically significant. Subgroup analysis including patients with ISS ≥ 16 showed that patients in the goal-directed group had significantly fewer consumption of total blood products than patients in the control group (7[6.1, 47.0]U vs 37.6[14.5, 89.9]U, $p = 0.015$). No differences were found in mortality at 28d, length of stay in intensive care unit and hospital between the two groups.

Conclusions: Goal-directed transfusion protocol via standard TEG was achievable in patients with abdominal trauma. The novel protocol, compared to conventional transfusion management, has the potential to decrease blood product utilization and prevent exacerbation of coagulation function.

Keywords: Transfusion, Thrombelastography, Trauma-induced coagulopathy, Abdominal trauma

Introduction

Uncontrollable hemorrhage is a major cause of early death in trauma patients [1]. Hemorrhage may occur due to direct injury, and is frequently complicated by coagulopathy [2,3]. Post-injury coagulopathy may exacerbate hemorrhage and contribute to poor outcome and an increased transfusion requirement [4,5].

Blood transfusion is an essential component in trauma management. The goal of transfusion includes improvement of tissue oxygen delivery by replacing red blood cell, as well as prevention and correction of coagulation dysfunction by supplementing appropriate blood components. However, the optimal transfusion protocol for trauma patients remains unknown. In lack of guidance by rapid and comprehensive tools monitoring coagulation status, current transfusion protocols are unable to utilize blood products according to individual demands. As a consequence, these protocols are likely to lead to inappropriate and excessive administration of blood products, which is associated with increased burden of

* Correspondence: liys@medmail.com.cn
†Equal contributors
[1]Department of Surgery, Jinling Hospital, Nanjing University School of Medicine, Nanjing, China

blood product supply and risk of transfusion-related morbidity.

In recent years, viscoelastic hemostatic assays (VHA), including thrombelastography (TEG) and thrombelastometry, have been demonstrated to be ideal methods of monitoring coagulation function in trauma patients [6,7]. Furthermore, several studies have suggested the potential of VHA tests to guide component blood transfusion in a variety of patient groups [8-12]. In particular, a recent study by Kashuk et al. [13] showed that goal-directed transfusion based on rapid TEG was useful in managing trauma-induced coagulopathy, with the potential to reduce blood product administration in trauma patients.

A goal-directed transfusion protocol via TEG was implemented in our department since 2010 [14]. In the present study, we assessed the utilization of the protocol in abdominal trauma management by comparing outcomes of patients admitted before and after implementation of the protocol. We aimed to determine if the novel transfusion protocol could be successfully integrated in abdominal trauma management, and identify potential benefits of the protocol compared to conventional transfusion management.

Materials and methods

This cohort study analyzed the prospectively collected data of patients with abdominal trauma at Department of General Surgery, Jinling Hospital. The study was approved by the ethics committee of Jinling Hospital. Waiver of informed consent from patients was approved because of the observational nature of the study. Jinling Hospital is a tertiary teaching hospital in Nanjing, China. The Department of General Surgery is responsible for medical and surgical care of patients with abdominal trauma admitted to the emergency department (ED) of the hospital. At ED, a consulting surgeon judges the need for emergency laparotomy of the abdominal trauma patient. The patient is subsequently transferred to one of the two surgical intensive care units (SICU) of our department from ED if emergency laparotomy is not needed, or from operation room after emergency laparotomy. Non-operative care is provided by a team of surgeons and SICU specialists following previously published guidelines [15].

Study population

We searched the abdominal trauma database to identify potential patients between November 2008 and October 2012. Inclusion criteria were age older than 18 years, abdominal abbreviated injury scale ≥2, and requirement of 2 or more units of red blood cell (RBC) transfusion within 24 hours of ED admission. Exclusion criteria included time interval between injury and ED admission >24 hours, major traumatic brain injury (head abbreviated injury scale ≥3), end-staged liver disease, pregnancy, and history of anti-coagulation therapy in the latest 3 months.

All included patients were subsequently divided into 2 groups according to the time of admission. Patients between November 2008 and October 2010, who received conventional transfusion management, were assigned to the control group, whereas patients between November 2010 and October 2012, who were managed with the goal-directed transfusion protocol, were assigned to the goal-directed group.

Transfusion protocol

At ED, patients with abdominal trauma might receive preemptive transfusion of 2 units of RBC and 2–4 units of fresh frozen plasma (FFP) following initial fluid resuscitation when hemoglobin level was below 90 g/L or showed active bleeding signs. Once the patient was planned to be transferred to our department, subsequent transfusion decisions were made by the treating surgeon or SICU specialist.

Patients in the control group received conventional transfusion management, which was based on individual experience and interpretation of conventional coagulation testing results of the treating surgeon or SICU specialist. RBC and FFP were delivered at a ratio of 1:1–1:2. Platelet and cryoprecipitate were administrated in selected cases.

The TEG 5000 thrombelastograph hemostasis analyzer system (Haemoscope Corporation, Niles, USA) was initially introduced to our department for monitoring post-operative coagulation function. The device enables point-of-care coagulation assay of whole blood at the patient's temperature. The device undergoes quality control daily according to the manufacturer's instructions. TEG analysis is carried out within 4 minutes of blood sample collection. The whole blood sample is placed in a manufacturer-supplied vial containing kaolin, and 0.35 ml of the blood sample is added to a cup, followed by adjustment of the temperature setting to the patient's temperature. TEG assay is then started and stopped when reaching full tracing. A number of parameters are generated from the TEG tracing, each representing an aspect of hemostasis. The R value is the time from the beginning to the onset of clot formation, representing the activity of enzymatic clotting factors. The α angle is the angle between the tangent line and the horizontal line of the tracing, representing the activity of fibrinogen. The maximal amplitude (MA) is the overall clot strength, indicating the platelet activity.

Patients in the goal-directed group were managed with goal-directed transfusion protocol based on TEG results (Figure 1). The protocol was developed by a group of surgeons, SICU specialists, and transfusion specialists, and was introduced to all surgeons and SICU specialists of our department before its implementation in November 2010. The algorithm of the protocol was shown as hard copies in SICU, and two attending surgeons and two SICU specialists ensured utilization of the protocol as the leaders of abdominal trauma management. In specific, standard TEG test was ordered by the treating surgeon or SICU specialist when the patient with abdominal trauma was admitted to SICU, or had active bleeding at ED, operation room (OR), or SICU. Whole blood sample was transferred immediately to the SICU of our department, where it was analyzed. Results were fed back via in-hospital communication system to the treating surgeon or SICU specialist, who determined further transfusion management according to the goal-directed transfusion protocol. The goal-directed transfusion might occur at ED, OR, or SICU. Subsequent TEG tests were ordered until the patient had no active bleeding or coagulopathy.

Data collection

Data of all included patients from ED, SICU, OR, blood bank, and laboratory were linked. Demographic characteristics (age and gender), injury severity indices (injury mechanism, injured organs, injury severity score [ISS], abdominal abbreviated injury scale [AIS]) were collected. Administration of component blood products within 24 hours of ED admission was also recorded. Clinical and laboratory parameters of interest included vital signs (body temperature, heart rate, and systolic blood pressure), arterial blood gas results (pH, lactate, and base excess), blood cell counts (hemoglobin concentration, RBC count, and platelet count), albumin and calcium concentration, international normalized ratio (INR) and activated partial thromboplastin time (aPTT) at ED admission and 24 h. TEG parameters (R value, α angle, and MA value) of the first TEG test and the follow-up one between 24–48 hours after the first one were collected from patients in the

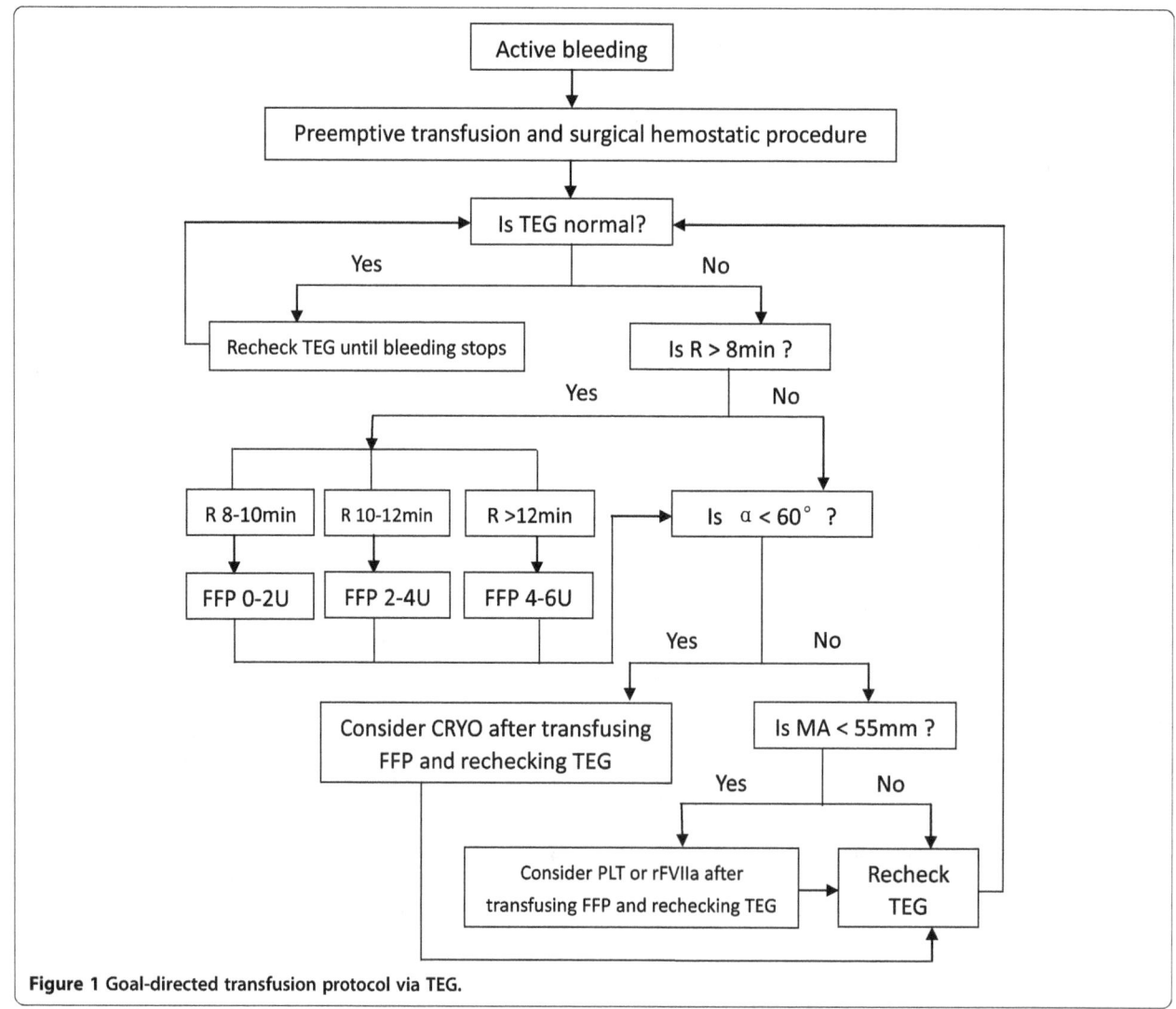

Figure 1 Goal-directed transfusion protocol via TEG.

goal-directed group. In addition, mortality at 28d, length of stay in ICU and hospital were noted. An independent investigator checked the accuracy of collected data before analysis.

Statistical analysis

We used SPSS software (v19.0 for Windows, IBM Corporation, USA) for statistical analysis. Normality of distribution was analyzed by Kolmogorov-Smirnov test. Continuous variables with normal distribution and skewed distribution were analyzed using Student's t test and Mann–Whitney u test, respectively. Categorical variables were analyzed using chi-square test. Significance was considered as $p < 0.05$.

Results

Patient characteristics

A total of 150 patients with abdominal trauma were admitted between November 2008 and October 2012, of whom 98 met the inclusion criteria. Thirty-eight patients were excluded due to prolonged time interval between injury and ED admission (n = 36), end-staged liver disease (n = 1), and major traumatic brain injury (n = 1), leaving 60 patients for final analysis (Figure 2).

There were 31 patients in the control group and 29 in the goal-directed group. The two groups were comparable in terms of age and gender. The control group and the goal-directed group had similar ISS (14.3 ± 5.7 vs 16.2 ± 8.0, p = 0.28) and abdominal AIS (3.1 ± 0.7 vs 3.1 ± 0.9, p = 0.86). There were, however, more frequent patients with pancreatic injury in the goal-directed group than the control group (44.8% vs 16.1%, p = 0.015). All but 3 patients (2 in the control group and 1 in the goal-directed group) underwent emergency operation for control of intra-abdominal bleeding or repair of intra-abdominal organ injury (Table 1).

Administration of blood products

Administration of blood products within 24 hours of ED admission was presented in Table 2. No significant differences were found in the proportion of patients receiving FFP (100% vs 96.8%, p = 1.0), platelet (13.8% vs 29.0%, p = 0.15), and cryoprecipitate (24.1% vs 29.0%, p = 0.67) between the goal-directed group and the control group. Administration of RBC, FFP, platelet, cryoprecipitate, and total blood products was fewer in the goal-directed group than the control group, but this did not reach

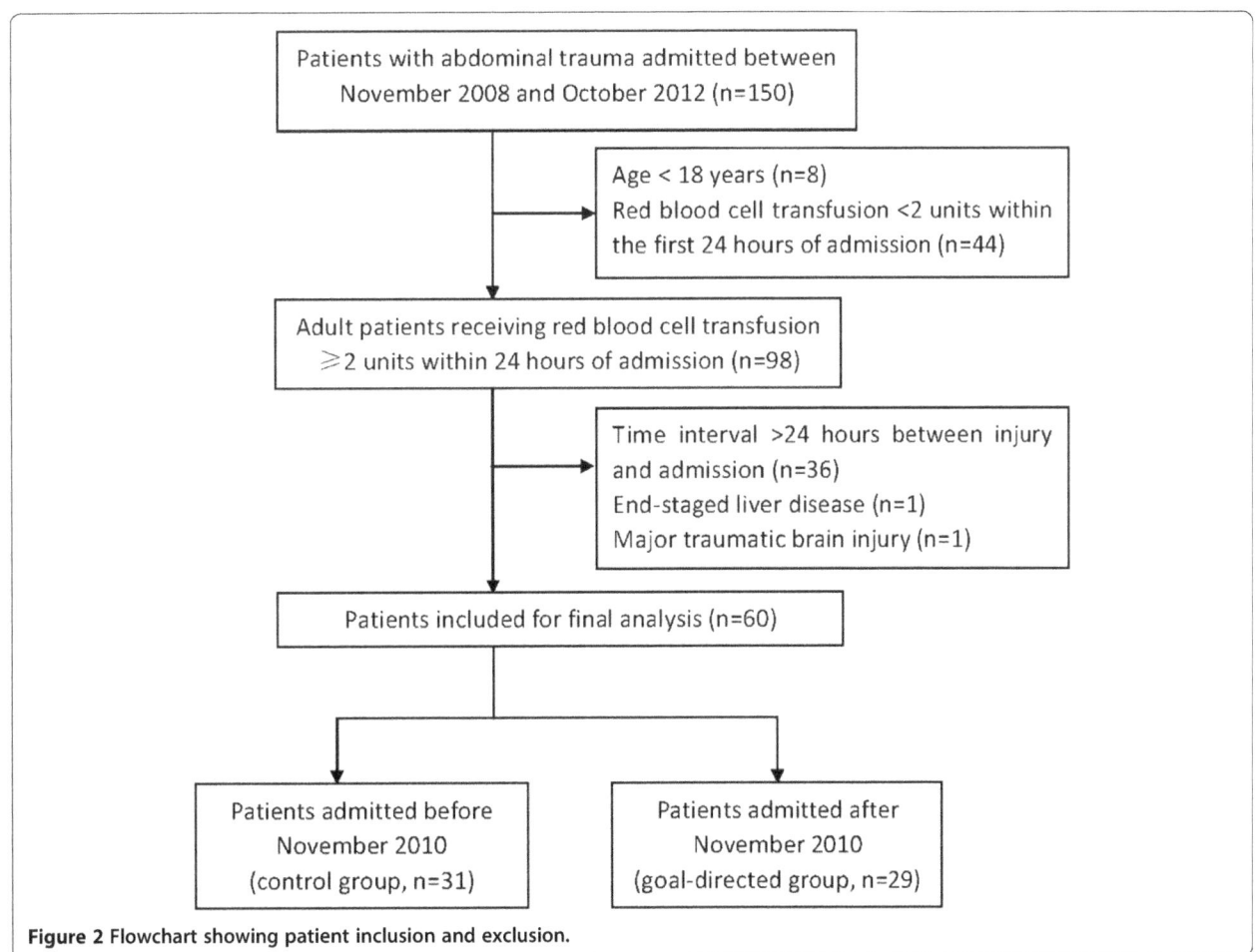

Figure 2 Flowchart showing patient inclusion and exclusion.

Table 1 Patient characteristics[a]

	Overall (n = 60)	Control group (n = 31)	Goal-directed group (n = 29)	p
Age (year)	41.7 ± 14.2	42.8 ± 15.6	40.5 ± 12.8	0.53
Gender				
Male	49(81.7)	26(83.9)	23(79.3)	0.65
Female	11(18.3)	5(16.1)	6(20.7)	
Mechanism of injury				
Blunt	50(83.3)	27(87.1)	23(79.3)	0.64
Penetrating	10(16.7)	4(12.9)	6(20.7)	
ISS	15.2 ± 6.9	14.3 ± 5.7	16.2 ± 8.0	0.28
Abdominal AIS	3.1 ± 0.8	3.1 ± 0.7	3.1 ± 0.9	0.86[b]
Involved abdominal organ				
Spleen	24(40.0)	15(48.4)	9(31.0)	0.17
Liver	14(23.3)	9(29.0)	5(17.2)	0.28
Pancreas	18(30.0)	5(16.1)	13(44.8)	0.015
Vessel	5(8.3)	4(12.9)	1(3.4)	0.39
Stomach	4(6.7)	1(3.2)	3(10.3)	0.35
Duodenum	6(10.0)	4(12.9)	2(6.9)	0.73
Intestine	12(20)	5(16.1)	7(24.1)	0.44
Colon	14(23.3)	6(19.4)	8(27.6)	0.45
Rectum	2(3.3)	1(3.2)	1(3.4)	1.00
Emergency operation	57(95)	29(93.5)	28(96.6)	1.00
ICU stay (day)	10.1 ± 9.2	8.1 ± 5.5	12.2 ± 11.8	0.28[b]
Hospital stay (day)	13.4 ± 10.0	11.3 ± 6.2	15.6 ± 12.7	0.10
Mortality at 28d	5(8.3)	2(6.5)	3(10.3)	0.94

[a]Data are presented as mean ± SD or number(%).
[b]Mann–Whitney u test.
ISS, injury severity score; AIS, abbreviated injury scale, ICU: intensive care unit.

statistical significance. We further performed subgroup analysis including patients with ISS ≥16. The results showed that patients in the goal-directed group (n = 16) had significantly fewer consumption of RBC (4[3,11.5]U vs 14[7.5, 32]U, p < 0.01), FFP (4[2.9, 9.8]U vs 10.5[5.6, 15.7]U, p = 0.036) and total blood products (7[6.1, 47.0] U vs 37.6[14.5, 89.9]U, p = 0.015) than patients in the control group (n = 13), whereas consumption of platelet and cryoprecipitate was not significantly different. Furthermore, the cost of total blood product appeared to

be lower in the goal-directed group than the control group ($227.5[152.9, 1221.7] vs $329.0 [197.2, 2904.8]), but this was not significantly different (p = 0.156).

Clinical and laboratory parameters

Clinical and laboratory parameters of interest at ED admission and 24 h were summarized in Table 3. Patients in the goal-directed group had significantly higher systolic blood pressure at ED admission (121.8 ± 23.1 mmHg vs 102.7 ± 26.5 mmHg, p = 0.005) and lower pH (7.39 ± 0.06

Table 2 Administration of blood products at 24 h[a]

	Control group (n = 31)			Goal-directed group (n = 29)			p
	Number	Median	IQR	Number	Median	IQR	
RBC (U)	31	6.5	4-14	29	5	3-13	0.22
FFP (U)	30	6.1	4-10.7	29	5.7	3.4-10	0.54
PLT (U)	9	0	0-10	4	0	0-0	0.15
CRYO (U)	9	0	0-10	7	0	0-5	0.68
Total (U)	31	14.8	8.3-37.6	29	10.2	7.0-43.1	0.28

[a]Data were analyzed using Mann–Whitney u test.
RBC: red blood cell; FFP: fresh frozen plasma; PLT: platelet; CRYO: cryoprecipitate; IQR: interquartile range.

Table 3 Clinical and laboratory parameters

| | At ED admission | | | | | At 24 h | | | | |
| | Control group (n = 31) | | Goal-directed group (n = 29) | | p | Control group (n = 31) | | Goal-directed group (n = 28) | | p |
	Number	Mean ± SD	Number	Mean ± SD		Number	Mean ± SD	Number	Mean ± SD	
Temperature (°C)	31	36.4 ± 0.3	29	36.4 ± 0.3	0.98	31	37.2 ± 0.7	28	37.2 ± 0.6	0.84
HR (/min)	31	100.3 ± 19.5	28	91.8 ± 18.7	0.09	31	101.4 ± 18.6	28	96.9 ± 18.3	0.35
SBP (mmHg)	31	102.7 ± 26.5	28	121.8 ± 23.1	0.005	31	122.4 ± 16.8	28	122.6 ± 14.7	0.97
Hb (g/L)	30	121.1 ± 20.6	28	122.5 ± 24.0	0.82	31	105.5 ± 15.2	27	106.6 ± 18.9	0.8
RBC (×10^{12}/L)	30	3.9 ± 0.6	27	4.1 ± 0.7	0.27	31	3.4 ± 0.5	27	3.5 ± 0.6	0.69
PLT (×10^9/L)	30	186.2 ± 52.9	28	181.1 ± 59.0	0.73	31	113.0 ± 45.1	27	116.6 ± 47.7	0.77
pH	16	7.38 ± 0.05	14	7.38 ± 0.04	0.66	25	7.41 ± 0.04	27	7.39 ± 0.06	0.048
Lactate (mmol/L)	16	2.8 ± 1.5	14	3.1 ± 2.4	0.68	25	2.6 ± 1.7	27	2.1 ± 1.4	0.18[a]
BE (mmol/L)	16	(−3.9) ± 3.4	14	(−3.0) ± 3.5	0.48	25	(−2.7) ± 4.6	27	(−2.4) ± 2.5	0.75
Albumin (g/L)	28	38.3 ± 6.1	28	38.1 ± 7.3	0.92	31	33.2 ± 5.8	27	33.6 ± 4.5	0.79
Calcium (mmol/L)	25	2.1 ± 0.2	27	2.1 ± 0.2	0.91	31	2.0 ± 0.2	27	2.0 ± 0.2	0.28
INR	27	1.1 ± 0.2	28	1.1 ± 0.1	0.73	26	1.2 ± 0.2	24	1.2 ± 0.2	0.97
aPTT (s)	27	28.4 ± 6.4	28	25.7 ± 4.8	0.09	26	58.6 ± 36.6	24	39.2 ± 16.3	0.044[a]

[a] Mann-Whitney u test.

vs 7.41 ± 0.04, p = 0.048) at 24 h than patients in the control group. In addition, aPTT at 24 h was significantly shorter in the goal-directed group compared to the control group (39.2 ± 16.3 s vs 58.6 ± 36.6 s, p = 0.044), while admission aPTT was similar (25.7 ± 4.8 s vs 28.4 ± 6.4 s, p = 0.09). No significant differences were observed in other parameters between the two groups.

The first TEG test in the goal-directed group showed R value of 10.1 ± 4.7 min, α angle of 44.1 ± 16.1, and MA value of 50.0 ± 12.1. A follow-up TEG test between 24–48 hours after the first TEG test was available from 21 patients, with improved R value of 8.5 ± 4.7 min (p = 0.037), α angle of 51.1 ± 11.5 (p < 0.001), and MA value of 52.0 ± 13.3 (p = 0.11).

Clinical outcomes

There were 3 deaths (1 for exsanguination at 24 h, 1 for multiple organ dysfunction at 72 h, 1 for coagulopathy at 14d) in the goal-directed group and 2 deaths for coagulopathy (1 at 48 h and 1 at 72 h) in the control group. No significant differences were found in mortality at 28d, length of stay in ICU and hospital between the two groups.

Discussion

This cohort study showed that goal-directed transfusion protocol via TEG was applicable in patients with abdominal trauma, and was associated with a trend towards fewer blood product utilization and better coagulation profile at 24 h compared to conventional transfusion management. The results support the use of TEG in guiding transfusion management in patients with abdominal trauma.

First, this study provides supplemental evidence for using TEG to guide transfusion management in the trauma setting. TEG has been shown to be helpful in detecting post-injury coagulopathy and directing transfusion management in patients with severe multiple trauma [13], but the use of TEG in patients with lower injury severity has not been thoroughly investigated, which may be due to the relatively low incidence of coagulopathy in moderately injured patients [2]. In this study, the majority of included patients sustained moderate abdominal injury, as suggested by mean ISS of 15.2 and mean abdominal AIS of 3.1. Despite the relatively low injury severity, our patients were still exposed to risk of coagulation dysfunction, as suggested by aggravation of INR and aPTT during the first 24 hours of ED admission. The exacerbation of coagulation function might be associated with primary injury, second hit of operation, blood loss, and massive fluid resuscitation [16]. We found that TEG had reasonable value in monitoring coagulation function in these patients, and goal-directed transfusion protocol via TEG could be successfully implemented.

Second, our results showed that goal-directed transfusion protocol via TEG had the potential to reduce administration of component blood products. Although not statistically significant, patients managed with goal-directed transfusion protocol received fewer component blood products, especially RBC and FFP than patients receiving conventional transfusion management. In subgroup analysis including patients with ISS ≥ 16, we showed that goal-directed transfusion protocol led to significant reduction in administration of RBC, FFP, and total blood products. These results are consistent with the findings of several previous studies [8,11,13]. Moreover, we found that the reduction in blood product administration did not compromise perfusion status and oxygen delivery capacity, as evidenced by similar lactate level, hemoglobin concentration, and RBC count at 24 h between the two patient groups. The reduction of blood product administration is important in two aspects. First, it relieves the burden of blood product supply, and may have the potential to decrease the cost of blood products for patients. Second, it is likely to lower transfusion-related morbidity, such as coagulopathy, transfusion-related acute lung injury, and infection [17]. However, these findings must be interpreted with caution given the small sample size of the study and subgroup analysis.

Third, goal-directed transfusion protocol appears to be better than conventional transfusion management in preventing coagulation function exacerbation after transfusion. In recent years, there is improving understanding in acute traumatic coagulopathy (ATC), which is resulted from tissue injury and hypoperfusion due to trauma. Subsequent medical interventions, such as massive transfusion, may further exacerbate coagulation dysfunction and lead to trauma-induced coagulopathy (TIC) [18]. In this study, we observed that patients in the goal-directed group had better coagulation profile at 24 h, as indicated by shorter aPTT, than patients in the control group. Furthermore, the TEG parameters were significantly improved in patients managed with goal-directed transfusion protocol. There are two possible explanations for these findings. First, goal-directed transfusion protocol could prevent coagulation function worsening through supplementing appropriate blood component according to individual requirement. Second, the reduction of blood product utilization, as a result of the use of goal-directed transfusion protocol, might lower the risk of TIC secondary to massive transfusion. However, these findings needed to be interpreted carefully, since aPTT can represent only part of the coagulation system, and is affected by multiple factors [19]. Moreover, although aPTT results were available in more than 83.3% and follow-up TEG results were available in 72.4% of patients, missing data might reduce the power of the results.

The present study did not observe benefits of goal-directed transfusion protocol on mortality, which is not surprising because of the small sample size and moderate injury severity in overall. The previous study by Kashuk et al. [13] did not conclude the effect of goal-directed transfusion management on mortality either, because of incomparable injury severity between the patient groups. Considering the potential of goal-directed transfusion protocol in decreasing transfusion-related morbidity and correcting post-injury coagulopathy, it would be justified to infer that goal-directed transfusion protocol might improve mortality of trauma patients. Further studies are needed to investigate this issue.

Several limitations are worth considering when interpreting the results of this study. First, this is a retrospective study with small sample size. Due to the retrospective nature, we could not achieve two identical patient groups, as manifested by different admission systolic blood pressure between the two groups. Second, we did not abandon conventional coagulation tests after implementation of TEG. Therefore, the influence of conventional coagulation testing results on goal-directed transfusion management could not be eliminated and should be taken into consideration. Third, we were using standard TEG to guide transfusion, rather than rapid TEG. Moreover, we were not able to perform "baseline TEG", which was shown to be important for patients receiving TEG monitoring, since we were studying trauma patients in this study. Finally, this single institution experience may not be generalized because of different strategies in resuscitation, transfusion, and operation between trauma centers.

Conclusions

In summary, the present study showed that goal-directed transfusion protocol via TEG was feasible in patients with abdominal trauma, and was better than conventional transfusion management in reducing blood product utilization and preventing coagulation function exacerbation. The results are in favor of implementation of goal-directed transfusion protocol in trauma patients. Further studies are needed to confirm the benefits of the novel transfusion strategy in the trauma setting.

Abbreviations
VHA: Viscoelastic hemostatic assay; TEG: Thrombelastography; ED: Emergency department; SICU: Surgical intensive care unit; RBC: Red blood cell; FFP: Fresh frozen plasma; OR: Operation room; ISS: Injury severity score; AIS: Abdominal abbreviated injury scale; INR: International normalized ratio; aPTT: activated partial thromboplastin time.

Competing interests
The authors declare that they have no competing interests.

Authors' contributions
JY and ZZ initiated the idea, carried out the study, and drafted the manuscript. JW, DY, and SZ helped collect and analyze data. YL and WY participated in the design of the study. NL and JL participated in the coordination of the study and helped to draft the manuscript. All authors read and approved the final manuscript.

Authors' information
Jianyi Yin and Zhenguo Zhao are joint first authors.

Author details
[1]Department of Surgery, Jinling Hospital, Nanjing University School of Medicine, Nanjing, China. [2]Department of General Surgery, The Affiliated Jiangyin Hospital of Southeast University Medical College, Jiangyin, China.

References

1. Sauaia A, Moore FA, Moore EE, Moser KS, Brennan R, Read RA, Pons PT: **Epidemiology of trauma deaths: a reassessment.** *J Trauma* 1995, **38**:185–193.
2. Brohi K, Singh J, Heron M, Coats T: **Acute traumatic coagulopathy.** *J Trauma* 2003, **54**:1127–1130.
3. MacLeod JB, Lynn M, McKenney MG, Cohn SM, Murtha M: **Early coagulopathy predicts mortality in trauma.** *J Trauma* 2003, **55**:39–44.
4. Maegele M, Lefering R, Yucel N, Tjardes T, Rixen D, Paffrath T, Simanski C, Neugebauer E, Bouillon B: **Early coagulopathy in multiple injury: an analysis from the German Trauma Registry on 8724 patients.** *Injury* 2007, **38**:298–304.
5. Brohi K, Cohen MJ, Ganter MT, Matthay MA, Mackersie RC, Pittet JF: **Acute traumatic coagulopathy: initiated by hypoperfusion: modulated through the protein C pathway?** *Ann Surg* 2007, **245**:812–818.
6. Holcomb JB, Minei KM, Scerbo ML, Radwan ZA, Wade CE, Kozar RA, Gill BS, Albarado R, McNutt MK, Khan S, Adams PR, McCarthy JJ, Cotton BA: **Admission rapid thrombelastography can replace conventional coagulation tests in the emergency department: experience with 1974 consecutive trauma patients.** *Ann Surg* 2012, **256**:476–486.
7. Tauber H, Innerhofer P, Breitkopf R, Westermann I, Beer R, El Attal R, Strasak A, Mittermayr M: **Prevalence and impact of abnormal ROTEM(R) assays in severe blunt trauma: results of the 'Diagnosis and Treatment of Trauma-Induced Coagulopathy (DIA-TRE-TIC) study'.** *Br J Anaesth* 2011, **107**:378–387.
8. Johansson PI: **Goal-directed hemostatic resuscitation for massively bleeding patients: the Copenhagen concept.** *Transfus Apher Sci* 2010, **43**:401–405.
9. Wang SC, Shieh JF, Chang KY, Chu YC, Liu CS, Loong CC, Chan KH, Mandell S, Tsou MY: **Thromboelastography-guided transfusion decreases intraoperative blood transfusion during orthotopic liver transplantation: randomized clinical trial.** *Transplant Proc* 2010, **42**:2590–2593.
10. Schochl H, Nienaber U, Hofer G, Voelckel W, Jambor C, Scharbert G, Kozek-Langenecker S, Solomon C: **Goal-directed coagulation management of major trauma patients using thromboelastometry (ROTEM)-guided administration of fibrinogen concentrate and prothrombin complex concentrate.** *Crit Care* 2010, **14**:R55.
11. Shore-Lesserson L, Manspeizer HE, DePerio M, Francis S, Vela-Cantos F, Ergin MA: **Thromboelastography-guided transfusion algorithm reduces transfusions in complex cardiac surgery.** *Anesth Analg* 1999, **88**:312–319.
12. Johansson PI, Stensballe J: **Effect of haemostatic control resuscitation on mortality in massively bleeding patients: a before and after study.** *Vox Sang* 2009, **96**:111–118.
13. Kashuk JL, Moore EE, Wohlauer M, Johnson JL, Pezold M, Lawrence J, Biffl WL, Burlew CC, Barnett C, Sawyer M, Sauaia A: **Initial experiences with point-of-care rapid thrombelastography for management of life-threatening postinjury coagulopathy.** *Transfusion* 2012, **52**:23–33.
14. Yao D, Li Y, Wang J, Yu W, Li N, Li J: **Effects of recombinant activated factor VIIa on abdominal trauma patients.** *Blood Coagul Fibrinolysis* 2014, **25**:33–38.
15. Stassen NA, Bhullar I, Cheng JD, Crandall M, Friese R, Guillamondegui O, Jawa R, Maung A, Rohs TJ Jr, Sangosanya A, Schuster K, Seamon M, Tchorz KM, Zarzuar BL, Kerwin A, Eastern Association for the Surgery of Trauma: **Nonoperative management of blunt hepatic injury: an Eastern Association for the Surgery of Trauma practice management guideline.** *J Trauma Acute Care Surg* 2012, **73**:S288–S293.
16. Frith D, Brohi K: **The pathophysiology of trauma-induced coagulopathy.** *Curr Opin Crit Care* 2012, **18**:631–636.
17. Sihler KC, Napolitano LM: **Massive transfusion: new insights.** *Chest* 2009, **136**:1654–1667.
18. Frith D, Davenport R, Brohi K: **Acute traumatic coagulopathy.** *Curr Opin Anaesthesiol* 2012, **25**:229–234.
19. Brohi K, Cohen MJ, Davenport RA: **Acute coagulopathy of trauma: mechanism, identification and effect.** *Curr Opin Crit Care* 2007, **13**:680–685.

Permissions

All chapters in this book were first published in WJES, by BioMed Central; hereby published with permission under the Creative Commons Attribution License or equivalent. Every chapter published in this book has been scrutinized by our experts. Their significance has been extensively debated. The topics covered herein carry significant findings which will fuel the growth of the discipline. They may even be implemented as practical applications or may be referred to as a beginning point for another development.

The contributors of this book come from diverse backgrounds, making this book a truly international effort. This book will bring forth new frontiers with its revolutionizing research information and detailed analysis of the nascent developments around the world.

We would like to thank all the contributing authors for lending their expertise to make the book truly unique. They have played a crucial role in the development of this book. Without their invaluable contributions this book wouldn't have been possible. They have made vital efforts to compile up to date information on the varied aspects of this subject to make this book a valuable addition to the collection of many professionals and students.

This book was conceptualized with the vision of imparting up-to-date information and advanced data in this field. To ensure the same, a matchless editorial board was set up. Every individual on the board went through rigorous rounds of assessment to prove their worth. After which they invested a large part of their time researching and compiling the most relevant data for our readers.

The editorial board has been involved in producing this book since its inception. They have spent rigorous hours researching and exploring the diverse topics which have resulted in the successful publishing of this book. They have passed on their knowledge of decades through this book. To expedite this challenging task, the publisher supported the team at every step. A small team of assistant editors was also appointed to further simplify the editing procedure and attain best results for the readers.

Apart from the editorial board, the designing team has also invested a significant amount of their time in understanding the subject and creating the most relevant covers. They scrutinized every image to scout for the most suitable representation of the subject and create an appropriate cover for the book.

The publishing team has been an ardent support to the editorial, designing and production team. Their endless efforts to recruit the best for this project, has resulted in the accomplishment of this book. They are a veteran in the field of academics and their pool of knowledge is as vast as their experience in printing. Their expertise and guidance has proved useful at every step. Their uncompromising quality standards have made this book an exceptional effort. Their encouragement from time to time has been an inspiration for everyone.

The publisher and the editorial board hope that this book will prove to be a valuable piece of knowledge for researchers, students, practitioners and scholars across the globe.

List of Contributors

Ramon Vilallonga
General Surgery Department. Endocrine, bariatric and metabolic Unit Universitary Hospital Vall d'Hebron. Autonomous University of Barcelona, Spain

Vicente Pastor
General Surgery Department. Universitary Hospital Vall d'Hebron. Autonomous University of Barcelona, Spain

Laura Alvarez
HBP Surgery and Transplants Department. Universitary Hospital Vall d'Hebron. Autonomous University of Barcelona, Spain

Ramon Charco
HBP Surgery and Transplants Department. Universitary Hospital Vall d'Hebron. Autonomous University of Barcelona, Spain

Manel Armengol
General Surgery Department. Universitary Hospital Vall d'Hebron. Autonomous University of Barcelona, Spain

Salvador Navarro
General Surgery Department. Universitary Hospital Parc Tauli. Autonomous University of Barcelona, Spain

Yasser Abbas, Vanitha Devi, Kumarapuram Venkatachalam Souriarajan Prasad, Kameel Narouz Rizk and Permasavaran Padmanathan Nair
Surgery Department, Khoula Hospital, Muscat, Sultanate of Oman

Mohsin Raza
4/894, AikMinar Enclave, Near Shaukat Manzil, Dodhpur, Aligarh, UP 202002, India

Clay Cothren Burlew, Lucy Z Kornblith, Ernest E Moore, Jeffrey L Johnson and Walter L Biffl
From The Department of Surgery, Denver Health Medical Center, Denver CO, USA

Clay Cothren Burlew
Surgical Intensive Care Unit, Trauma & Acute Care Surgery Fellowship, Department of Surgery, Denver Health Medical Center, 777 Bannock Street, MC 0206, Denver, CO 80204, USA

Eric Irwin and Robert Roach
Department of Trauma, North Memorial Medical Center, Robbinsdale, MN, USA

Molly James and Patrick K Horst
Division of Critical Care and Acute Care Surgery, University of Minnesota, Minneapolis, MN, USA

Matthew C Byrnes
North Memorial Medical Center, Division of Trauma, 3300 Oakdale Avenue, Robbinsdale, MN 55422, USA

Antonio C Marttos and Fernanda M Kuchkarian
University of Miami Miller School of Medicine, Surgery Department (D40), Miami, FL 33101, USA

Phillipe Abreu-Reis
Federal University of Parana, Rua XV de Novembro, 1299, CEP 80.060-000, Curitiba, Parana, Brazil

Bruno MT Pereira and Gustavo P Fraga
University of Campinas (Unicamp), Faculty of Medical Sciences, Division of Trauma Surgery, (FCM/Unicamp), R. Alexander Fleming, 181, Cidade Universitaria "Prof. Zeferino Vaz", CEP: 13.083-970, Campinas, São Paulo, Brazil

Francisco S Collet-Silva
Hospital das Clínicas da Faculdade de Medicina Universidade de Sao Paulo, Av. Dr. Arnaldo, 455, Cerqueira Cesar, CEP: 01.246-903, São Paulo, Brazil

Raimundas Lunevicius and Klaus-Martin Schulte
Major Trauma Centre, King's College Hospital NHS Foundation Trust, King's Health Partners Academic Health Sciences Centre, Denmark Hill, London, SE5 9RS, UK

Osvaldo Chiara, Anna Mariani and Stefania Cimbanassi
Trauma Team Dip. DEA-EAS, Ospedale Niguarda Ca'Granda, Piazza Ospedale Maggiore 3, 20162, Milan, Italy

Sofia Lelli
Quality Department, Ospedale Niguarda Ca'Granda Milan, Milan, Italy

Cristina Mazzali
Universita' di Milano, Dip, Scienze cliniche Luigi Sacco, Milan, Italy

Ajith Sankarankutty
Faculdade de Medicina de Ribeirão Preto, Universidade de São Paulo, Brazil

Bartolomeu Nascimento and Luis Teodoro da Luz
Trauma Program, Sunnybrook Health Sciences Centre, University of Toronto, Canada

Sandro Rizoli
Departments of Surgery and Critical Care Medicine, Sunnybrook Health Sciences Centre, University of Toronto, Canada

Faris Azar, Elisha Brownson and Tracey Dechert
Department of Surgery, Boston University Medical Center, 850 Harrison Avenue Dowling 2 South, Boston, MA 02118, USA

Leonardo Centonze, Lorenzo Valesini, Gabriele Campana and Claudio Modini
Emergency Department, Division of Emergency Surgery and Trauma, Policlinico "Umberto I", Rome, Italy
Umberto I General Hospital, University of Rome "Sapienza", Rome, Italy

Mario Corona
Department of Radiological Sciences, Vascular and Interventional Radiology Unit, Policlinico "Umberto I", Rome, Italy

Marco Assenza
Surgical Research Fellow, Via Demetriade 58, Rome 00178, Italy

Fikri M Abu-Zidan
Head Trauma Group, Faculty of Medicine and Health Sciences, UAE University, Al-Ain, UAE

Mohamed I Abusharia
General Surgeon, Al-Ain Hospital, Al-Ain, UAE

Katharina Kessler
Visceral, and Proctology Surgeon, Al-Ain Hospital, Al-Ain, UAE

Jacqueline JEM van Laarhoven, Steven Ferree, Falco Hietbrink and Luke PH Leenen
Department of Surgery, University Medical Center Utrecht, Heidelberglaan 100, 3584, CX Utrecht, The Netherlands

R Marijn Houwert and EgbertJan MM Verleisdonk
Department of Surgery, Diakonessenhuis Utrecht, Bosboomstraat 1, 3582, KE Utrecht, The Netherlands

Cino Bendinelli and Andrew Martin
Department of Traumatology, John Hunter Hospital, Newcastle, NSW, Australia

Shane D Nebauer and Zsolt J Balogh
University of Newcastle, Newcastle, NSW, Australia

Afshin Mohammadi
Department of Radiology, Urmia University of Medical Sciences, Urmia, West-Azerbaijan, Iran

Mohammad Ghasemi-rad
Student research committee, Urmia University of medical Sciences. Urmia, Iran

Pradeep Navsaria, Andrew Nicol and Donald Hudson
Department of Surgery, Groote Schuur Hospital, University of Cape Town, Cape Town, South Africa

John Cockwill
Smith & Nephew, St Petersberg, Florida, USA

Jennifer Smith
Smith & Nephew, 101 Hessle Road, Hull HU3 2BN, UK

Yoshimitsu Izawa, Tomohiro Muronoi, Keisuke Yamashita and Masayuki Suzukawa
Department of Emergency Medicine, Jichi Medical University, Tochigi, Japan

Taka-aki Nakada and Koichiro Shinozaki
Chiba University Graduate School of Medicine, 1-8-1 Inohana, Chuo, Chiba 260-8677, Japan

Shuji Hishikawa and Alan T Lefor
Department of Surgery, Jichi Medical University, Tochigi, Japan This manuscript was presented in part at the World Society of Emergency Surgery 1st World Congress on 2nd July 2010 in Bologna Italy

Bonnie Tsang and Sandy L Widder
Department of Surgery, Faculty of Medicine and Dentistry, University of Alberta, 2D WMC, 8440-112 Street NW, Edmonton, AB T6G 2B7, Canada

Jessica McKee
Alberta Centre for Injury Control and Research, School of Public Health, University of Alberta, Edmonton, AB, Canada

Paul T Engels and Damian Paton-Gay
Department of Surgery and Division of Critical Care, Faculty of Medicine and Dentistry, University of Alberta, Edmonton, AB, Canada

Masashi Taniguchi, Taka-aki Nakada, Koichiro Shinozaki, Yasuaki Mizushima and Tetsuya Matsuoka
Senshu Trauma and Critical Care Center, 2-23 Rinku Orai Kita, Osaka 598-8577, Japan

Gokhan Aksel and Betul Akbuga Ozel
Emergency Department, Baskent University Faculty of Medicine, Ankara, Turkey

Omer Salt
Emergency Department, State hospital, Yozgat, Turkey

M Serkan Yilmaz, Tamer Durdu and Cihat Yel
Emergency Department, Numune Training and Research Hospital, Ankara, Turkey

Ali Demir
Emergency Department, Yenimahalle State hospital, Ankara, Turkey

Gulsüm Kavalci
Anesthesia Department, Yenimahalle State hospital, Ankara, Turkey

Ertugrul Altinbilek
Emergency Department, Şişli Hamidiye Etfal Training and Research Hospital, İstanbul, Turkey

Polat Durukan
Emergency Department, Erciyes University Faculty of Medicine, Kayseri, Turkey

Bahattin Isik
Emergency Department, Keciören Training and Research Hospital, Ankara, Turkey

Chun-Yi Wu, Shang-Ju Yang, Chih-Yuan Fu, Chien-Hung Liao, Shih-Ching Kang, Yu-Pao Hsu, Being-Chuan Lin, Kuo-Ching Yuan and Shang-Yu Wang
Department of Trauma and Emergency Surgery, Chang Gung Memorial Hospital, Chang Gung University, 5, Fu-Hsing Street, Kwei Shan Township, Taoyuan, Taiwan

Wai Hung Chan, Yao-Li Chen and Chien-Pin Chan
General Surgery Division, Surgery Department, Changhua Christian Hospital, Changhua City, Taiwan
Trauma Division, Surgery Department, Changhua Christian Hospital, 500 No. 135, Nanxiao Street, Changhua City, Taiwan

Ying-Cheng Chen
Cardiovascular Division, Surgery Department, Changhua Christian Hospital, Changhua City, Taiwan

Ping-Yi Lin
Transplant Medicine and Surgery Research Centre, Changhua Christian Hospital, Changhua City, Taiwan

Pei-Hung Wen
Surgery Department, Cishan Hospital, 84247 No. 60, Zhongxue Rd., Cishan District, Kaohsiung City, Taiwan

Engin D Arslan, Alper G Solakoglu, Fevzi Yilmaz, Evvah Karakilic, Tamer Durdu and Muge Sonmez
Emergency Department, Ankara Numune Training and Research Hospital, Altındağ, 06100 Ankara, Turkey

Cemil Kavalci
Emergency Department, Başkent Univercity Hospital, Çankaya, 06350 Ankara, Turkey

Erdal Komut
Radiology Department, Ankara Numune Training and Research Hospital, Altındağ, 06100 Ankara, Turkey

Ajeet Ramamani Tiwari and Jayashri Sanjay Pandya
Department of General Surgery, Topiwala National Medical College and Bai Yamunabai Laxman Nair Charitable Hospital, Mumbai Central 400008, India

Matthias Kuster
Department of Visceral and Transplant Surgery, Bern University Hospital, Bern, Switzerland

Aristomenis Exadaktylos
Department of Emergency Medicine, Bern University Hospital, Bern, Switzerland

Beat Schnüriger
Department of Visceral Surgery and Medicine, Bern University Hospital, Bern, Switzerland

Alberto Aiolfi, Emanuele Asti and Luigi Bonavina
Department of Biomedical Sciences for Health, University of Milan, IRCCS Policlinico San Donato, Piazza Edmondo Malan, 1, 20097 Milan, Italy

Kenji Inaba, Gustavo Recinos, Desmond Khor, Elizabeth R. Benjamin, Lydia Lam, Aaron Strumwasser and Demetrios Demetriades
Division of Trauma and Surgical Critical Care, LAC+USC Medical Center, University of Southern California, 2051 Marengo Street, Los Angeles, CA 90033, USA

Takayuki Irahara
Graduate School of Emergency and Critical Care Medicine, Nippon Medical School, Tokyo, Japan

Norio Sato
Department of Primary Care and Emergency Medicine, Kyoto University, Kyoto, Japan

Yuuta Moroe, Reo Fukuda, Yusuke Iwai and Kyoko Unemoto
Emergency and Critical Care Center, Nippon Medical School Tama- Nagayama Hospital, Tokyo, Japan

Miklosh Bala and Gidon Almogy
Department of Surgery and Shock Trauma Unit, Hadassah-Hebrew University Medical Center, Jerusalem, Israel

Jeffry L Kashuk
Director of Surgical Research and Academic Development, EM Care Acute Care Surgery, Dallas, Texas, USA

Dafna Willner and Dima Kaluzhni
Department of Anesthesiology and Intensive Care Unit, Hadassah-Hebrew University Medical Center, Jerusalem, Israel

Tali Bdolah-Abram
Department of Social Medicine, Hadassah-Hebrew University Medical Center, Jerusalem, Israel

Federico Coccolini and Luca Ansaloni
General Emergency and Trauma Surgery, Bufalini Hospital, Viale Giovanni Ghirotti, 286, 47521 Cesena, Italy

Derek Roberts
Department of Surgery, Foothills Medical Centre, Calgary, Canada

Rao Ivatury
Virginia Commonwealth University, Richmond, VA, USA

Emiliano Gamberini
ICU Department, Bufalini Hospital, Cesena, Italy

Stefania Cimbanassi
Emergency and Trauma Surgery Department, Niguarda Hospital, Milano, Italy

Jeffry L. Kashuk
General Surgery Department, Assuta Medical Centers, Tel Aviv, Israel

Martha Larrea
General Surgery, "General Calixto García", Habana Medicine University, Havana, Cuba

Juan Alberto Martinez Hernandez
General Surgery, Medical Faculty "General Calixto Garcia", Habana Medicine University, Havana, Cuba

Alain Chichom Mefire
Department of Surgery and Obs/Gyn, Faculty of Health Sciences, University of Buea, Buea, Cameroon

Ken Boffard
Milpark Hospital Academic Trauma Center, University of the Witwatersrand, Johannesburg, South Africa

Lena Napolitano
Acute Care Surgery, Department of Surgery, University of Michigan Health System, Ann Arbor, MI, USA

Fausto Catena
Emergency and Trauma Surgery, Parma Maggiore Hospital, Parma, Italy

Hang-Tsung Liu, Chi-Cheng Liang, Shiun-Yuan Hsu and Ching-Hua Hsieh
Department of Trauma Surgery, Kaohsiung Chang Gung Memorial Hospital and Chang Gung University College of Medicine, No. 123, Ta-Pei Road, Niao-Song District, Kaohsiung City 833, Taiwan

Cheng-Shyuan Rau
Department of Neurosurgery, Kaohsiung Chang Gung Memorial Hospital and Chang Gung University College of Medicine, No. 123, Ta-Pei Road, Niao-Song District, Kaohsiung City 833, Taiwan
Department of Neurosurgery, Kaohsiung Chang Gung Memorial Hospital and Chang Gung University College of Medicine, Kaohsiung, Taiwan

Ali Demir, Muhittin Serkan Yilmaz, Fevzi Yilmaz, Tamer Durdu, Mehmet Ali Ceyhan, Fatih Alagoz and Cihat Yel
Emergency Department, Numune Training and Research Hospital, Ankara 06370, Turkey

Cemil Kavalci
Emergency Department, Baskent University Faculty of Medicine, Ankara 06450, Turkey

Jung-Fang Chuang, Hang-Tsung Liu, Yi-Chun Chen, Shiun-Yuan Hsu, Hsiao-Yun Hsieh and Ching-Hua Hsieh
Department of Trauma Surgery, Kaohsiung Chang Gung Memorial Hospital and Chang Gung University College of Medicine, No.123, Ta-Pei Road, Niao-Sung District, Kaohsiung City 833, Taiwan

Shao-Chun Wu
Department of Anesthesiology, Kaohsiung Chang Gung Memorial Hospital and Chang Gung University College of Medicine, Kaohsiung, Taiwan

Jianyi Yin, Yousheng Li, Jian Wang, Danhua Yao, Shaoyi Zhang, Wenkui Yu, Ning Li and Jieshou Li
Department of Surgery, Jinling Hospital, Nanjing University School of Medicine, Nanjing, China

Zhenguo Zhao
Department of General Surgery, The Affiliated Jiangyin Hospital of Southeast University Medical College, Jiangyin, China

Index